THE UNITY
OF THE SENSES

Interrelations
among the Modalities

ACADEMIC PRESS
SERIES IN COGNITION AND PERCEPTION

SERIES EDITORS:
Edward C. Carterette
Morton P. Friedman
Department of Psychology
University of California, Los Angeles
Los Angeles, California

Stephen K. Reed: *Psychological Processes in Pattern Recognition*

Earl B. Hunt: *Artificial Intelligence*

James P. Egan: *Signal Detection Theory and ROC Analysis*

Martin F. Kaplan and Steven Schwartz (Eds.): *Human Judgment and Decision Processes*

Myron L. Braunstein: *Depth Perception Through Motion*

R. Plomp: *Aspects of Tone Sensation*

Martin F. Kaplan and Steven Schwartz (Eds.): *Human Judgment and Decision Processes in Applied Settings*

Bikkar S. Randhawa and William E. Coffman: *Visual Learning, Thinking, and Communication*

Robert B. Welch: *Perceptual Modification: Adapting to Altered Sensory Environments*

Lawrence E. Marks: *The Unity of the Senses*

THE UNITY
OF THE SENSES

Interrelations
among the Modalities

LAWRENCE E. MARKS

John B. Pierce Foundation Laboratory
New Haven, Connecticut
and Yale University

ACADEMIC PRESS
New York   San Francisco   London   1978
A Subsidiary of Harcourt Brace Jovanovich, Publishers

The top part of Figure 3.10 is reprinted from *Gestalt Psychology* by Dr. Wolfgang Köhler. By permission of Liveright Publishing Corporation. Copyright 1947 by Liveright Publishing Corporation. Copyright renewed 1975 by Lili Köhler.

ACADEMIC PRESS, INC.
111 Fifth Avenue, New York, New York 10003

United Kingdom Edition published by
ACADEMIC PRESS, INC. (LONDON) LTD.
24/28 Oval Road, London NW1 7DX

Library of Congress Cataloging in Publication Data

Marks, Lawrence E.
The unity of the senses.

(Cognition and perception series)
Bibliography: p.
Includes indexes.
1. Senses and sensation. 2. Intersensory
effects. 3. Poetry--Psychological aspects.
4. Music--Psychological aspects. I. Title.
II. Series.
BF233.M27 152.1 77-25625
ISBN 0-12-472960-6

PRINTED IN THE UNITED STATES OF AMERICA

To Liza and Laura

Contents

vii

Preface

What is "the unity of the senses"? Simply stated, it is the thesis that the senses have a lot in common. Different senses often assist one another in the perception of objects and events. Different senses often share common phenomenological attributes. Different senses often obey similar laws, often employ similar or common mechanisms. My intent in this book is to bare the kinship among the various sense departments by exploring their similarities and interrelations.

The unity of the senses is perhaps a theory, but even more importantly is a way of looking at sensory functioning: It is a viewpoint that pulls together a host of phenomena. To be sure, many of its doctrines are not wholly new. Bits and pieces have appeared from time to time, notably in the works of Erich von Hornbostel, Georg von Békésy, and S. S. Stevens. My goal is to assemble all of its parts, to show how the unity of the senses expresses itself in perception, in phenomenology, in psychophysics, in neurophysiology.

And in cognition, too. Although most of this book treats similarities and interrelations (correspondences, for short) that are found in sensory and perceptual processes, a major impetus to putting it together was my discovery that certain correspondences also show themselves in language. That curious sensory phenomenon known as synesthesia, where, for instance, sounds take on visual qualities, has a counterpart in language: A synesthetic factor—the metaphorical combination of words describing sensations of different modalities—infiltrates both the language of the common man and the language of the poet.

As a consequence, the book divides into two parts—the first six chapters treating sensory and perceptual phenomena per se, the last two treating the expression of some of these phenomena in language and literature. The first part includes a chapter on each of four central doctrines: One deals with the common perceptual function of the senses—how the senses combine information about spatial and temporal characteristics of objects and events. Another deals with similarities in sensory experiences—with those attributes of sounds, lights, touches, tastes, and smells that resemble each other. A third recounts similarities in psychophysical behavior—similarities in the quantitative rules that describe how sensory responses depend on stimulation. A fourth examines possible similarities in the neural mechanisms that underlie sensory performance. The sum of these four doctrines constitutes the scientific theory of the unity of the senses.

The second part examines two ways that the unity of the senses manifests itself in language, especially in poetry. One is through sound symbolism, where speech sounds in and of themselves convey meanings. The other is through synesthetic metaphor, the verbal expression of analogies among different sense qualities.

In order to handle the subject matter in a reasonable fashion, which is to say, to set out the arguments and evidence in a manageable package, I had to deal primarily with the high points. A truly comprehensive evaluation of all of the doctrines of sensory correspondence requires a full account of all the dissimilarities as well as all the similarities. Such an account could easily swell so as to encompass everything that is known about sensory functioning. The urge to tell all was resisted. All human works are necessarily selective, and the present volume is no exception.

A final point: The theme of this book is similarity among the senses. While writing the book, I became aware (at first only dimly, but gradually more clearly) of the importance and scope of the very concept of similarity itself. Yes, similarity is the book's theme. But it is the theme in at least two distinct ways. First of all, many of the phenomena that come under scrutiny are perceptual similarities; the existence of synesthesia—both in sense perception and in verbal metaphor—implies that people comprehend resemblances between superficially different sensory experiences. But similarity also enters in another way—as a principle of scientific investigation. To subscribe to any or all of the doctrines of the unity of the senses means, in part, to search out similarities among the senses, to devise analogous accounts of the mechanisms and processes that operate in different modalities. But this metascientific imperative applies generally to the scientific endeavor. Analogy and resemblance are part and parcel of the scientific enterprise. To evaluate the unity of the senses is, therefore, to bring to a focus the dual role of similarity, and ultimately to help disclose the basic complementarity of observed and observation in the science of psychology.

The doctrine of the unity of the senses extends into a manifold of subjects, including psychology, physiology, philosophy, and the arts. In particular, the present work will be of interest to psychologists and physiologists concerned with sensation, perception, and language, and to students of epistemology, esthetics, and philosophy of science.

I wish to thank Marc Bornstein for an acute, critical review of the entire manuscript, Barry Green and Wesley Lynch for comments on selected chapters, Marian Hubelbank for typing the manuscript, Wayne Chappell for drafting the figures, and my wife, Joya, for her patient support. The dedication belongs to my two wonderful daughters, who demonstrate the unity of life through love.

1

Introduction

Who has not been enthralled by the splendor of dawn, as when the golden-red sun climbs up from behind a rolling hill or emerges from under the sea, assaulting sleepy eyes in an outburst of pageantry that awakens the now visible world in its glow? Painters have often essayed to represent such dawns in form and color on canvas, poets to express and interpret the visual experience in words. Rudyard Kipling attempted to communicate certain characteristics of an oriental sunrise of this sort when he wrote, "the dawn comes up like thunder."[1] Kipling's phrase has seen such frequent repetition that one may hardly be aware of its multimodal nature; apparently, this image linking two sense modalities has, through overuse, been sapped of much of its poetic meaning. For to say that the dawn rises up like thunder is to say that an event perceived through one sense modality—here, vision—can resemble a seemingly very different event perceived through quite another modality—hearing. In short, Kipling's simile is synesthetic: It expresses, or perhaps forges, a relationship between features of experience that properly belong to different senses.

[1] "Mandalay."

To appreciate the resemblance between the visual perception of dawn and the auditory perception of thunder is to acknowledge that every sense modality is not an island, entire of itself; it is to comprehend, albeit implicitly, that there are correspondences between dimensions of auditory and visual experience; it is to discern, however dimly or remotely, that amidst the diversity of sensory perception there is unity.

Unity and Diversity

The senses form the subject matter of this book, and the unity of the senses forms its theme. There is an old motto, a motto that used to be the byword of adherents to one school of thought—and perhaps still is for some diehards—that states that all human knowledge comes from the senses. Now, this is not the place to argue either the epistemological or psychological merit of such a radical empiricism. The dictum is repeated here mainly because quoting it provides an opportunity to point out the primary and central role that the senses play in so much of human activity. The senses are channels for information, devices for communication, organs for pleasure and pain in a plethora of variety.

It is hardly disputable that there are seven different external senses—more or less. The senses of sight, hearing, taste, smell, and pain make five; if we lump touch, warmth, and cold together into a single somesthetic sense, the total is six (less), but if we take the three separately, the total is eight (more). At first blush, a most salient characteristic of these six or eight or however many senses is their dissimilarity: The qualitative, phenomenal experience of sight seems to have little in common with that of hearing, and hearing to have little in common with taste. But a little further thought—the second blush—tells us otherwise. If there is a yin that reflects the qualitative differences amongst the senses, there is also a complementary yang that incorporates a number of domains of similarity. And it is each of these domains that the present work seeks to explore.

I have already introduced one type of similarity, namely the common dimensions that befall the variegated sensory experiences themselves: Qualitatively distinct and dissimilar sorts of sensation, say of sight and sound, may link up because both are intense. The sun's brightness at dawn resembles thunder's loud roll and crack. Another domain consists of all the ways that different senses can provide information about the same objects and events in the world: Sizes and shapes can be felt and seen. Finally, there are similarities among the principles that underlie the processes by which various sensory systems operate. Common and analogous processes exist both at the psychophysical level (describing the relation between physical stimuli and the corresponding perceptions) and at the neurophysiological level (describing the relations between stimuli and neural responses and between neural responses and sensations).

Questions about what is common to different senses have received notice and theoretical consideration since the beginnings of interest in sensation itself. Doctrines of the unity of the senses can be traced at least as far back as the Greek philosopher Democritus, who in the fifth century B.C. theorized that all of the senses are modes of touch; the same notion was espoused later by Thomas Hobbes (1651), among others. According to Democritus, excitement of a sense organ—any sense organ—comes from its contact with a stream of atoms. About 100 years after Democritus, Aristotle (*ca.* 350 B.C.) developed the notion of a *sensus communis,* a common sense that integrates the activity of several senses.

The theory of sensory correspondences—or, more generally, the observations and doctrines of sensory similarities and interrelations—has been around for a very long time. It pops up time and again, here and there, in psychology and in metaphysics, in religion and in literature. Like other phenomena and activities that play a significant role in mental life, sensory correspondences are more than categories to be entered into a scientific ledger, more than abstract grist for a scientist's experimental or theoretical mill. Because all human experience is, by its very nature, colored with the stuff that sensations are made of, the sensory qualities pervade thought as well as perception. In particular, properties of sensory experience wend their way through language—permeating that most human manifestation and expression of thought.

Benjamin Lee Whorf (1956) is well known for his proposal that the structure of a language determines, in part, the cognitive processes of the language user. Perhaps this is so. But there is an alternative view, as some of Whorf's critics have countered, whereby language and linguistic structure are considered a reflection or manifestation of the cognitive processes, rather than vice versa. Regardless of the direction of the causal relation, verbal expressions surely do serve as representations and expressions of cognitive activities. To the extent that language reflects or at least parallels thought, and to the extent that sensory correspondences color thinking, interrelations among the senses that appear in perception will also find their way into speech and writing. An example is the synesthetic metaphor implicit in the expression "bright music"—this the verbal representation of a cross-modal relationship that complements Kipling's thundering dawn.

Overview

This work divides itself into two parts. Both parts deal with similarities and interrelations among the senses. The first considers these sensory correspondences as objects of scientific scrutiny, from the point of view of experimental psychology; the second looks at the ways that sensory correspondences reveal themselves in language, with particular emphasis on intersensory relationships in poetry.

For the sake of rationality, as well as convenience, let me take the first part first. There are five major scientific doctrines that I wish to describe. They overlap somewhat in their fundamental concepts, and often data relevant to one are also relevant to others; yet they are distinguishable enough to treat them at least somewhat independently.

Several of the doctrines of sensory correspondence can be subsumed under the aforementioned Aristotelian notion of a *sensus communis*. Aristotle, in his *De anima, De sensu, De memoria et reminiscenti, De iuventute et senectute,* and *De somno et vigilia,* postulated the existence of a common sense to serve eight important psychological functions. Among the responsibilities of this common sense were the finalizatiɔn (last stage) of sense perception, the consciousness of sense perception, the judgment and discrimination of percepts, and the appreciation of the so-called "common sensibles." The latter consist of all of the qualities of sensation that are general, that is, not particular to a single sense. The six common sensible attributes are, according to Aristotle: motion, rest, number, form, magnitude, and unity [*De anima,* 418a, 425a]. (In *De memoria et reminiscenti* [450a], Aristotle discussed time in relation to the common sense. However, he did not include duration in his major expositions on the common sense.) As a matter of fact, it was Aristotle's opinion that it is only the common sense that apprehends these six categories properly; the specialized senses like sight and touch apprehend them only accidentally [*De anima,* 425a]. Whereas color is appreciated only by the eye and taste only by the tongue, qualities like shape and number are appreciated properly by Aristotle's sixth or common sense, even though the latter qualities are also appreciated accidentally by the senses of sight and touch. Clearly, the *sensus communis* lies at a higher level than do the other five senses.

THE FIVE DOCTRINES

Let me briefly outline the five theories or doctrines of sensory correspondence. The first is the *Doctrine of Equivalent Information.* This doctrine is a contemporary formulation of Aristotle's common sensible attributes. Simply stated, it notes that different senses can inform us about the same features of the external world. One wall of my office is constructed of cinder block. The coarse texture of its surface is made known to me both visually and tactually. As Hornbostel (1925) wrote, "It matters little through which sense I realize that in the dark I have blundered into a pig-sty [p. 290]."

Not a heady theory, to be sure, the Doctrine of Equivalent Information, but nevertheless one that is incorrect if pressed too far. The philosophical implications of this doctrine are complex and tortuous. One philosophical offshoot is a brand of realism that treats equivalent information as the expected result of our perceptual encounter with an existent reality. Another is a brand of mystical correlationism that interprets the interrelation between the senses as symbolizing an arcane correspondence between the psychological and the physical realms.

Second is the *Doctrine of Analogous Attributes and Qualities*. Despite the salience of the phenomenal differences among qualities of various sense modalities, there are a few properties of sensation held in common. Some attributes are suprasensory. Suprasensory attributes are those categories or dimensions of experience that are not limited to a single modality, but that apply to most or to all modalities. Intensity is a classic example, to which duration must also be added. Size (extension), brightness, and hedonic tone are other candidates, though perhaps not universally applicable. It is presumably by dint of similarities mediated through analogous qualities that one can apprehend how "the dawn comes up like thunder."

A stronger version of this second doctrine states that *suprasensory dimensions are not only analogous, but identical*. Such a theory was propounded by Hornbostel (1931) with respect to the dimension of sensory brightness. Hornbostel argued that lights, sounds, odors, and touches all have brightnesses that can be said to be equal in an absolute manner. Actually, the dimension that has been studied most explicitly by experiment is that of sensory intensity.

A third doctrine states that *different senses have corresponding psychophysical properties*. By psychophysical is meant the functional relations between properties of sense perceptions on the one hand and the properties of physical stimuli that produce them on the other. Thus this theory proposes that at least some of the ways the senses behave and operate on impinging stimuli are general characteristics of sensory systems, similar from vision to hearing, from touch to olfaction. It is worth pointing out that the existence of common psychophysical processes is itself contingent upon the validity of either or both the first two doctrines. For in order to talk of similar quantitative laws governing the relation between sense perception and stimulus in different modalities, we must first indicate the analogous properties of sense perception—that is, there must be common or analogous sensory features or attributes.

In essence, then, this third doctrine proposes that there are general principles that govern sensory psychophysics, laws that are valid for all of the senses. Weber's law of discriminability (pp. 118–121) and S. S. Stevens's law of sensory intensity (pp. 127–132) come foremost to mind, but there are several other principles of sensory functioning common to more than one sensory system.

The fourth doctrine states that *similar or identical neurophysiological mechanisms* parallel the foregoing examples of sensory correspondence. All of the first three doctrines just enumerated are psychological; the fourth doctrine states that there is a neural analogue to each of the psychological doctrines. Hence this doctrine has three subspecies. One says that there are special neural mechanisms that integrate information from several senses. These mechanisms mediate equivalent information about space and time. Another part of this doctrine deals with the neural processes that are responsible for psychophysical processes, and it says that the neural processes are the same whenever the psychophysical properties are the same. Included are processes that underlie the detection of stimuli, the discrimination of one stimulus from another, the way stimuli are perceived to be located in space, and so on. The third part of the doctrine deals with neural coding, and it says that whenever sensory attributes of different modalities are the same, then some characteristics of the underlying neurophysiological responses are also the same. According to this theory, the neural code for sensory intensity might be frequency of neural discharge or number of active nerve fibers, but in any case it would be the same code in vision (brightness), hearing (loudness), and so forth.

The fifth and last theory is a full-blown *Doctrine of the Unity of the Senses,* which incorporates all of the first four theories, and in which the several senses are interpreted as modalities of a general, perhaps more primitive sensitivity. The differentiation from general into specific is presumed to take place both phylogenetically and ontogenetically. However, differentiation is incomplete, at least to the extent that all of the senses remain united in the ways stated by the other four doctrines. This Haeckelian theory is closely associated with the work of Heinz Werner (e.g., 1934, 1940).

Chapters 2–6 elaborate, in succession, the five doctrines of sensory correspondence. Each chapter therefore amalgamates one of the doctrines with empirical evidence that highlights it.

SENSORY AND PERCEPTUAL INTERACTIONS

Before going on, I would like to mention briefly one topic that has often been touted as a prime example of the nonindependence of different sensory channels. This is the topic of sensory interaction—the modification of responses to stimulation in one modality by concurrent or juxtaposed stimulation in another. This subject has an enormous experimental literature, dating back at least to the pioneer studies by Urbantschitsch (1888). Unfortunately, it is difficult to cull out of this literature very many satisfactory conclusions; although numerous studies report that senses interact with one another, some studies report that they function independently: And even when interactions appear, it is often difficult to decide whether the positive results actually reflect an effect of stimulating one sense on processes of another, or instead an effect on the subjects' expectations and hence on their judgments.

Perhaps the most crucial factor in determining the significance of any interaction is the objective relationship between the stimuli that are used. When stimuli presented to different senses bear no meaningful relation to each other, interaction often seems to be small or nonexistent. Trying to hear weak sounds in the light, when the sounds are played through earphones and hence are not correlated spatially with objects in the visual field, is not very different from trying to hear the same sounds in the dark. But meaningfully related stimuli are quite a different matter. The voice of a good ventriloquist sounds displaced in space, away from the ventriloquist's mouth, which does not move, toward the dummy's, which does. Meaningful *perceptual* interactions of this type can and do occur; they occur when concurrent *information* enters different sensory channels. Other examples are given in the next chapter.

SYNESTHESIA AND METAPHOR

Sensory correspondence is not a domain of inquiry restricted to scientists, a matter solely for experimental scrutiny and empirically based theory. The plain fact is that sensory analogies do exist; they are important to the ways that we sense, perceive, and cognize; they are significant properties of the bodies and minds of people. (They are probably also properties of the bodies and minds of animals, but this opinion is, at present, difficult to substantiate.) Furthermore, resemblances between one sense modality and another are profound and important aspects of our interactions with the world; our internal representations of the world, which develop through all of the senses—sight, hearing, smell, taste, touch—are colored by these correspondences.

What I am talking about here are intersensory correspondences that fall under the rubric of *synesthesia*. Synesthesia is a term that refers to the transposition of sensory images or sensory attributes from one modality to another, as where the mellow tones of a lover's voice flow in a kaleidoscope of color, or where the sundry flavors of dinner come alive in melody. Probably the most common form—certainly the most thoroughly studied—is visual hearing, where sounds take on the accoutrements of sight.

Relatively few people are truly synesthetic—rarely do sensory experiences of sight, sound, and taste actually arise, secondarily, from inappropriate stimuli; rarely do secondary images actually blend into primary sensations. Nevertheless, there is a universal synesthetic capacity to appreciate the closeness and richness of similarities among visual, auditory, and other sensory qualities, a capacity that is strongly aroused in particular by powerful sensory–esthetic experiences.

It is little wonder, then, that descriptions and expressions of sensory correspondence appear, occasionally even as doctrine, in the arts and in literature as well as in science. Art forms like opera and ballet are intrinsically synesthetic modes of expression. Even the words used to describe the visual and auditory converge, as when one speaks of a relationship between the line of movement and the corresponding musical line. To perceive ballet, it is necessary to integrate sight and sound so that, in John Keats's words, "eyes / And ears act with that unison of sense / Which marries sweet sound with the grace of form."[2] Divorce sound from sight or sight from sound, and only music or dance remains.

We may and do experience the correspondences of diverse senses, so it is little wonder that the ways we describe our sensory experiences with words also reflect intersensory analogies. Colors are not only bright or dark, deep or pale, but sometimes loud or soft, as well as warm or cool. The adjective "smooth" can be applied to a melody, to a taste, or to a texture that is seen or felt. It was only a few years ago that I first began to take serious notice of poetic metaphors and literary statements of sensory correspondence. But alas, it turned out, as I

[2] "Hyperion: A Vision."

should have foreseen, that my discovery was no discovery at all, not even a rediscovery, nor even, it would seem, a re-rediscovery. My kindled awareness of the doctrines of correspondence—for instance, in the poetry and prose of Charles Baudelaire—was predated 70 years by the discussion given by Clavière (1898), and later by Mahling (1926). Most certainly, there were others who saw possible relations between the scientific and the literary.

The language of poetry, and even the language of prose, is heavily laced with analogies between sensory qualities of different modalities. Our prosaic expressions contrast bright sounds with dull or dark sounds, loud colors with muted colors, sweet notes with sour notes. Such metaphors bespeak similarities and relationships, the connectedness of the mind's contents and activities. Unlike Leibniz's monads, metaphors are windows.

Poets tend to speak in even fuller and richer images. When the poet Dante Gabriel Rossetti borrowed a phrase from Job to write how "Her voice was like the voice the stars / Had when they sang together,"[3] he fulfilled Coleridge's criterion that "the poet must . . . understand and command what Bacon calls the *vestigia communia* of the senses, the latency of all in each, . . ., the excitement of vision by sound and the exponents of sound [1847, p. 142]." Sensory correspondences in poetry have received some attention in the past. For the most part, however, studies of synesthesia in literature have been undertaken primarily from a literary point of view. Chapters 7 and 8 of the present work examine, from a psychological point of view, expressions of sensory analogy and correspondence in literature, particularly in poetry of the nineteenth century.

---

[3] "The Blessed Damozel." The verse in Job [38:7], "The morning stars sang together," has been popular with poets. Witness also the opening line to "Singing God's Praise" by the Spanish Hebrew poet Judah Ha-Levi: "All the stars of the morning sing to you."

2

The Doctrine of
Equivalent Information

On Common Sensibles

There is no doubt that different senses can convey information about the same features of the environment. As John Locke (1690) pointed out, the senses assist one another in demonstrating the very existence of objects. Another person nearby may make himself or herself known in several ways: through sight, through the sound of his or her footstep or voice, through the odor of his aftershave lotion or her perfume. The poet W. H. Auden alluded to an "infirm king" to whom "eyes, ears, tongue, nostrils bring / News of revolt."[1] Objects that vary in size, texture, and shape are perceived as different from one another both when we touch them and when we see them. Yoshida (1968) found, for instance, that various materials such as fur, aluminum foil, cloth, and cotton differ perceptually from one another in the same manner and to the same degree when sensed by sight and by touch. Movement can be perceived by sight, by sound, or by touch, as Hornbostel (1925) noted.

---

[1] From "Paid on Both Sides" by W. H. Auden. In *Collected longer poems;* copyright 1969. Reprinted by permission of Random House.

Consider for a moment the perfectly ordinary activity of watching and hearing someone speak. The speaker's voice itself can be located in space, and under normal circumstances the voice appears to come from the speaker's mouth. We are well accustomed to the visual code for speech, that is, to the correspondence between the seen movements of the mouth and the sounds of speech. In the real world, speech sounds typically are synchronized perfectly with mouth movements, thereby providing an excellent sensory environment for learning the cross-modal equivalences—to the extent that learning is necessary. With practice, a person can become adept at "reading lips" even when speech is inaudible. Many deaf individuals do.

It is a common observation that the blind as well as the deaf appear to make extra use of the discriminative capacities of the senses that remain functioning. Leopold Bloom, the central character in James Joyce's *Ulysses* (1934), essayed to construct in his imagination how the blind Penrose perceived the world:

> How on earth did he know that van was there? Must have felt it . . . . Must be strange not to see [that girl]. Kind of a form in the mind's eye. The voice temperature when he touches her with fingers must almost see the lines, the curves. His hands on her hair, for instance. Say it was black for instance. Good. We call it black. Then passing over her white skin. Different feel perhaps. Feeling of white [pp. 178–179].

The way we perceive objects by means of different senses, for example by touch and vision, has been an issue of long-standing concern. To Hobbes (1656) and Locke (1690), among others, form or figural shape was a common attribute of sensation, an example of what Aristotle called the κοινὰ αἰσθητά, or common sensibles. One of the primary functions of the κοινὸν αἰσθητήριον or *sensus communis* in Aristotelian doctrine was the apprehension of the common sensible attributes: rest, motion, number, size, unity, and shape. For the most part, it seems fair to say that Aristotle tended to equate these sensory qualities with the corresponding stimulus qualities: "For the perception of magnitude, figure, roughness, smoothness, and sharpness and bluntness, *in solid bodies* [italics mine], is the common function of all the senses, and if not all, then at least the common function of sight and touch [*De anima*, 442b]."

Properties of objects like shape and texture, properties of events like movement and duration, can make themselves known through several sensory channels; the common sensibles appear to correspond closely with what philosophers like Locke later called *primary qualities.* Locke (1690) distinguished primary from secondary qualities of objects.

Primary qualities are those characteristics or properties of things, like their size and shape, that are wholly inseparable from them and that are perceived to be inseparable. Percepts of primary qualities, according to Locke, resemble the physical qualities themselves. A ball is spherical, and it is perceived as being spherical. Not so with secondary qualities: Percepts of secondary qualities do not resemble the corresponding physical qualities. A modernized Lockean example is the lack of resemblance between the wavelengths of light reflected by an object and the color that is perceived. Although both primary and secondary qualities refer to properties of objects (not to attributes of sensation), the distinction is based largely on the presumed relation between the qualities and the way the qualities are perceived. The distinction can itself be traced back to Aristotle's time. For Theophrastus [*De sensibus*, 69–70], in his discussion of Democritus's theory of sensation, implicity made the same dichotomy.

Galileo (1623) named four primary qualities—size, shape, quantity, and motion—whereas Locke (1690) later named five—solidity, size, shape, motion or rest, and number. These primary qualities are meant to contrast with secondary qualities, which are perceived as color, pitch, warmth, cold, taste quality, odor quality, and so forth. To repeat, the percepts of these latter qualities are solely properties of sense, and do not seem to be inherent in objects and events, at least not in the way that primary qualities like size and shape are. What is most relevant to the Doctrine of Equivalent Information is that each of the perceived secondary qualities is limited to a single sense, whereas primary qualities may be perceived through several or all, and, especially, if we follow Aristotle, through the common sense. Clearly, then, there is significant overlap between the Aristotelian set of common sensibles and the Galilean–Lockean list of primary qualities.

A case could be made for similar interpretation—in terms of common sensibles—of Immanuel Kant's (1781) position, even though Kant's transcendental analysis purports to be logical rather than psychological. This analysis begins with the role of extension and duration (space and time) in sense perception. According to Kant, space and time are general forms of perception, logically prior and applicable to all sensation. These perceptual forms link up, via what he called *Schemata*, to the *Categories of the Understanding;* the Categories, which include concepts like number and quantity, are to thought much as space and time are to perception. Space, time, number, and quantity are suprasensory in Kantian doctrine; their roles are in several respects different, however, from those played by common sensibles in Aristotelian doctrine. For one thing, the forms of perception and the categories of conception are purely phenomenal, that is, properties only of mind, not noumenal, properties of reality.

The philosophical tenability of the doctrine of primary qualities is moot. A skeptical argument, such as that made by David Hume (1739), is difficult to refute. According to Hume, it is impossible to go beyond sense data to objects and events themselves; hence no justification exists for distinguishing primary from secondary qualities, since there is no independent means to determine whether given perceived qualities are qualities of objects as well as qualities of sense. Bishop George Berkeley's (1710) analysis led to questioning the very existence of a reality independent of sensation. Be this as it may, from a non-philosophical point of view—and in particular from a psychological point of view—the distinction between primary and secondary qualities has value. For even if some philosophers cannot demonstrate the existence of an objective world, people—most people at least—behave as if one exists. And they behave as if common sensibles or primary qualities are indeed properties of objects and events, not merely properties of sense perception. The final section of this chapter will examine philosophical implications of this thesis.

To the extent that the common sensibles—or primary qualities, Schemata, Categories, or whatever else we may wish to call them—are attributes of objects, they play a central role in the Doctrine of Equivalent Information. To the extent that they are only attributes of sensations, on the other hand, they pertain to the doctrine considered in the next chapter, the Doctrine of Analogous Sensory Attributes.

The notion of common sensibles can be cast in a more modern and experimental mold. Then the questions that it raises concern the problems of cross-modality equivalence and transfer of information. For example, How well does the perception of size or form translate from vision to touch or from touch to vision? Do objects look the way they feel?

Cross-Modal Perception of Size

I reach into my pocket and, after fumbling through the coins, select the dime, nickel, or quarter that I desire. Occasionally, I err, picking out a penny instead of a dime, not noticing my error until I look at the coin. But most of the time my tactual identification of coins is fairly accurate. Sizes, shapes, lengths of familiar, everyday objects, indeed, the objects themselves, are perceived and identified quite well by the way they feel, though not always as well as by the way they look.

When I talk of "touch" or "feel" in this context, I do not mean merely the tactile sensation of pressure on the skin. Rather, I mean active touch, or haptic touch, as it is called—where the manipulation of objects leads to a perceptual unity of the tactile, kinesthetic, and proprioceptive, of pressure, movement, resistance, and position. Simple pressure on the skin alone provides scant information about objects in the environment. We have little capacity to identify shapes of objects when they are impressed on the skin (e.g., Zigler & Northrup, 1926). Indeed, sensations produced by steady, passive pressure on the skin quickly adapt and disappear (a phenomenon that is reminiscent of the disappearance of visual sensations when images are fixed on the retina, unmoved by movements of the eye). Much of the time we are hardly aware of the clothes we wear.

PERCEPTION OF LINEAR EXTENT

Scientific studies of cross-modal perception were conducted more than a century ago by Wundt (1862), who compared distances as they are perceived by vision and by touch, and later by Jastrow (1886), who compared distances perceived by three different modalities: vision, kinesthesis, and proprioception. Jastrow's study remains one of the most extensive and intensive empirical investigations of the perception of linear extent by different senses. He found that linear extents, sizes in one dimension, appeared greatest to the eye (visually), smaller to the moving arm (kinesthetically) and to the unmoving hand (proprioceptively—distance between thumb and forefinger). A most important point of these results—and of other results to be described— is that there may not always be a complete equivalence in the information provided by different senses.

Subsequent research confirmed Jastrow's finding of a significant difference between the visual perception of length and the proprioceptive perception of thickness, but contradicted his finding of a similar difference between visual length and kinesthetic distance. I will defer, temporarily, consideration of the former in order to take up the latter. Connolly and Jones (1970) and Jones and Connolly (1970) had subjects match visual length and distance of arm movement. The errors made in these cross-modality matches were quite small in size. Previously, Mme. Piéron (1922) showed that there is little if any difference between visual length and perceived extent of active and passive arm movements. Hence there is a rough equivalence between linear extents when they are sensed through vision and through kinesthesis (active and passive movements); this equivalence is depicted in Figure 2.1.

Because visually perceived length and kinesthetically perceived distance are equal to each other, it follows that both types of perceived linear extent must bear the same mathematical relationship to physical length. When subjects are called upon to make quantitative judgments of spatial extent, both visual length (S. S. Stevens & Guirao, 1963; M. Teghtsoonian & Teghtsoonian, 1965) and kinesthetic distance (Ronco, 1963) turn out to be directly proportional to physical length. These outcomes are shown in Figure 2.2.

As I mentioned before, Jastrow (1886) found that the same physical extent was perceived to be larger by vision than by proprioception. Proprioceptive length could differ from visual length in two ways. In the first way, both visual and proprioceptive length might be directly proportional to actual physical length, but not in the same proportion. Proprioceptively perceived length might be some constant fraction of visually perceived length. On the other hand, and in actual fact, the relation between proprioceptively perceived length and visually perceived length might be nonlinear.

Jastrow's data show a large relative difference between thickness that is felt and length that is seen when linear extents are small, but nearly complete equality between felt thickness and seen length when extents are greater. Given that visual length is proportional to physical length, as we have already noted, it follows that proprioceptive extent—thickness perceived through finger span—cannot also be. This

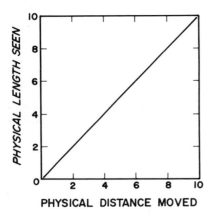

Figure 2.1. Lengths look approximately as long to the eye as distances feel to the moving arm.

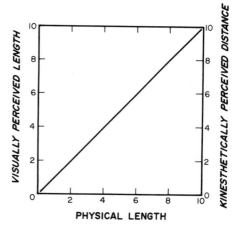

Figure 2.2. Through both sight (left-hand ordinate) and active touch (right-hand ordinate), people perceive lengths and distances to be just about proportional to the actual physical lengths and distances.

prediction is borne out by several studies. S. S. Stevens and Stone (1959), Mashhour and Hosman (1968), and R. Teghtsoonian and Teghtsoonian (1970) all examined quantitative judgments of finger span, the perceived distance between thumb and forefinger. Figure 2.3 summarizes the results, which are fully consistent with Jastrow's findings. Perceived finger span increases as a positively accelerated function of

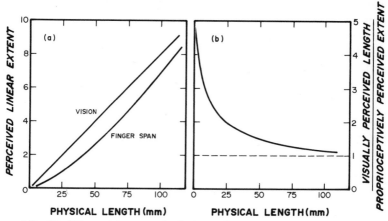

Figure 2.3. (a) When objects are looked at, their lengths appear proportional to physical length—when physical length doubles, visually perceived length doubles. But when objects are gripped between two fingers, their lengths do not appear proportional to physical lengths—when physical length doubles, proprioceptively perceived length more than doubles. (b) A very small object appears to the eye considerably larger than it feels when held between two fingers (ratio of proprioceptive to visual length is great). As the object increases in size, this discrepancy between lengths perceived by sight and by proprioception diminishes (ratio of proprioceptive to visual length near unity).

physical thickness (Figure 2.3a); the ratio of visually to proprioceptively perceived extent decreases as the physical length increases (Figure 2.3b).

It needs to be pointed out that perceived finger span is only one rather specialized type of proprioceptive distance and that nonlinearity and nonequivalence are not necessarily the rule with other types of proprioceptively perceived length. As a matter of fact, M. Teghtsoonian and Teghtsoonian (1965) compared lengths of rods as they were seen and as they were felt when touched by the index fingers of the out-stretched hands. By means of the method of numerical magnitude estimation, a procedure whereby subjects attempted to gauge the sensory magnitudes by assigning numbers to perceived extent, Teghtsoonian and Teghtsoonian showed that this sort of proprioceptively felt length is like visually perceived length. Both are fully proportional to physical length.

An important sensory mode for the perception of size is haptic touch. Under some, but not all conditions, haptic touch and vision appear to give equivalent information about the size of objects. Abravanel (1971b) showed that judgments of synthesized lengths can be about as accurate when vision and active touch are combined as when either modality is used alone. It is interesting to note that older children are more accurate than are young children in matching lengths cross-modally between touch and vision (Abravanel, 1968). This increase in accuracy with age may reflect either an ongoing developmental facilitation in cross-modal matching, or, more simply, an increasing accuracy in haptic perception itself. The latter is an important possibility, since haptic perception tends to be inferior to visual perception (e.g., Scholtz, 1958).

PERCEPTION OF EXTENT IN TWO DIMENSIONS

Equivalence between vision and haptic touch sometimes fails to obtain in the perception of two-dimensional size. Anstis and Loizos (1967) compared the sizes of holes perceived by sight and touch, in the latter case by the tongue, index finger, and little finger. Holes appeared about the same to the tongue as to the eye, but smaller to the fingers. This result is probably not surprising to anyone who ever discovered the discrepancy between how large a dental cavity feels to the tip of the tongue and how small to the tip of the finger.

Differences between visual and tactual sizes and between tactual sizes at different sites on the skin previously received the attention of Stout (1915) and of Waterman (1917). Waterman compared the sizes of circles (ends of tubes) placed on the palm of the hand and on the tongue to the sizes seen. Unlike Anstis and Loizos, Waterman found visual size to be greater than either tactual size; but like Anstis and Loizos, he found perceived size on the tongue to be larger than perceived size on the hand.

It is interesting to ask what happens if the same physical stimuli are presented simultaneously to different modalities—the visual and the tactual. R. Teghtsoonian and Teghtsoonian (1970) found the answer to be that visual length dominates proprioceptive (finger span). With concurrent stimulation, perceived length was wholly proportional to actual length, as it is when lengths are perceived only visually. Actually, the domination of vision over touch was already well known prior to the Teghtsoonians' (1970) study. If one wears distorting prisms that make straight edges look curved or that distort the shapes of objects, the edges also feel curved to the touch, and the objects' shapes feel the way they look (J. J. Gibson, 1933; Rock & Victor, 1964).

In a more naturalistic, less contrived situation—perception under water—objects are perceived in accordance with their optical size rather than with their tactual size; the effect on perceived size is predictable from the way that refraction by water increases the size of the optical image (Kinney & Luria, 1970). That is, in this case of conflicting information it is again the visual that dominates. In infants as young as 7 days old, vision was found to dominate touch in controlling the prehension of objects (Bower, Broughton, & Moore, 1970).

The domination of touch by vision helps to refute Bishop Berkeley's (1709) hypothesis that tactile–kinesthetic perception of spatial extension is primary, whereas visual perception of space is secondary. As Berkeley's doctrine is sometimes stated, "Touch teaches vision." This seems unlikely given the way that vision often dominates touch. If teaching is needed, the reverse of Berkeley's doctrine seems more likely, as Abbott (1864) considered.

Vision's capacity to override touch was even noted by Aristotle, in his discussion of the crossed-finger illusion [*De insomniis,* 460b]. When a single object, a pencil say, is held between crossed fingers, the tactile perception is of two objects. As Aristotle pointed out, if the pencil is seen as well as felt, the illusion disappears and the perception is of only a single object. The visual overrides, and in this case corrects, the tactile.

SENSORY NONCORRESPONDENCES

To sum up: Under many conditions, vision, kinesthesis, touch, and even proprioception yield equivalent and corresponding information about spatial extents and sizes of objects. Let us note here, though, an interesting feature about differences in perceived size—about the differences that do sometimes occur between exploring eye and spread fingers, between hand and tongue, between eye and tongue—namely that these differences remain in spite of our experience. After all, we live multimodally, with continuously correlated stimulation from several senses, and hence we have ample opportunity to learn which visual, proprioceptive, and haptic perceptions correspond to one another—to learn what might be called relative veridicality. Why are not all sense percepts "true" to their objects—or, if "untrue," at least all untrue in the same way? One might expect that any sort of discrepancy between modalities would wash out during perceptual development, that feedback from the world would tend to make the front teeth feel the same size to tongue and finger. Clearly, this scenario is not correct.

Similar discrepancies take place with other characteristics of objects and events. The roughness and smoothness of surfaces as they are perceived by touch are not proportional to textures perceived by sight (Björkman, 1967). Another example of a regular difference between two modes of perceiving the same dimension is the common finding that durations appear slightly longer to the ear than to the eye (e.g., Behar & Bevan, 1961; Goldstone & Goldfarb, 1963; S. S. Stevens & Greenbaum, 1966). A pulse of sound seems to last longer than an equally long flash of light. This discrepancy in time perception occurs despite our continuous, synchronized visual and auditory experiences. No matter the overwhelming number of occasions that we have seen mouths move in harmony with heard voices, the relatively simple dimension of duration fails to hook up perfectly between sight and hearing.

A conclusion is to be drawn: Although the organization of heteromodal information must be based upon experience, some characteristics of the environment lure different senses quite naturally into producing discrepant information; moreover, the discrepancies most certainly are not anything that themselves could be learned. Instead, they are cases of intrinsic sensory noncorrespondence.

The simplest hypothesis seems to be that size or extensiveness is a property of perception that, *contra* Berkeley, is common to the nature of several senses, including vision, touch, kinesthesis, and proprioception. The basis for whatever equivalences there are in size perception is most likely something that is, by and large, wired into the system. Unfortunately, not all of the wiring is precise or aligned, so cross-modal agreement is not perfect. If sensory systems do play the roles of teacher and pupil, then the educational system surely leaves much to be desired.

Cross-Modal Perception of Form

As I have already noted, the shape or form of objects holds a position of prominence not only on Aristotle's list of common sensible attributes, but also on Galileo's and Locke's list of primary qualities. Features of objects, like straightness and curvature, roundness and peakedness, regularity and irregularity, can be determined by several means—for instance by visual inspection and by tactile exploration. I see the pen that I am writing with—long, hexogonal in cross-section— and the visual perception agrees with the way the pen feels in my hand.

HOW EQUIVALENT ARE TACTILE AND VISUAL INFORMATION ABOUT FORM?

My children when they were younger enjoyed playing a simple game—sort of an attempt at ESP—where I flipped a coin into the air, caught it, and had them guess "heads" or "tails." I soon learned that if I caught the coin between thumb and index finger, then by means of a slight palpation I could identify the coin's surface position. This discovery enabled me to announce, in an appropriately grand manner, the outcome of each flip of the coin before anyone looked at it. Actually, any benefit of this prodigious feat was short-lived, for the children soon caught on to what I was doing. From this I concluded, first, that adults are capable of obtaining some of the same information about texture and shape through haptic touch and through vision, and second, that children at least as young as 6 years are capable of perceiving accurately when adults utilize such haptic or multimodal information.

The first of my conclusions, at least, was not original. J. J. Gibson (1962) reported that young adults can make error-free cross-modal identifications of the same objects by vision and by active touch, given sufficient practice at the task. Similarly, good transfer of identification takes place between equivalent visual and tactile forms (Krauthamer, 1968). Lobb (1965) showed that eighth-grade children were able to identify by one modality (vision or touch) random shapes presented to the other; however, he did note that visual matching to visual stimuli excelled cross-modal matching.

Intramodal transfer of form discrimination (transfer within a single modality) often is found to be superior to cross-modal transfer (Abravanel, 1971a; Cashdan, 1968). Thus, tactile information and visual information about the shape or figure of an object are not always completely equivalent, certainly not identical. Part of the reason for this may reside in a basic, inherent inferiority of haptic touch as compared to vision in its capacity to process information (cf. Abravanel, 1971a; Cashdan, 1968; Rudel & Teuber, 1964).

We are usually just better at perceiving form with our eyes than with our hands. Because cross-modal tasks must perforce employ touch, cross-modal matching between vision and touch will necessarily be inferior to intramodal visual matching. If this were the whole story, then we would expect intramodal tactual matching to be the poorest of all, that is, poorer than, or at least not better than, cross-modal matching. This is precisely what Rudel and Teuber (1964), Lobb (1965), and Abravanel (1971a) found. Even so, this does not mean that the inferiority of haptic perception must shoulder the whole blame for the inferiority of cross-modal matching compared to intramodal visual matching. Alternatively, or concomitantly, there may be some loss of information where visual and haptic information are correlated, that is, some loss within the *sensus communis*.

Despite the quantitative difference in the capacities of sight and touch to perceive and discriminate forms, cross-modal translation of information does occur. And it occurs very early in life. Bruner and Koslowski (1972) showed infants (8–22 weeks old) two balls; one was small in size and graspable, the other large and not. Before the infants were able to reach the balls, they made appropriate grasping motions only to the one that was graspable. Visual information about size seems to be coordinated with prehaptic activity even before action arises.

Children 4 to 5 years old are able to match shapes from touch to vision and from vision to touch; again, we have an example of the visual modality dominating perception, in that when stimuli are available to both modalities, the tactile information often is ignored (Abravanel, 1972). Between the ages of 5 and 11 years, there is a regular improvement in children's capacity to match shapes presented visually, haptically, and kinesthetically (Birch & Lefford, 1963), but even at age 5, cross-modal matching is good. In this respect, cross-modal matching of form resembles cross-modal matching of length (Abravanel, 1968). Again, this outcome may reflect, at least in part, the way that cross-modal matching ultimately depends on haptic form perception. Milner and Bryant (1970) showed that improvement with age in intramodal matching of forms parallels improvement in cross-modal matching. This finding conforms to the hypothesis that there is no special improvement with age in cross-modal matching. In fact, children as young as age 3 can do as well cross-modally (visual–tactile) as intramodally (visual–visual, tactile–tactile) in the matching of shape and of texture as long as there is no demand placed on memory (Rose, Blank, & Bridger, 1972).

MUST CROSS-MODAL EQUIVALENCE
BE DEVELOPED?

Interest in the visual and tactile identification of objects actually has a long and eminent history, tracing back at least to John Locke (1690), who reported a query raised by his friend William Molyneux. Molyneux asked whether a person blind from birth but suddenly given sight could distinguish immediately by vision between a sphere and a cube (assuming, of course, that the person had previously learned to make the discrimination by touch). Locke agreed with Molyneux that such a person could not. Thus both men took an empiricist viewpoint concerning the origin of this particular function of the *sensus communis*. The capacity to transfer information from one sensory modality to another requires experienced association, so Locke's hypothesis goes, the simultaneous or contiguous stimulation of the two modalities. Almost 2½ centuries later, Senden (1932) reviewed many if not all of the extant reports on the initial vision of people given sight (by removal of cataracts) after congenital blindness. His summary suggests that Locke's and Molyneux's conjecture was basically correct. Cross-modal identification does take time to develop after vision is first instated. Visual perception and identification of simple geometrical shapes is at first very poor. In fact, sometimes different shapes are not even perceived immediately as different.

Gregory and Wallace (1963) described the visual discriminations made by a man who had become blind at a very early age—about 9 months—but whose sight was restored in adulthood. Right after restoration of sight, some visual form perception was evidenced. For example, the man could identify correctly the colored numerals on isochromatic plates that are typically used to test for color blindness. An obvious visual deficit appeared in the man's perception of depth. Gregory and Wallace concluded that early touch experience can transfer to vision many years later. But it must be pointed out that the subject did have sight during the first 9 months of his life, so common visual and tactile information was available and presumably used. Although it is unlikely that specific cross-modal connections made in infancy were still available to mediate cross-modal transfer many decades later, nevertheless it is conceivable that some sort of multimodal stimulation was necessary in order to permit subsequent multimodal organization.

The conclusion from studies of restored sight seems to be that some experience or practice is necessary before significant cross-modal transfer from touch to vision can manifest itself. At first glance this conclusion may appear to contradict the picture that emerges from developmental studies (Bower *et al.*, 1970; Bruner & Koslowski, 1972), which suggest the primacy of vision over touch. But the two are not necessarily at odds. Objects' shapes and sizes can be perceived through both vision and touch. To utilize fully either sense takes time and, undoubtedly, some practice. The mastery of fine cross-modal integration must, perforce, require at least as much. The relatively slow accretion, under normal circumstances, of haptic skills—and, concomitantly, of cross-modal skills—attests to that modality's slow development. With congenital or early blindness, the haptic sense advances perhaps a bit more quickly; once sight is instated or restored, visual development—and hence cross-modal development—shows itself, as best it can under the circumstances.

DOES LANGUAGE MEDIATE CROSS-MODAL TRANSFER?

A basic question to be asked of cross-modal transfer is, Where does the transfer take place? or, in other words, What mediates transfer? What are the crucial properties or features of the *sensus communis*? One possibility is verbal mediation. This is to say that translation between modalities may depend on language, may require linguistic coding of critical features of the stimulus. In order to transfer from vision to touch the identification of a triangular solid, it might be necessary to code properties such as the shape and size in words—"as large as my hand," "four points," "straight edges," "smooth surface," etc. Under this interpretation, verbal tags—words—bridge gaps among the senses. Language acts as an internal medium of communication among different modalities.

Evidence favoring such an explanation is scanty, though the explanation is suggested, for example, by a study conducted by Gaydos (1956). Subjects learned to identify forms either by touch or by vision and then were tested on the other modality. Some transfer was evident, but the important point here is that Gaydos reported that verbal descriptions were commonly used; this implies that the subjects used language to code and identify the forms.

Several lines of evidence militate against the generality of the hypothesis of verbal mediation. Rudel and Teuber (1963) examined the perception of length in the well-known Müller–Lyer illusion (see Figure 2.4). Adding angled corners to a line modifies the line's apparent length; furthermore, the illusion occurs when the line is perceived

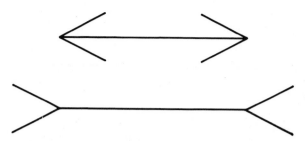

Figure 2.4. The Müller-Lyer illusion. The two horizontal lines are equally long. But the lower line, with the outwardly flaring wings, looks longer. The illusion also operates tactually, when the shapes are explored with the fingers.

tactually (through passive exploration by the fingers) as well as when the line is perceived visually. Now, the magnitude of the illusion decreases over time, as the stimuli are repeatedly exposed; moreover, this adaptation-like decrement is found in both the visual and tactile modes. This is itself an interesting analogy between the two senses. But what is even more striking and significant is Rudel and Teuber's finding that the decrement can transfer from touch to vision, and, to a lesser degree, from vision to touch. That is, repeated trials with the tactile form reduced the size of the visual illusion. It is noteworthy that the subjects in the experiment gave no indication of being aware even of the occurrence of the illusion, to say nothing of its decrement. Hence linguistic mediation of the cross-modal transfer seems extremely unlikely.

Other evidence that verbal labels are not always necessary for cross-modal transfer or identification comes from examining the behavior of infants. Bryant, Jones, Claxton, and Perkins (1972) found that children as young as 8 to 9 months of age displayed, at a simple level, almost as much cross-modal transfer (tactile to visual) as intramodal transfer; that is, the children reached for objects they had touched. Blank and Bridger (1964) decided that language is not always important or necessary for transfer to occur because their subjects (3- and 4-year-old children) did not explicate verbally the basis for their cross-modal (visual and tactile) transfer of shape. Blank and Klig (1970) arrived at the same conclusion for the transfer of form and texture information by 4-year-olds.

Obviously, failure to verbalize does not preclude implicit verbal mediation. However, a similar conclusion—that verbalization is not necessary—was also reached by Rudel and Teuber (1964), who found cross-modal equivalence of shape could be as efficient as intramodal equivalence in children as young as 3 years. Transfer from visual to visual and from tactual to visual forms were best, from visual to tactual and from tactual to tactual, worst. Aside from the inferiority inherent in our ability to use tactual information, Rudel and Teuber concluded: "The problem of perceptual equivalence across sense modalities thus does not seem to be too different from the problem of equivalence within a particular modality. There is some common aspect of perceptual activity which permits one to utilize information from within a sensory channel or from several sensory channels in such a way that invariant properties of objects are extracted . . . [1964, p. 6]." This statement describes a modern version of Aristotle's *sensus communis* where the "invariant properties of objects" play the role of κοινα αἰσθήτα.

In order to evaluate further the hypothesis of verbal mediation, it is worthwhile to look also at studies of how infrahumans transfer information across modalities. Since at present only humans have a well-developed system of abstract language, evidence of cross-modal transfer in infrahumans would imply that verbal mediation is not a requisite for transfer to take place. In fact, some experiments, such as those of Ettlinger (1960, 1961), failed to demonstrate cross-modal transfer of training in monkeys. Ettlinger reported that rhesus monkeys, trained to discriminate visually between different shapes and different sizes, failed to demonstrate any gains during subsequent training when the stimuli were presented tactually. The conclusion was that language may be necessary for transfer of information about shape and size.

Two points are worth making. First, failure to demonstrate cross-modal transfer in infrahumans does not prove that language is needed. Second, transfer of training is not always the best paradigm for demonstrating cross-modal translation, even in humans. For example, Lobb (1970) showed that learning shapes by vision improved subsequent learning by touch, but not vice versa, and Shaffer and Howard (1974) found little evidence of transfer from touch to vision or vision to touch with dot patterns.

It is not surprising, then, that many studies on infrahumans fail to show cross-modal transfer of training. Rhesus monkeys trained to discriminate between two temporal rates of interruption of a light did not transfer the learning to an auditory stimulus (Burton & Ettlinger, 1960). Ettlinger and Blakemore (1967) tried to teach rhesus monkeys to match objects cross-modally, using touch and vision. The attempt failed; in general, the monkeys tended to ignore the tactually presented stimuli. (Recall a similar finding that human children ignore tactual in favor of visual information [Abravanel, 1972].) In fact, discrimination of objects by sight and by touch may proceed quite independently. Rhesus monkeys were taught to discriminate a cone from a pyramid in the dark (by touch), then the pyramid from the cone in the light (by sight), apparently with no interaction between the two learning experiences (Moffett & Ettlinger, 1966). W. A. Wilson, Jr. and Shaffer (1963) confirmed Ettlinger's (1960) finding that rhesus monkeys do not transfer information about shape, but found that they do transfer information about length. W. A. Wilson, Jr. (1965) surmised that the reason that shape information was not transferred may be that the two sense modalities use different cues (features of the stimuli). For instance, edges might be used as discriminal cues for touch, vertices as cues for vision.

Perhaps part of the problem is phylogenetic: Monkeys—lower primates—just may not be able to do what higher primates can. Actually, even monkeys can demonstrate some capacity for cross-modal transfer of shape and size, albeit the transfer may be subtle and small in degree (Blakeslee & Gunter, 1966). But higher primates do better. Apes (chimpanzees and orangutans) can match, that is, select by active touch, objects presented visually that were previously unfamiliar: The objects included handles, clamps, and springs (Davenport & Rogers, 1970). Furthermore, after extensive training with such matches, the apes showed immediate transfer upon presentation of novel stimuli. In a subsequent study, Davenport and Rogers (1971) reported that apes can even select by haptic touch objects that match photographs. These experiments suggest "the presence in apes of a metamodal concept of stimulus equivalence which is based on a mediation process independent of verbal language [Davenport & Rogers, 1970, p. 280]."

CROSS-MODAL TRANSFER BY DETECTION
OF COMMON FEATURES

Clearly, language is not requisite to cross-modal equivalence, although there is little doubt that language can help to mediate transfer of information from sense to sense and may play a prominent role in the cross-modal transfer by humans. After all, language is there, it is convenient and most useful as a cognitive shorthand. Language is not necessary for transfer, but it is sufficient to permit transfer. Language may as a matter of empirical fact be necessary, however, to the mediation of more complex or abstract cross-modal relations, such as "number" (cf. Blank & Bridger, 1964).

One alternative—or concomitant—to verbal mediation is the possibility that certain distinctive feature of objects "register" directly in perception, regardless of the modality of presentation. Given a direct realist view of perception, a particular property of an object, say its size, is apprehended directly, as a property of the object, and is so apprehended regardless of the particular modality through which the property is sensed. This hypothesis derives from the theory of J. J. Gibson: "There must be [a] simple type of perceptual development, the registering of the concurrent covariation from different organs . . . . Insofar as this linkage is invariant, the information is the same in all of them, that is, the systems are equivalent [1966, p. 289]." E. J. Gibson (1969) pointed out that, under such an hypothesis, the term "transfer" is itself inappropriate. Transfer implies a process of mediation, of going from one modality to another through or by means of still something else. The hypothesis of invariant features, on the other hand, requires no extraneous intermediary to fill a gap between modailties. The only intermediaries are the features of the objects themselves.

Some support for this position is provided by results of A. D. Pick, Pick, and Thomas (1966), who examined transfer of form discrimination between touch and vision. Subjects were first-grade children who were presented meaningless forms (similar to letters of the alphabet). Identification took place cross-modally, and the results suggested that what the children had learned were the important dimensions, or distinctive features, by which the forms differed—for example, features like rotation and size. The identification of visual forms by adults is readily transferred to tactile equivalents in a way that suggests stimulus features are learned independently of modality (Shaffer & Ellis, 1974). Owen and Brown (1970a) asked subjects to judge the complexity of random forms, which were perceived either by sight or by touch. The judgments themselves and the time required to make the judgments suggested that the two senses processed similar informational features. On the other hand, Shaffer and Howard (1974) found no evidence of transfer of distinctive features when the stimuli consisted of patterns of dots.

In this context, some striking results were obtained by Holmgren, Arnoult, and Manning (1966). In their experiment, subjects first learned to associate nonsense syllables with either auditory patterns (temporal sequences of different sound frequencies) or visual patterns (spatial sequences of the corresponding sinusoids). This initial learning was followed by a transfer task in which the subjects had to learn associations to the stimuli of the other modality. When the visual and auditory patterns were analogous, that is, had the same structure optically as acoustically, positive transfer ensued; that is, learning was superior to that of control groups. When the patterns were structurally different, negative transfer ensued; that is, learning was inferior to that of control groups. What was most striking about the findings was that the subjects seemed to be totally unaware of any structural similarity between the auditory and visual patterns! Whatever mediated the cross-modal transfer must have been subtle indeed.

In conclusion, it seems fair to suggest that the *sensus communis* is probably rather broad in its functional scope. Both linguistic and non-linguistic mechanisms are surely involved in the mediation of cross-modal translation and equivalence (and here I use "mediation" broadly enough to include "registration" of common features). The failure of several attempts to demonstrate cross-modal matching or transfer in infrahumans most likely indicates a paucity—though certainly not a complete lack—of complex mediating mechanisms in lower animals.

Cross-Modal Perception of Space

The topic of space perception both incorporates the subject matter of the last two sections—size and shape—and transcends it. Not only must we consider extension of objects in space, but the relations of objects in space to one another and to the perceiver. Kant (1781) theorized that space is an a priori form of perception. By this, Kant meant that, from a logical point of view, the property of spatiality precedes the contents of sensory experience. Jumping off from this, we may take a psychological tack and ask whether there exist several spaces or just one, a spatiality proper to each sense or a single space common to several. Attneave and Benson (1969) reported a study in which subjects first were taught to discriminate among several vibratory stimuli placed in different spatial locations, then were required to transfer the discriminations from one hand to the other. Subjects succeeded, both when they had to transfer responses to the same locus in space (spatial learning) and when they had to transfer responses to the analogous finger (stimulus–response learning). Transfer occurred both with and without visual cues. The authors concluded that spatial information is represented in a common space, and the results indicated that the common space to which tactual and kinesthetic information is transfered is intrinsically visual.

To repeat, the concept of spatiality encompasses the extension or size of objects, but includes much more. We perceive that there is a physical space in our universe within which we move about; as we move, we change our relative positions over time with respect to various objects in the environment. And in this environment the objects themselves also may move relative to each other as well as relative to us. Objects heard and felt, as well as objects seen, are perceived as external, as existing out in space. When a blind person explores a portion of the external world with his cane, what he feels is an external array of surfaces and substances, a world outside of him, not an array of sensations in his hand and arm.

Objects can be localized in space by means of several senses, by hearing as well as by vision and touch, for example, though it should be noted that auditory spatial localization is sometimes rather crude. S. S. Stevens and Newman (1936) had subjects try to localize sounds in space by pointing to the source of the source of the sounds in a free field. The subject's head was held stationary. This procedure yielded rather large errors in spatial acuity, with deviations between actual location and indicated location of 10° and greater. Much smaller errors—about 1° in size—are made when the subject's task is simply to detect a change in the spatial position of a sound source, rather than to identify the absolute position itself (Mills, 1958).

Our ability to localize sounds in space is based primarily on what are called interaural time cues: These are the very small differences between the times that the sound waves arrive at the two ears. (Differences in intensity are also important, mainly when sound frequency is high.) Acoustical signals impinge on the two ears in a temporal relation that depends on the spatial location of the sound source. Whichever ear is closer to a source of sound gets the sound first. For instance, a sound that comes from one's left side reaches the left ear before it reaches the right ear, and this temporal asynchrony contains the information needed to determine the sound source's position. The first full statement of this view was presented by Hornbostel and Wertheimer in 1920. In real life, auditory spatial localization is an active process; by moving our heads about in relation to sound sources we effect changes in the temporal relations between the signals that reach the two ears, thus enabling us to localize sounds with greater accuracy than would be possible if we were to keep our heads stationary.

How is auditory space related to visual space? It is useful to begin from a functional point of view, from the observation that people behave in general as if there is a single space. When my alarm clock wakens me, I reach over to turn it off without looking at it; when I hear someone speak, the voice is heard, indeed almost seen, to come from the speaker's mouth. It may be that there is only one space, one psychological representation that incorporates visual, proprioceptive, kinesthetic, tactile, and auditory information. Or it may be that there are several modally distinct spaces, several psychological representations—one visual, another proprioceptive, still others kinesthetic, tactile, and auditory—but these are well enough coordinated to permit ready cross-migration and translation of information, so that in their joint operation they resemble a single psychological space.

Berkeley (1709) proposed that there exists a primary psychological space and that this space is given through kinesthesis and haptic touch. Visual and auditory cues, according to this theory, become tied to the kinesthetic through association: The visual world changes as we move ourselves and objects through space. We learn to see or hear one distance as twice as far as another by the process of pacing out twice as many steps.

> Sitting in my Study I hear a Coach drive along the Streets. I look through the Casement and see it. I walk out and enter into it. Thus, common Speech wou'd incline one to think, I heard, saw, and touch'd the same Thing, *viz*. the Coach. It is, nevertheless, certain, the *Ideas* intromitted by each Sense are widely different, and distinct from each other; but having been observed constantly to go together, they are spoken of as one and the same thing [pp. 51–52].

I find myself somewhat loath even to bring up Berkeley's hypothesis: Little can be said in its favor, whereas much can be said against it. Berkeley's position would seem to require the primacy of haptic space in infancy, yet even in 1-week-old infants vision predominates over touch (Bower *et al.*, 1970). When the spatial representations of vision and touch are put into battle—when the world is viewed through prisms that optically displace the retinal image of the visual world—it is vision that dominates touch, and, as the new visual representation becomes coordinated again with the proprioceptive–tactile representation, it is the latter that changes, not the former (C. S. Harris, 1965).

To return to the major point, under normal circumstances spatial information obtained from different senses is coordinated. Auerbach and Sperling (1974) concluded that perceived direction in vision and perceived direction in hearing derive from a single, common spatial representation. Subjects were required to discriminate between spatial directions of two sound stimuli, of two light stimuli, and of a sound stimulus and a light stimulus. Analysis of the results suggested little or no variability in judgment that could be attributed to translating from one spatial representation to another; that is, both auditory and visual sensations appeared to be referred to a single perceptual space.

What sort of learning, if any, is involved in developing this multimodal spatial representation remains unclear. Evidence has been presented to suggest that infants as young as 30 days of age manifest a common auditory and visual space (Aronson & Rosenbloom, 1971);

infants displayed noticeable distress when their mother's voice was spatially displaced from her visual image. Unfortunately, an attempt, with additional controls, to replicate this finding failed (McGurk & Lewis, 1974). Should the original result be confirmed, though, verbal mediation again would seem to be precluded, this time as an explanation for the coordination of multimodal space.

We have already noted several instances—with regard to form perception as well as to space perception—where vision dominates touch when conflicting information is made available to subjects. There seems to be going on something like a "law of minimal perceptual effort" or what information theorists might call a "maximization of redundancy." Put simply, people try to make sense out of what they sense, and make simple sense at that. When making simple sense requires the resolution of a conflict, something has to give. What gives, though, is typically not vision. Apparently, seeing is believing.

In the perception of space, vision dominates other modalities besides touch. Witkin, Wapner, and Leventhal (1952) measured how far a sound must be displaced from the midline in order for a person to tell that it is off center. The displacement had to be made much larger when the sound source appeared visually at the midline: We tend to hear sounds where we see them. This is a one-way street, though; whereas auditory localization is strongly influenced by visual displacement of a stimulus (for instance, as produced by a prism), visual localization is hardly influenced by auditory displacement (H. L. Pick, Jr., Warren, & Hay, 1969). It is a good thing that hearing and sight interact in the way they do, else ventriloquists would be without employment.

Cross-Modal Perception of Time, Motion, and Number

Aristotle did not include time in his discussion of the *sensus communis;* nevertheless, time is surely deserving of at least brief mention. If there is any attribute that truly deserves to be called a common sensible, any attribute of objects or events that really can manifest itself through *all* of the senses, it is time. Duration is unquestionably universal.

Mention has already been made of the fact that auditory intervals appear to be slightly longer than visual intervals of the identical real duration (Behar & Bevan, 1961; Goldstone & Goldfarb, 1963; S. S. Stevens & Greenbaum, 1966). This effect is illustrated in Figure 2.5. Another interesting fact is that temporal intervals that contain sensory events appear to be longer than intervals that are empty of sensory

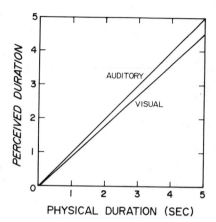

Figure 2.5. To both ear and eye, the perceived duration of a stimulus grows just about in proportion to its physical duration. But any given physical duration seems longer when heard than when seen.

events (Goldstone & Goldfarb, 1963). The magnitude of this curious effect appears to depend somewhat on the number of sensory elements that fill the interval: The larger the number of sensory elements, the longer the interval appears to last (Buffardi, 1971). This filled-interval illusion, as it is called, in which perceived time stretches out, is independent of sensory modality. The illusion occurs regardless of whether the sensory elements in the interval are visual, auditory, or tactile. Hence this illusion of time may be one that arises in the "common sense."

Behar and Bevan (1961) noted that categorical judgments of the duration of sounds were influenced by the visual stimuli presented as end-points of the rating scale, and judged durations of lights were influenced by auditory end points. From this result they concluded that duration is supramodal, that is, judged by a central process. That a single, common mechanism mediates the perception of visual and auditory time was also concluded by Eijkman and Vendrik (1965), who investigated the ability of subjects to discriminate small differences in the durations of two lights and of two sounds. Their first experiment showed that the ability to detect small differences in visual duration is identical to the ability to detect small differences in auditory duration; hence the mediating mechanism may be similar, perhaps identical, in the two modalities. It is their second experiment that is critical; this experiment measured sensitivity to differences in duration given simultaneous visual and auditory stimulation. It turned out that the fluctuations in sensitivity to duration in the two modalities were perfectly correlated. But if the modalities acted independently—with regard to the perception of duration—the fluctuations should have been uncorrelated. From this outcome one may conclude, as the authors did, "that discrimination of duration of auditory and visual stimuli is done by the same 'duration center' [Eijkman & Vendrik, 1965, p. 1109]."

Motion obviously bears a close relation to both time and space, since movement consists of a change in spatial position over time. The intersensory cues to motion can be complex. Consider the way we perceive an oncoming police car or ambulance, with its lights flashing and its siren blaring. The visual image appears and, optically, the visual angle subtended by the car enlarges as it approaches. Our perception of the car's size does not increase accordingly, but instead remains relatively constant—this is the phenomenon called *size constancy*. If visual fixation falls on some other object in the field, one whose position stays constant, the image of the car will sweep across the visual field; we are more likely, though, to follow the car with our eyes, so the image remains fairly well located in central vision. (The way we do this is itself worthy of a chapter!) Once the car passes, the optical image now begins to decrease in size—though again the perceived size remains roughly constant—until finally the car is gone.

Changes in the sound of the siren complement the visual transformations. The car's approach is marked by increases in both the siren's loudness and its pitch: Loudness increases because loudness depends on sound energy, which in turn depends on distance from source—the relationship between intensity and distance obeys the famous inverse-square law; pitch increases because pitch depends on sound frequency, which in turn increases as a sound-emitting object moves nearer—the relationship between frequency and motion is known as the Doppler effect. Once the car passes and recedes into the distance, both loudness and pitch decrease. Thus sound energy and sound frequency both change over time in an orderly manner. These acoustical variations, together with changing interaural time cues, are normally correlated with correspondingly orderly variations in the size of the retinal image, and these systematic changes in auditory and visual stimulation serve as common sources of information about movement of objects in the environment.

Objects or events that are discontinuous in space, time, or both are countable or denumerable. That is, discontinuous events or objects provide the raw stuff that makes the contents of the concept of number. It is more than just a matter of linguistic convenience that I use the phrase "concept of number," for number appears in some way to be even more an abstraction than is, for example, either space or time. To be sure, Aristotle included number among his common attributes of sensation, and Locke included it among the primary qualities; nevertheless, the truth of the matter may lie as well with Kant (1781), who placed number among the Categories of the Understanding. The distinction may be relevant to a result of Blank and Bridger (1964), who found that although 3- and 4-year-old children were capable of directly transferring information about the shape of objects from vision to touch, the children had difficulty in similarly transferring the concept of number ("oneness, " "twoness" of lights and sounds). To appreciate that the same number of items in two sensory modes were equivalent seemed to demand the use of verbal mediation; indeed, the discrimination of one item from two within a single modality seemed to depend on verbalization. This outcome led Blank and Bridger to distinguish between cross-modal equivalence (e.g., form) on the one hand and cross-modal concepts (e. g., number) on the other. The mediation of concepts demands more than just registering perceptual features.

Perhaps one reason that number sometimes seems better described as a concept than as a percept is that the same value on this dimension (that is, the same number) can apply to objects or events perceived by different modalities even when the objects or events are not themselves identical. Two sounds form an event that is like two flashes of light, even when the sounds do not come from the light source. It becomes both valuable and important to distinguish between two roles that nunber can play in the present scheme: One role is as a common sensible attribute that pertains to the same objects, regardless of sense modality through which the objects are perceived; the other is as a suprasensory attribute, a dimension of experience that is appropriate to all modalities, but one that does not take on the functional role of specifying common properties of stimuli. A few examples will make the distinction clear. I hold several coins in my hand: Two, three, four—the number is perceptible by active touch and by sight. A spatial array of objects can be counted, probably with about equal accuracy, by feel and by look. In this instance, number is a common sensible.

By way of contrast, consider a similar spatial array of sounds, perhaps several voices heard at once. How many different voices can we pick out? Two, three, four? Perhaps a few more, but not many. The auditory system has only a feeble capacity to determine number—when the several sounds are heard at once. Only when events are separated in time, as when soldiers "count off," does hearing become a good modality for conveying information about number. But now we are more properly talking about number of events than of number of objects: tenuous is the claim that hearing provides information about number that is equivalent to the information that sight and touch provide. Unlike the visual sense, where spatial position dominates, in the auditory sense temporal position dominates (O'Connor & Hermelin, 1972). Denumerability is an attribute of hearing as well as of seeing, but primarily through time for the former, through space for the latter.

This distinction helps clarify and understand empirical findings concerning the perception of number in different modalities. White and Cheatham (1959) determined the relationship between the perceived number of events and the actual physical number of events that were presented, where the stimuli were pulse sequences of light, of sound, and of touch. That is, in all three modalities the discontinuities were temporal. With both hearing and touch, perceived number was directly proportional to actual number, that is, the perception of number was veridical. With vision, however, the sense we just denoted as "spatial," White and Cheatham found systematic underestimation of perceived number, even though the actual numbers of pulses were small (only up to eight). (It should be noted that the visual and tactile pulses were presented at a rate of 30/sec, whereas the auditory pulses were presented at a rate of 10/sec.) Were the visual display represented spatially rather than temporally, for example, as up to eight spots of light in a line, it is hardly conceivable that people would underestimate such small numbers of items. Lechelt (1974) too found marked underestimation when the eye was stimulated by sequences of flashes of light; he noted also that touch showed some underestimation, and, furthermore, that the degree of underestimation in both vision and touch depended systematically upon pulse rate. To the ear, however, perceived number was always directly and fully proportional to actual number. This is as we might expect in such a temporal paradigm.

That vision, hearing, and touch fail to display complete equivalence in psychophysical tasks on the perception of number reflects the fact that there are real and significant differences among them in sensory functioning, but does not necessarily mean that different senses fail to provide equivalent information about objects or events in the environment. The senses surely can provide equivalent information, as when we both see and hear several people speak in succession; they can provide complementary information, as when we either see or hear them; and they can provide independent information, as when we see and hear one person speak several times in succession.

Some Philosophical Considerations

What is the nature and meaning of this first doctrine of sensory correspondence? Even given the occasional examples of sensory noncorrespondence, the several senses usually succeed admirably in cooperating. What, we may ask, do they cooperate about? Obviously, or so it would seem, they cooperate in telling us about objects and events in the real world. Is such an interpretation tenable?[2]

THE SKEPTICAL ARGUMENT

A couple of centuries ago the Scottish philosopher David Hume (1739) argued forcefully that we can never learn what the real world is, or if in fact there is one; epistemologically, all we have are our sensations. We can never know what, if anything, underlies or causes sense perception, because no matter where we look or listen or feel, all we can obtain is more sensation. Given that sensory experience not only does provide, but must provide, the threads we have to weave our mental tapestries of the world, then, so the argument goes, all that we can justifiably say we know is the sensory experience. Like molten shadows poured by twilight—shadows that fall, to use T. S. Eliot's words, " between the idea and the reality"[3]—try as we may to grasp them, we manage only to cast more shadows. Between the external world and our understanding of it looms the impassable gulf of perception.

This skeptical argument is often regarded as the culmination of the thought of the British empirical school that is usually said to have begun with John Locke. But if one accepts the skeptical approach, it becomes difficult to accept also the interpretation given above of the first doctrine of sensory correspondence. For if we can never know anything about the real world, then there is no way to ascertain what it is that the different senses reflect in common.

Such a dismaying conclusion is ultimately derived by relentlessly applying a radical empiricism to Locke's epistemology. Because the skeptic's departure from Locke's theory comes just at the point where the Doctrine of Equivalent Information appears, it is pertinent to examine this point of departure in some detail.

Throughout this chapter I have repeatedly evaluated the Doctrine of Equivalent Information in terms of Aristotle's notion of common sensible attributes, a notion that, in turn—I have also repeatedly noted—seems closely allied to Locke's formulation of the theory of primary qualities. Let me reclothe Locke's position in modern garb: There exists an external world of matter and motion (which can be described in physical terms). Whatever it is that we know about this world—veridical knowledge, to use a seemingly redundant expres-

---

[2] For other approaches to several of the issues discussed in this section, the reader is directed to the collection of articles in Weimer and Palermo (1974).

[3] From "The Hollow Men" by T. S. Eliot. In *Collected poems* 1909–1962, Harcourt Brace Jovanovich, Publishers.

sion—comes ultimately through the senses; in Locke's words, all of our ideas come from "sensation and reflection." To be more specific, certain inherent properties of the physical world—the primary qualities of objects such as their shape, size, number, motion—have the power to act on the senses so as to produce perceptual attributes that resemble the physical properties. Other inherent properties of objects—the secondary qualities—act so as to produce perceptual attributes that do not resemble their causes. Warmth, sweetness, pain are not copies of the physical properties that cause them. In the words of Democritus, "Sweet exists by convention, bitter by convention, color by convention; atoms and void (*alone*) exist in reality [Freeman, 1948, p. 93]."

Perceptions that do resemble their causes in the external world can arise from more than one sense modality. This is how the Doctrine of Equivalent Information ties in with the theory of primary qualities: Different senses inform us, veridically, about the same properties of the external world.

Unfortunately, Locke's theory of primary qualities has been difficult to defend philosophically, for it is not clear, prima facie, how to demonstrate, either empirically or logically, which sensory attributes reflect primary qualities, which secondary qualities of things—an objection made by Berkeley (1710) and Hume (1739). How can it be shown that there are physical qualities similar to perceptual ones, if all that we have is perception to go on? Everything that we know, in sum, derives from our perceptions, which in turn must always appear at the interface between us and the external world. To take this last step is to succumb to the skeptic's brief.

The skeptical argument can be pushed even further—to solipsism, to denying the very existence of an external reality, or at least to questioning whether its existence can be demonstrated. So the spirit of skepticism can carry one to an unreasonable conclusion. Because it is unreasonable, I will reject the solipsism that the skeptical route so readily leads to and instead take up the more fruitful topic of whether (or how) perceptions resemble their objects. The minimal assumption that will be made, then, is the patently reasonable one that there does exist an external reality capable of providing stimulation to the senses. The issue to be investigated is now slightly different: It is not whether we glean information about reality—the assumption is that we do—but rather how closely perception hews to reality. A sensory system can channel information about objects and events, indeed different senses can channel convergent or equivalent information about the same objects and events, without the resulting percepts resembling their causes.

In this regard, it is important to separate two distinct questions. One asks how well perception resembles reality; the other asks how much the mind itself contributes to perception. The former question is the issue under prime consideration: An alternative to Locke's formulation of resemblance says that percpetion consists only of mental qualities, that is, attributes of sensation, which must by their nature differ from physical properties and hence can never be shown to resemble them.[4]

Both of the alternatives just described are, or at least can be, attributed to the empiricist position that all knowledge comes from experience. Both Locke and Hume (or Berkeley), who, respectively, held and denied the Principle of Resemblance, are usually placed in the empiricist tradition. This brings us to the second issue: An alternative to the empiricist's claim that all knowledge comes from experience is the rationalist's counterclaim that some knowledge comes from the activity of the mind itself.

By one of the curious ironies of philosophy, the skeptical extension of the empiricist approach can lead directly to a rationalism. Take Locke's position as a starting point and look carefully at the ontogenesis of relationships like space, time, and causality. Where do these come from? They seem to have no external justification. In Hume's famous analysis, for example, causality reduces to repeated conjunctions of perceptions; causality itself is never perceived. But if the concept of causality does not come from without, it must come from within. Thus Kant (1781) was led to conclude that space and time in perception, causality and number (among others) in conception, are logically prior to the contents of perception and thought, therefore are the mind's own contribution. Actually, it is not necessary to go to Kant in order to uncover such a rationalistic constructionism. Hume's (1739) *Treatise on human nature* contains the ingredients of an epistemology in which some of the components arise from the mind itself (examine, for example, Hume's notion of "natural belief" in causality, and his analysis of time).

Both rationalistic and nonrationalistic approaches may be constructionistic. Constructionism view perception as the building of models, and it may postulate either a set of empiricist principles—that the

---

[4] Johannes Müller's (1838) doctrine of "specific energies of nerve," as he called it, translates this alternative to the level of the nervous system: When we perceive, we are aware only of the state of sensory neurons, not of the objects that are the ultimate causes of neural activity, not even of the stimulus energies that are the proximal causes. Although Müller's doctrine is sometimes said to be an expression of Locke's theory, it is in my opinion more nearly an expression of Berkeley's or Hume's. Locke's theory makes room for some resemblances between sensations and causes, whereas Müller's excludes any.

mental constructions are erected from sensory inputs plus memories, unconscious inferences, and the like—or rationalist ones—that mental constructions are erected from sensory inputs as these are molded by intrinsic constraints of the perceptual and cognitive apparatus. At first glance, constructionism of either sort seems inimical to Locke's Principle of Resemblance. But to repeat an old saw, appearances can be delusive.

THE REALIST ARGUMENT

Implicitly if not explicitly opposed to the Humean sort of skepticism is the approach to sensory perception taken by James J. Gibson (1966), an approach entrenched in direct realism. Gibson, who prefers the "common-sense" epistemology of Thomas Reid (1764), argues that the senses do more than just give sensations. Rather, they—the senses—are systems organized to enable us to obtain information about the world, to perceive *objects.* Now the epistemology is reversed: Instead of starting with sensation and attempting to arrive at perception of an existent reality, which is an approach doomed to fail, we start with the existent reality—objects and events that are sources of stimulation.

Perceptions are invariant across transformations of stimulus energies, whereas sensations are not. We can recognize the same book regardless of its orientation in space, we can recognize the same pig-sty regardless of the sensory system that is stimulated. In a way, Gibson's approach is strongly reminiscent of Aristotle's, in that perception, comparison, integration of information are suprasensory: Gibson's (1966) view that "Texture, consistency, shape, size, and granularity are qualities of objects, not qualities of sense [p. 140]" echoes Aristotle's view that "the perception of magnitude, figure, roughness, smoothness, sharpness and bluntness, in solid bodies, is the common function of all the senses." The alternative view—that perception is only phenomenal, rather than informational—is actually the later one, deriving from the British philosophy of the seventeenth and eighteenth centuries.

How does Gibson's view compare with Locke's? Are they truly so different? A close look shows that, despite important differences, their starting points are similar. Both commence by postulating an external world that has certain physical characteristics; these characteristics can be detected by sensory systems—and several of them can be detected by more than one sense. In indicating this similarity between the theories, I am ignoring the enormously greater sophistication contained in Gibson's approach. The physical characteristics of prime import to his theory comprise what he calls "higher-order variables," such as ratios of stimuli, gradients, etc. Probably the most important difference between the theories is, in summary, that Gibson identifies the stimuli as the objects and events in the world, rather than as the stimulus energies that serve as the medium for perception. Because higher-order variables specify objects and events, the latter are perceived directly. They need not be constructed. Nonetheless, there is in Gibson's view, as in Locke's, a primitive Principle of Resemblance.

The philosopher Rogers (1975) has attempted an epistemological synthesis of, on one hand, the Lockean view that objects in the physical world generate stimulus energies that in turn cause sensations and perceptions, and, on the other hand, the direct realist view that what is perceived is the physical world. In a nutshell, Rogers hypothesizes that perceiving is like recording; that is, to perceive is to copy an event. What is perceived is caused by objects and events in the world; in Rogers's view what is perceived is perceived *as* the cause of perception.

An admitted limitation to this synthesis is its lack of verification. To be sure, one can start with a theory of direct perception, in which some features of the world are impressed on the mind without any intervening constructional process, and from such a theory generate a reasonable set of principles to govern perceptual functions, It is not difficult, for instance, to predict the Doctrine of Equivalent Information.

But even if some perceptual dimensions do directly reflect "primary qualities," can the one be said to copy the other? Surely it is true that sensory systems are inherently selective. Not all of the physical characteristics of objects are accessible to perception—to give a few simple examples, ultraviolet and infrared radiation are, in essence, invisible; sound waves of extremely low or high frequencies are, in essence, inaudible. (Chapter 4 gives an account of the senses' passively selective or band-pass character.) Much of the discipline of psychophysics devotes itself to a systematic study of such selective processes in sensation and perception; psychophysics tries to account for the ways that sensory systems tune in on a limited portion of the physical universe.

This restriction in the input available to the senses suggests, for one, that the process of perception cannot be well analogized by a process of recording or copying, unless the limitations of the latter are made explicit. After all, a black-and-white photograph of a rustic village is not the same as a color photograph of the same scene, nor, in fact, will color photographs produced with different films (that is, with different wavelength-sensitive pigments and dyes) be identical. Even if, in some sense modalities, percepts are copies of reality, they are at the same time constructed representations. Though a series of "elemental" musical notes may be directly recorded, it is perception that puts them together into tunes.

Once we begin to attend the melodies played by perception, we find ourselves drawn along the path toward the skeptic *cum* pied piper. His route seems always to lead back to the same ineluctable question: Can it be demonstrated that perception copies reality? Despite all of the merit in synthesizing causal theory with direct perception, there still seems to be a philosophical impasse. That such an impasse does appear, that the question is not easily answered—and may not in fact be satisfactorily answerable—is, however, no reason for despair. Asking the epistemological question is important, even if no reply can persuade the relentless skeptic. Perhaps there is another question that should be asked, one that may turn out to be far more significant and as fundamental as the epistemological one: Why is it so important to show the correspondence between perception and external reality?

A MODEST PROPOSAL

Can we circumvent the reductionistic dilemma and its seemingly inescapable path to skepticism, if not solipsism? Psychologically, there is something compelling about the Lockean view. After all, most people believe not just that the world exists, but also that objects in the physical world have sizes, shapes, and textures that are like the sizes, shapes, and textures that they normally see and feel; that substances really are gaseous, liquid, or solid, as they feel; that even if no person existed to perceive it, a lilac would not only exist in the garden, but each conical blossom would continue to send forth the molecules that have the power to arouse its fragrance. What I have described in this way is close to J. S. Mill's (1865) definition of reality as the "permanent possibility of sensation."[5]

To "common sense" the continual and independent existence of the physical world is evident despite any perverse philosophical acrobatics to the contrary. The contents of perception do not typically appear to arise inside the head or in the sense organs, but outside—in the world. When we feel an object we do just that; we perceive its shape and size, its weight and texture as external to the hand, not as a spatio-temporal pattern of pressure on the skin. The same shape can be

---

[5] One may also come to believe in a reality that is itself "permanently impossible as sensation"— for example, in the physicists' "quarks," those theoretically most fundamental of subatomic particles. But I suspect the compelling belief in the perceived world goes far deeper.

felt by stroking the object with the back or front of the hand, or even by exploring it with a hand-held probe, as when a dentist, pick in hand, searches out cavities. The sensory patterns are quite different, but the object—and in a way the perception—is the same.

This last point may be extended by noting that the same shape or form can be seen as well as felt. Not only does perception externalize objects, but the same objects, and some of the same properties of objects, are perceived in concert through different senses. That we can feel as well as see a coffee cup, smell the coffee's aroma, and feel and taste its hot bitterness, is powerful psychological evidence for the existence of a certain object of a certain shape in a certain place at a certain time. Of course, not all of this information comes redundantly. Some of the perceptual information derived from different senses, though integrated into a unified whole, is not mutually confirming. The coffee could be cold, taste bitter–sweet if sugar were added, or mostly sweet if it were root beer instead. Nonetheless, some properties of reality do produce correlated information: The shape of the cup and the liquidity of its contents are essentially the same to sight and to touch. And it is these properties that "common sense" tells us are in the world as well as in perception. Multimodal concurrence becomes a possible criterion for distinguishing primary from secondary qualities.

This argument does not constitute a philosophical justification for resemblance. Logically, the agreement of perceptual evidence from different senses no more demands the existence of physical *analogues* to the perceptual attributes than does the evidence from a single sense, no better parries the blows of a skeptic demanding certainty than does the latter. But what are the alternatives? Either some percepts resemble their physical objects—in which case multimodal concurrence reflects an intrinsic correspondence between perception and reality—or they do not—in which case multimodal concurrence is partly a mirage. The justification, if that is the proper term, is fundamentally psychological. It emerges from what is part and parcel of the human makeup. There is a psychological persuasiveness to the agreement of information from different sensory channels that helps engender in most of us an unshakable personal epistemology.

Before trying to tread deeper water, it is important to elucidate what is meant when it is said that perception resembles or copies reality. How close to the original must the facsimile be in order to be called a copy? To the forger of a Great Master or of paper currency it obviously needs to be nearly identical (anything else is deemed a "bad copy"). But when I make a handwritten transcription of typed text, it suffices to take down all of the same words and punctuation. That the original is in print, the copy in script, is not particularly germane. What about perception? Is perception like forgery or like transcription? The question may be turned around: How close must the relationship be in order to say that percepts resemble reality? Is the pitch of a sound enough akin to its acoustical frequency to be said to copy it? What of an object's perceived size and physical size?

J. L. Austin (1962) raised an intriguing question, When (at what distance) does an object look its real size? First of all, we should distinguish two conditions. In one, perceived size remains constant, independent of an object's distance from the perceiver; in this case, the question can have one of only two answers: always or never. In the second condition, perfect size constancy does not obtain; here, the answer is: perhaps at one distance, perhaps never. A partial solution emerges from what may be termed a rule of "relative veridicality." Object A looks (or feels) its real size only when A's perceptual size bears the same relationship to the perceptual sizes of B, C, etc., that the actual sizes of A, B, C, etc., bear to one another. That is, in order for objects to be perceived at their real size, perceived size must be wholly proportional to physical size. An example is given in Figure 2.1, p. 16, which shows the psychophysical relationship that governs linear extent. When physical length is augmented or diminished, perceived length follows suit. The criterion of relative veridicality does not require that any object look any particular size, only that the quantitative structural relationship between different perceptual sizes match the relationship between different physical sizes. When size constancy fails, and an object appears to change its size with distance, the object cannot always look its real size. Resemblance demands that there be a fundamental equivalence between two sets of structural relationships, one in the perceptual domain and the other in the physical.

Does structural identity suffice to account for the intuitive notion of resemblance? From a person's interaction with the environment emerges perception, which is a representation of certain properties—by definition, salient properties—of that environment. The environment is cohesive, its cohesiveness an outcome of the regularity and stability that is described by macroscopic laws of the physical universe; and so, accordingly, is the representation generated from the perceptual interaction. Both percept and perceptible comprise articulated structures, and these structures may be isomorphic to one another in several ways. Regardless of the type of isomorphism, one particular relationship must hold—external arrays map onto percepts in a many-to-one manner. Not all physically differentiable arrays are discriminable (because the senses are both selective and imperfect), and even discriminable arrays may be lumped together perceptually so as to form a smaller number of categories.

At one end of the continuum that defines the possible range of similarity between percepts and objects, the many-to-one correspondences are purely informational. To construct a rather extreme but nonetheless pertinent example, the physical sizes of objects could be marked perceptually by hues—for instance, as its size increased, an object could yield a percept that shifted in color from yellow to red. Differences in size could translate into differences in hue, such that, in principle, as much information were conveyed by hue as is actually conveyed by what we experience as perceived size.

Perhaps an even better example would be to recode size as perceived brightness. Again, the perceptual dimension could, in principle, provide sufficient information; there could be a discriminal brightness for what is presently every discriminal perceived size. Of course, in order to devise a system that behaved in such a fashion and that was coherent, all of the spatial attributes of the physical world would presumably have to be coded differently from the way they actually are. In order to perceive a variety of objects simultaneously, all of them would have to be given in perception at their individual brightness levels (thus indicating their relative physical sizes). No spatial feature would exist in perception, however, to code the relative positions of objects. In some essential respects, then, vision would not be vision as we know it. Perhaps it would be more like hearing: For instance, position in space might be given perceptually as variations in a psychological dimension that is similar to auditory pitch!

One of the interesting aspects of this imaginary example is the primitive analogy that actually exists between size and brightness. To some extent, both attributes seem intrinsically quantitative in nature. Imagine, for example, a device that produced a "percept" whose brightness doubled every time the size of a stimulus object doubled. Such a device would satisfy the requirement of structural identity.

In order for a perceptual system of this type to work in a way that is analogous to the way our senses really do, there would also have to be a tactile mode of size perception. Specifically, in our imaginary example, there would have to be a tactile dimension of brightness that mapped fairly precisely onto the corresponding visual dimension.

Might it be that this imaginary example actually provides a correct account of the relation between percept and perceptible? To argue so is to say that perceived size, as we know it, no more resembles physical size than brightness does. A counterargument is that perceived size does resemble physical size in that both are extensive, whereas bright-

ness does not resemble physical size in that brightness is only intensive. But, retorts the skeptic in turn, it is possible that perceived size
seems to be extensive only because it is the psychological correlate to an
extensive physical dimension. Against this retort it might be argued
that extensiveness in perception, rather than in physical objects, is the
primary given. What this dispute eventually boils down to is the question whether extensiveness is quintessentially physical or perceptual.

That visual (and tactile) perception is phenomenologically
spatial—that this spatiality itself helps make vision the sort of experience that it is—suggests that extensiveness is given both in objects *and*
in perception. Even insofar as perception is a constructed representation, it is a representation that matches (resembles) certain properties of
the external world.

Because the question of resemblance is so clearly linked to the
distinction between primary and secondary qualities, any evidence that
helps to substantiate that distinction may also help to support the
notion of resemblances. Direct realism—J. J. Gibson's (1966) version,
for example—tries to do away with the distinction on the grounds that
it is a vestigial relic of the view that sensations intervene in the perceptual process. In Gibson's theory, perception is direct, not constructed
from sensory elements. But the distinction between primary and secondary qualities does not go away so easily. Though he eschewed the
terms "direct perception" and "indirect perception," Austin (1962) espoused a sort of direct realism in *Sense and sensibilia*. There, he asked
the same sorts of questions about the "real nature" of sensations of both
secondary and primary qualities. One such question was, "What is the
real taste of saccharine?" This might contrast with a question such as,
"What is the real shape of a penny?" As Austin rightly noted, asking
about the real anything of anything requires that one specify what sort
of answer is desired—to use one of his examples, the real color of
someone's hair might refer to its color before it was dyed. In the case of
saccharine, Austin pointed out that the taste depends on the concentration. Saccharine may taste sweet at low concentrations, bitter at high.

But the problem goes deeper than this. Even if all people with
maverick taste buds are eliminated from consideration, and even if only
one concentration of saccharine is employed, there is no single answer
to the question. For some individuals will find sweet the same saccharine that others find bitter (see Theophrastus [*De sensibus*, 69]). Now,
this outcome creates no problem at all as long as one does not try to put
the taste of saccharine in the saccharine itself. The taste—sweet or
bitter—comes from a perceptual encounter, the interaction between
person and sapid environment. To some individuals saccharine and

sugar solutions will taste identical, whereas to others they will taste quite different. To ask whether sugar and saccharine have the same real tastes is only meaningful vis-à-vis a sapient organism.

Similarly color: Husband and wife may disagree whether the color of his tie is turquoise or blue, though they presumably would not disagree as to the physical specification of the wavelength spectrum of the light reflected by the tie (as well as that of the surrounding, which may influence the tie's perceived color). The spectrum is verifiable in a way that the color is not. Not so the shape of a penny: The question of its real shape arises when it does not look round. That the question does arise is predicated on the possibility of ascertaining that it is round. Perhaps from an oblique vantage it looks elliptical. Unlike the taste of saccharine, the real shape of the penny can be determined by changing its orientation—or that of the perceiver. (This is to say nothing of the opportunity to ascertain the shape by touch.) As Austin noted, verification of this sort is virtually always possible.[6]

To summarize, perception—notably, multimodal perception—has the ability to produce a belief not only in the existence of external objects and events, but also in the existence of certain properties of them. These are spatial and temporal properties and they correspond closely to Locke's class of primary qualities. The distinction between primary and secondary qualities has some value, even though it is often considered philosophically disreputable. The close resemblance between certain perceptual dimensions and the correlated physical properties cannot be shown to be the outcome of a simple photographic-like process; the process of perception may be largely one of constructing isomorphic representations, which, in the case of primary qualities, by chance or by design closely resemble their objects. In part, the correspondence is one of structural relationships: Quantitative relationships among properties of objects match the analogous quantitative relationships among percepts. But the correspondence that underlies resemblance goes deeper than this; it delves into the very heart of the perceptual experience itself. The correspondences may be philosophically arcane, but they are psychologically pellucid.

Thus the senses do tell us about the real world: the real world—the noumenal world—not merely the phenomenal world. This seems to be precisely what Charles Baudelaire wrote of in his famous poem "Correspondances":

---

[6]This is not to deny that a similar situation can arise with regard to color. A question about "real color," Austin noted, may refer to an object's color under a different illumination.

La Nature est un temple où de vivants piliers
Laissent parfois sortir de confuses paroles;
L'homme y passe à travers des forêts de symbols
Qui l'observent avec des régards familiers.

Comme de longs echos qui de loin se confondent
Dans une ténébreuse et profonde unité,
Vaste comme la nuit et comme la clarté,
Les parfums, les couleurs et les sons se répondent.

Il est des parfums frais comme des chairs d'enfants,
Doux comme les hautbois, verts comme les prairies,
—Et d'autres, corrompus, riches, et triomphants,

Ayant l'expansion des choses infinies,
Comme l'ambre, le musc, le bejoin et l'encens,
Qui chantent les transports de l'esprit et des sens.

Not only do odors, lights, sounds correspond to one another, but they also point to the noumena underlying the phenomena (cf. MacIntyre, 1958).

3

The Doctrine of Analogous Sensory Attributes and Qualities

On Common Qualities

A few years ago, a remarkable item in a local newspaper captured my attention. The item appeared in an article that described Vienna's Wettheimstein Park, and in particular a section of the park whose use is restricted to the blind. The article quoted a woman's account of her attempt to describe a rose to a young girl. The woman once had sight, but subsequently lost it, whereas the girl had been blind from birth:

> "She has never seen a rose . . . . I have seen a rose and remember what it looks like . . . . How do you tell someone what a rose looks like in plain words if they [sic] cannot see it?" she asked. "I am trying to describe the colors of the flowers in this garden to this young friend of mine. Red or yellow—like the warmth of the sun. Blue like the coolness of the water that splashes in that fountain over there. Green like the freshness of the grass under your feet or the taste of mint. I can remember these colors because I was not always blind."[1]

Red and yellow like warmth, blue like coolness, green like the texture of grass and the taste of mint: A result of memory and associa-

[1] *New Haven Register*, July 19, 1972, p. 16.

tion? To be sure. A result of memory and association alone? Perhaps not. Implicit in the older woman's attempt to describe, by means of cross-modal surrogates, the colors of flowers to her friend is an assumption that these correspondences are intrinsic properties of sensory experience, that they are not merely the outcome of habitual experience and association. For if the cross-sensory correspondences had to be learned, how could she expect that her congenitally blind friend would comprehend them?

Regardless of where they come from or how they come about, cross-modal correspondences such as these—analogies between the perceptions of sight and perceptions of temperature, touch, and taste—do exist. Their reality and significance to the older blind woman is clear. Indeed, to the older woman the feelings and tastes are in some manner equivalent to the sights, for she believed that feelings and tastes could convey visual meanings to someone who had never seen. If this were literally true, we would have here an expression of one version of the Doctrine of Equivalent Information, similar to that suggested by Baudelaire in his poem "Correspondances"; not just shapes and sizes, but colors, smells, and tastes would resemble their "primary qualities" in the world. But I believe such an interpretation goes too far. The red warmth of the sun, the green taste of mint express a second doctrine—a different doctrine—the Doctrine of Analogous Sensory Qualities.

The Doctrine of Correspondence among Sensory Attributes states that certain dimensions of sensory experience are similar or even identical in different modalities. A feather brushes the skin like a beckoning whisper; a pungent food attacks taste buds like a flash of lightning. Similarities such as these are of foremost concern to the present work. Resemblances among colors, sounds, tastes, smells, and touches can be solely phenomenological, which is to say that similar qualities need not refer back to common objects or events in the physical world, need not provide equivalent information. Aristotle's notion of common attributes of sensation may, accordingly, be interpreted more broadly, so as to incorporate the Doctrine of Analogous Attributes as well as the Doctrine of Equivalent and Complementary Information. The κοινα αἰσθήτα then are treated in phenomenal terms—as analogous attributes or qualities of sensation *qua* sensation.

To take an example of this duality: Sounds have several spatial characteristics, for instance their apparent location. People have the capacity, albeit limited, to identify where a sound comes from. This subject came up in the last chapter. But sounds have another characteristic of location—one that is independent of where the sound comes from—namely the dimension of high versus low that is commonly called pitch. This is no mere spatial metaphor: Sounds that differ in pitch appear to come from different heights, even when the sounds actually come from the same spot. Roffler and Butler (1968) studied this phenomenon extensively; they found that perceived height correlated directly with pitch in the congenitally blind as well as the sighted and in children so young that they seemed not to command the verbal concepts of high and low pitch. High and low pitch in sounds represent purely phenomenal characteristics of sensation, not spatial characteristics of the corresponding stimuli.

Not everyone will agree wholly with the distinction just made. Stern commented, "Color and sound, hardness and warmth, are not only attributes of things, given in sensation, but the veil through which the sensible content, the inner dynamic arrangement, of the *object* presents itself to us [1938, p. 161]." For Stern, it would seem, as for Baudelaire, all sensory qualities contain information about features of noumenal reality.

Külpe (1893) argued that there are three universal suprasensory attributes, that is, three properties or dimensions that apply to sensory experience of all modalities. These three are intensity, quality, and duration, to which Külpe added a fourth and somewhat less general attribute, namely extension. According to this scheme, all sensations have some degree of intensity, from weak through moderate to strong; have some quality, whether red or green, blue or yellow, high or low pitched, salty, sweet, sour, or bitter, pungent, fragrant, or rancid, soft or hard, warm or cold; have some span in time, from brief to long. Külpe's list provides a reasonable scheme of universal sensory attributes. Given this notion, we might say that the several senses display a fundamental unity in part because a class of suprasensory attributes pertains to sensations on all modalities.

What this all boils down to in phenomenal terms is the notion that sensations of sight, sound, taste, smell, touch, and temperature are, in certain ways, similar to each other. To be sure, some modalities are more similar to each other than are others. Sensations of taste and smell are frequently confused, which may, in part, reflect the fact that they are frequently fused: It is a noteworthy characteristic of odors and tastes to merge into flavors whose olfactory and gustatory components may at times be difficult to distinguish. Confusions can also occur between other modalities. It has been reported that when they are presented with "alternating auditory and cutaneous stimuli, [subjects] often report that a pulse on the fingertip resembles a sound, and, similarly, that a weak auditory click resembles a cutaneous tap [Gescheider & Niblette, 1967, p. 313]."

Analogies among sensory qualities are both explicit and implicit in Platonic doctrine. Plato [*Timaeus*, 64–68] invoked a corpuscular model to explain the arousal of sensation. He believed that large particles contract the visual substrate, producing the sensation of black, and contract the skin, producing the sensation of cold; small particles dilate, producing white and warmth, respectively. Hence there are analogies between white and warm on the one hand, and between black and cold on the other. Plato implicitly extended these two analogies to taste, where sweet would correspond to the white–warm pair, bitter to the black–cold. And it is noteworthy that Aristotle [*De anima*, 421; *De sensu*, 443] gave sweet, bitter, pungent, harsh, acid, and succulent as the qualities of both smell and taste. In a more contemporary vein, Crocker and Henderson (1927) proposed a fourfold classification of odor qualities— fragrant, acid, burnt, and goaty—that parallels the modern, fourfold system of taste qualities—sweet, sour, salty, and bitter.

The present chapter will focus on four sensory dimensions: extension, intensity, brightness, and quality. The first three are eminent candidates for status as suprasensory analogues: extension—the apparent spatial magnitude of sensations; intensity—the apparent strength of sensations; and brightness—the apparent piquancy of sensations. Quality, the fourth characteristic, is more dubitable as a suprasensory analogue. Brightness, which did not appear on Külpe's list of suprasensory attributes, is added, but duration, which did appear on Külpe's list, was already taken up in Chapter 2 and hence is omitted here. Duration is properly treated as a feature of events, not just of sensation, and thus falls outside the scope of the present chapter.

Extension

The psychological attribute of extension or size plays a rather curious double role, first as a common, cross-modal feature of environmental stimuli (see Chapter 2, pp. 14–20) and second as a suprasensory attribute. In its first role, the perception of spatial extent provides the means by which the sizes of objects become known to us, primarily by way of the senses of vision and touch. It is its second role that I shall consider here: size *qua* size. The major point is that sensations from modalities besides vision and touch also exhibit a spatial attribute. There exists, for instance, a property of sounds that is usually called apparent volume, which is not the same thing as loudness. Sounds differ not just in their subjective intensity, or loudness, but also in the degree to which they appear to fill up space. Loud, low pitched sounds appear most massive and seem to fill up large volume, whereas soft, high pitched sounds appear most thin, small, and seem to take up only small volume. Perhaps the majesty of deep, rich organ music resides in part on its seeming to encompass all the listener's subjective space. Moul (1930) claimed that both pure tones and colored lights yield sensations that can be said to have "thickness." He concluded that "We are dealing not with unrelated perceptions of visual depth and auditory volume, but with an aspect of experience which is fundamentally the same whether mediated by the eye or by the ear [p. 559]."

There is, to be sure, some correlation between the perceived size of a sound and the actual size of the object producing it: Large objects, when set into resonant motion, tend to produce low frequency sounds (hence low pitched and voluminous sounds), whereas small objects tend to produce high and small ones. An orchestra of 100 instruments may actually give cues to its spatial extent. Moreover, the orchestra will also produce a more powerful acoustical signal than will a solo instrument, and accordingly will appear to the ear to take up a larger space. But the correlations between perceived auditory size and physical size are far from perfect. Auditory volume is not primarily a feature of object size the way that tactual and visual size are.

It is interesting to note that sensations produced by repetitive stimulation of the skin can also vary in phenomenal extent, and they do so in ways that are remarkably similar to sensations of sound. A mechanical vibration or an alternating-current electrical stimulus applied to the skin will feel large or small depending on the stimulus frequency. Parallels among the auditory and skin senses are shown in Figure 3.1, taken from data of Békésy (1957a). To a first approximation, the phenomenal sizes of sounds, vibrations, and electric shocks are all inversely proportional to the frequency of the stimulating sine wave. Double the physical frequency of the stimulus and the apparent size drops by one-half.

Intensity

The subjective strength of a sensation is one of its most salient dimensions. Lights, sounds, touches, smells, tastes, pains—all of these can run the gamut from mild to strong, from feeble and barely detectable to overwhelming and unpleasant. The almost delicate pain from a small scratch, the faint flicker of light seen from the corner of the eye,

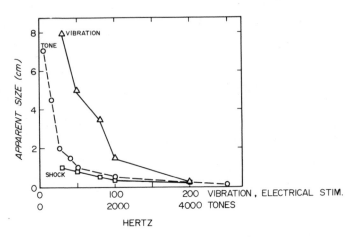

Figure 3.1. The phenomenal size of vibratory stimuli presented to the ear and to the skin. Tones, vibrations, and shocks all produce sensations that vary in size, in inverse proportion to the frequency of the sinusoid—when frequency doubles, size drops by one-half. Based on data in Békésy (1957a).

the muted whisper spoken from a distance that gently caresses the ear, all of these speak of softness—and thereby contrast with their opposites, the agony of sharp and severe abdominal pain, the dazzling brightness of the sun to sleepy eyes, the din of an argument next door that swallows up all other thought as well as sound.

There are several ways to investigate scientifically the cross-sensory equivalences of the attribute of perceived intensity. One psychophysical means is to ask subjects to assess the perceived intensities of stimuli taken from two or more domains (Melamed, 1970). Another approach is to ask subjects to equate directly the perceived intensities of sensations from different modalities (e.g., S. S. Stevens, 1959).

Cross-modality matching of sensory intensity presents subjects with the task of adjusting stimulus intensity on one physical dimension (for example, sound energy) so the sensation that is aroused "matches" that produced by a stimulus on another physical dimension (such as light energy). S. S. Stevens (1959) and others (e.g., J. C. Stevens, Mack, & Stevens, 1960) have demonstrated a high degree of internal consistency (transitivity) of matches performed on very many sensory continua. If subjective values on Modality A match others on Modality B, and those on B match others on C, then the original values on A should match the final values on C. Subjects have little difficulty understanding the instructions or effecting the matches between sensations of

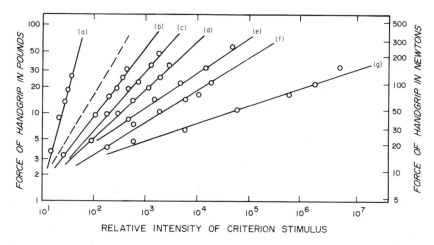

RELATIVE INTENSITY OF CRITERION STIMULUS

Figure 3.2. Cross-modality matching of the effort perceived in squeezing a hand dynamometer to each of seven other perceptual continua: (a) electric shock to the fingers; (b) lifted weights; (c) pressure on the palm; (d) vibration to the fingertip; (e) white noise; (f) 1000-Hz tone; (g) white light. The graph shows the average force in pounds (left ordinate) and newtons (right ordinate) matched to various levels of the criterion stimulus. The dashed line indicates a proportional relation between the physical intensities of the matching continua. None of the matching functions obeys this relation, which means that the psychophysical function relating intensity of sensation to intensity of stimulation differs in different sense modalities. These results are consistent with S. S. Stevens's law—that sensation grows as a power function of stimulation, with power–function exponents that vary from one continuum to another. After J. C. Stevens, J. D. Mack, and S. S. Stevens, Growth of sensation on seven continua as measured by force of handgrip, *Journal of Experimental Psychology*, 1960, *59*, 60–67. Copyright 1960 by the American Psychological Association. Reprinted by permission.

different modalities. Typically, the cross-modal relationship seems to the subject quite a natural one, as natural, I would presume, as it seemed to the poet Swinburne when he wrote: "Soft and strong and loud and light / Very sound of very light." [2]

Figure 3.2 displays results that were obtained when groups of subjects matched the perceived force of muscular exertion (handgrip) to seven other perceptual continua (J. C. Stevens *et al.*, 1960). Plotted are the average physical force levels produced, versus the corresponding physical intensities of the stimuli presented on the other continua. The points that lie along any one function give the pairs of stimulus intensities that produced matching subjective intensities. As will be made

[2] "A Child's Laughter."

clear in the next chapter (pp. 132–134), the mathematical form of these cross-modality functions has an important implication for the psychophysical processes that describe how sensory systems transform stimulus energies into sensation magnitudes. To anticipate that discussion, these cross-modality matching functions support the notion that there is a single, general mathematical law governing the way subjective intensity grows with physical intensity on virtually all sensory continua: On any continuum, S. S. Stevens's law states that equal stimulus ratios give rise to equal sensory ratios.

Brightness

The notion of *identity* among attributes of several sense modalities belongs to Erich von Hornbostel (1925, 1931), who promulgated the idea that *brightness* is a universal sensory dimension. According to Hornbostel, the brightnesses of lights, touches, sounds, odors are not only analogous to each other, but can be equal and identical.

The experiment that Hornbostel (1931) conducted to confirm his theory went as follows. First, his subjects attempted to match the lightness of a gray surface to the brightness of an odor—this step resulted in an equation between a mixture of 40% white, 60% black on the one hand and benzol on the other. Second, the subjects attempted to match the brightness of a tone to that of the same odor—this resulted in an equation between a 220-Hz tone and the benzol. The final match was gray surface to tone, and it produced values—an equation between 41% white, 59% black and a 220-Hz tone—that were almost identical to those of the first two parts. Hornbostel took this round-robin transitivity as strong support for his theory of the unity of the senses. Hartmann (1935) reported Hornbostel's preliminary attempt at verification as follows:

> Among the Berlin *cognoscenti* the story goes that when Hornbostel first had the idea in embryo, he telephoned his friend, the late *Musikwissenschaftler*, Otto Abraham, and inquired what note on the piano corresponded to the odor of violet. When this extraordinary question was answered in a way that Hornbostel expected if the theory were sound, he was almost beside himself with joy [p. 143].

Interestingly, at about the same time that Hornbostel conducted his experiments, Juhász (1926) reported a study of *Geruchshöhe* or odor pitch. This attribute Juhász likened to *Tonhöhe* or auditory pitch. To give some examples, amyl acetate (odor of banana) was said to be high in odor pitch, eugenol (oil of cloves) lower, and geraniol (an alcohol often described as rosy) still lower. Odor pitch likely correlates closely with Hornbostel's odor brightness.

Schiller (1933) reported results of an experiment—on fish!—that was claimed to support the cross-modal generality of the attribute brightness. He first trained the fish to discriminate visual brightness from darkness, then tested transfer of the discrimination to two chemicals: musk and indol. The fish demonstrated preferences that were not apparent before the visual training, in that they responded to musk as they had been trained to respond to light, to indol as to dark. Because humans describe the odor of musk as brighter than that of indol, Schiller (1935) took his results as evidence of cross-modal equivalence, and, he argued, as did Hornbostel (1931) and Börnstein (1936), that brightness is an attribute of all sensory modalities.

The possibility that brightness serves as a universal sensory attribute was also noted on the western side of the Atlantic. John Paul Nafe (1927) undertook an introspective examination of the somesthetic qualities—the qualities of the skin sensations. The response category common to all of the introspective reports given by his subjects was brightness. Tactile and thermal sensations alike were characterized by patterns of brightness: Subjects described cold, sting, and weak pain as bright, warmth and pressure as dull. "The aspect of brightness or sharpness is reported throughout as the only qualitative aspect of felt experiences; but this brightness, if it is the qualitative aspect of these experiences, varies as pitch or brightness in audition or as brightness in vision rather than as colors in vision [Nafe, 1927, p. 382]." And later in the same paper Nafe commented, "It has often been remarked that auditory experiences terminate, at the lower end, in a pressurelike, dull, flat quality, and at the upper end, in distinctly painful bright tones. This in itself is a relationship between the senses. . . [p. 383]."

It is likely that Nafe's neurovascular theory of thermal sensation grew, to some extent, out of observations that sensations of warmth and cold have tactile (pressure) qualities. The theory (Nafe, 1929) proposes that thermal sensations arise from mechanical stimulation of neural endings located in small blood vessels: Warmth results from stimulus patterns produced by expansion of vessels, cold results from contraction of vessels. Thus, Nafe's theory assumes the mediation of temperature sensation to be mechanical, as is the mediation of touch proper. It is of historical interest to note that a theory relating warmth to expansion and cold to contraction of the skin was previously proposed by Plato in his *Timaeus*.

Nafe's (1927) results on somesthetic sensations fit neatly into Hornbostel's (1931) scheme:

Bright	Dull
smooth	rough
hard	soft
sharp	blunt
light	heavy
cold	warm

Intense lights and high frequency sounds were also categorized as bright by Nafe (1927) as well as by Hornbostel.[3]

Hornbostel's theory of universal brightness was picked up and extended by Börnstein (1936). According to Börnstein, sharp touch and cold are bright, warmth is dark; the tastes of urea (bitter) and sucrose (sweet) are bright, that of magnesium sulfate (sour–bitter) is dark. He speculated on a possible physiological underpinning to these differences: Stimuli that excite brightness are, Börnstein hypothesized, ones that heighten body tone. Thus the brightness dimension is universal because there exists a fundamental biological process, namely brightness excitation, that encompasses the entire organism. As a basic phenomenon, body tone, he argued, manifests itself as the root of thought itself (Börnstein, 1970). Heinz Werner (1934) also propounded the notion that there is a generalized body reaction to stimuli, and, he argued, this generalized reaction underlies many intersensory correspondences—as displayed, for example, in synesthesia.

At some point it becomes necessary to come to grips with the question of what is meant by this attribute, brightness. What property of sensory experience is signified by the brightness of touches, sounds, and odors? The brightness of lights poses no problem, for, in this instance, brightness refers to subjective intensity. Specifically, the brightness of a light refers to the subjective intensity of a visual stimulus viewed in the dark; the magnitude of the sensation varies from dim to bright. Visual brightness should properly be distinguished from lightness, which is as attribute of surface colors—for instance, the dimension that describes the variation from black to white.

But what is meant by the brightness of a sound? Surely auditory brightness is not, like visual brightness, the same as subjective intensity. Loudness is.

[3] Irwin's (1974) analysis of Greek poetry shows a similar scheme. She concluded that "the Greek poets saw [a unity] between high, clear sounds, fine, delicate surfaces, and 'whiteness' or 'lightness' [p. 213]."

Hornbostel, it may be recalled, had his subjects manipulate auditory brightness by varying sound frequency; he took advantage of the fact that high frequency sounds are bright, low frequency sounds dark or dull. Several commentators, like Rich (1919), Hartshorne (1934), and to some extent Nafe (1927), identified brightness with pitch. But the brightness of a sound is not just its pitch, as Troland (1930) and Boring and Stevens (1936) noted. A complex sound, composed of several sound frequencies, appears to be less bright than a pure tone of the same fundamental pitch and overall loudness. Clearly, what is needed to evaluate auditory brightness is a psychophysical analysis of all the relevant acoustical dimensions.

When I asked a dozen subjects to judge the brightness of pure tones, brightness correlated both with increasing pitch and with increasing loudness, as can be seen in Figures 3.3 and 3.4. The brightest sounds are high pitched and loud; the darkest or dullest are low pitched and soft. From these results, one can predict, at least qualitatively, how subjects should match the brightnesses of sounds and lights. If pitch is held constant, subjects should increase loudness in order to match increasing visual brightness. If, on the other hand, loudness is held constant, subjects should increase pitch in order to match increasing visual brightness. Experimental results that I obtained are shown in Figure 3.5, and they bear out these predictions. People are able to match

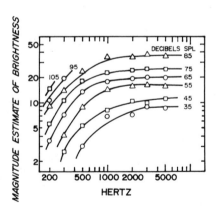

Figure 3.3. Magnitude estimates of the brightness of pure tones, plotted as a function of sound frequency. As frequency increases, tonal brightness increases. Each curve represents a constant sound pressure level.

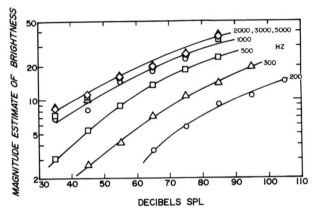

Figure 3.4. The same magnitude estimates as in Figure 3.3, plotted here as a function of sound pressure level in decibels. As sound pressure increases, tonal brightness increases. Each curve represents a constant sound frequency.

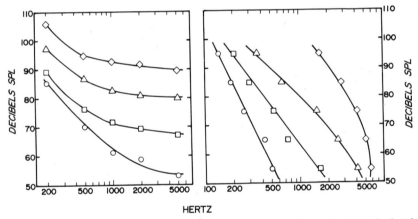

Figure 3.5. Curves of constant brightness. The subjects' task was to match the brightness of a pure tone to the brightness of a white light. In one part of the experiment, sound frequency was held constant on each trial, and the subjects adjusted sound pressure level; these results appear in the left-hand panel. In the other part of the experiment, sound pressure was held constant on each trial, and the subjects adjusted sound frequency; these results appear in the right-hand panel. Each curve represents the combinations of sound frequency and sound pressure matched to a given luminance of the white light: Circles, squares, triangles, and diamonds represent luminances of 1, 10, 100, and 1000 candelas/m², respectively. At a constant sound pressure, brightness increases with frequency, and at a constant frequency, brightness increases with sound pressure. To offset increases in frequency, subjects decreased sound pressure. Hence sound frequency and sound pressure combine their effect to produce a tonal analogue to visual brightness.

the brightness of a pure tone to the brightness of a white light, and in doing so confirm that tonal brightness is neither pitch nor loudness alone, but comprises both.

Hornbostel (1931) tried to demonstrate that brightness is a suprasensory attribute that pertains to at least three modalities: vision, hearing, and smell. Nafe (1927) and Börnstein (1936) made similar suggestions. It is perhaps too easy to dismiss the theory that brightness is a universal sensory dimension. Additional evidence in support of the notion that a dimension of brightness links several senses will be described later in this chapter in the section on synesthesia. For the present, let it suffice to say that evidence from the realm of visual hearing demonstrates a correspondence between the brightness of sounds and the brightness of the secondary visual images that the sounds produce.

Suprasensory Equivalence: Absolute or Relative?

Hornbostel believed cross-modal brightnesses to be more than merely analogies: "Brightness is not just an analogy, but is an identical side of phenomena of different sensory realms [1931, p. 519]." His claim did not go long unchallenged. Cohen (1934) attempted to replicate Hornbostel's result, but reported failure to get agreement between initial and final cross-modal matches in which pure tones were compared to odors. Actually, the discrepancies Cohen found were not so very large. One subject gave a value of 159 Hz initially, 267 Hz finally; the other gave 300 Hz, then 804 Hz. Thus agreement was quite good for the first subject. In neither case was the difference extremely large when one considers the enormous frequency range of human hearing—effectively from 20–20,000 Hz. All of the sounds judged to match benzol were relatively low in frequency and presumably, therefore, low in brightness.

Cohen argued that context plays a significant role in determining the exact matching values, hence that the matching values between different modalities are defined by relative, not absolute positions on their respective scales. To decide whether cross-modal matches are relative or absolute is difficult. Variability or response bias might easily tend to distort results that could otherwise support absolute equivalence.

The same question of absolute versus relative judgment has been raised with regard to cross-modality matching of subjective intensity.

Krantz (1972) argued that such matches are only relative. One can begin a cross-modality matching study by selecting, more or less arbitrarily, the initial pair of stimuli, one from each of the two physical domains. For instance, in the matching of loudness and brightness, the experimenter might select the first pair of stimuli to consist of a tone of sound energy E_1 and light of luminance L_1. But the experimenter could just as well select another luminance, L_2, two or three times as great as L_1, to go with sound energy E_1. Given either pair of stimuli to start with (E_1 and L_1 or E_1 and L_2) subjects are able to make cross-modal matches to subsequent stimuli. Triple the sound energy, and the subject will approximately triple the matching luminance. Apparently, then, the argument goes, the absolute sensation values that make up the initial pair matter only little if at all. This outcome is consistent with Krantz's view that what really matters are *relations*, for example, ratios, among sensory intensities, not the absolute values of individual sensations.

An alternative view of cross-modality matching asserts that indeed there are absolute equalities of sensory brightness or intensity across different modalities. This view suggests that a certain visual brightness truly does *equal* a certain auditory brightness or loudness. Accordingly, the fact that subjects can give consistent and reliable results when they perform cross-modality matching with an arbitrary selection of initial stimulus values only reflects the fact that subjects can respond in a relational manner if they are forced to. But absolute matches may exist nonetheless. A mathematical model consistent with absolute, rather than relative, matching has been proposed by Levine (1974).

Both of these viewpoints probably contain some truth. Correspondences between individual sensations on different modalities seem not to be exact, but neither are they wholly relative. In a cross-modality matching experiment that compares loudness to brightness, a given subject might accept a finite range of sound energies to match a particular luminance. But there is little doubt that some particular level of sound energy—or at least, some range of sound levels—is better than others. If the luminance selected falls only a small factor above the absolute visual threshold, and its brightness is therefore relatively low, then sound energies relatively close to auditory threshold will yield better matches than will sound energies that are much greater. A dim light more closely resembles a whisper than a jackhammer.

It may be difficult to prove that a particular sound energy actually matches a particular luminance (more precisely, that a particular loudness equals a particular brightness). Nevertheless, there seem to be somewhat limited regions of matching stimulation and sensation. A sound of moderate loudness should attract only a small range of matching brightnesses, and these too should come from near the middle of the subjective range. Indeed, when brightness and loudness are matched by means of a procedure that permits the subject to select both the visual and the auditory stimuli, and thus minimizes some of the external constraints, precisely this result obtains (Marks & Stevens, 1966).

Quality

STRUCTURE OF SENSORY QUALITY

Sensory quality is the dimension that appears to show the fewest similarities from modality to modality. Although one can make the perceived intensity of a light "match" that of a briny taste, it is much harder to make the light's color "match" the salty quality. Is salt a "warm" taste? If so, then the appropriate matching color might be orange–red. Or perhaps salty is cool, and better matched with blue–green, the color of the sea. My own feeling is that yellow agrees best, but I am reluctant to foist my preference in analogy upon anyone else.

When Hornbostel (1931) argued that brightness is not merely a cross-sensory analogy, but represents an identical aspect of sensations, he did not by that mean that modalities are identical. The essential differences among modalities were, it may be presumed, as apparent to Hornbostel as they are to the rest of us. To say that olfactory brightness is identical to auditory brightness is not at all to say that the smell of musk is identical to the sound of a whistle. Quite the contrary: To say that their brightnesses are the same is to signify that other characteristics are not.

I do not mean to deny any similarities at all among qualities themselves. One sort of parallel may be seen in a principle that applies to different qualities within a given modality—to the way that the qualities of each modality relate to one another. In several modalities, sensations seem to arrange themselves so as to form opposing pairs, as Aristotle noted: "All sensible objects contain the principle of opposition [*De anima*, 442b23]." White is psychologically opposed to black, red to green, yellow to blue, warm to cold. Pikler (1922) and later Hartshorne (1934) suggested the existence also of two sets of opposites in both taste and in smell: sweet versus salty and bitter versus sour in both senses. Again, individual phenomenologies may vary. To the present author, it seems more appropriate to form an opponent pair out of sweet and bitter, at least in taste. Some others, at least, doubtless agree. Witness the verse in Isaiah [20: 5]: "Woe unto them that call evil good, and good evil; that put darkness for light, and light for darkness; that put bitter for sweet, and sweet for bitter!"

CROSS-MODAL COMPARISONS
OF SENSORY QUALITY

The entire area of cross-modality comparisons of sensory quality has hardly been explored experimentally, although a few occasions have brought out guesses about the chart of analogies. Cross-modal comparisons are implicit in Plato's psychophysical doctrine as outlined above; to repeat, Plato hypothesized that contraction produces sensations of black, cold, and bitter, whereas dilation produces white, warm, and sweet. Comparisons are explicit in Aristotelian doctrine. According to Aristotle, odors, like tastes, can be sweet, harsh, pungent, succulent (oily), or rancid–bitter [*De anima* 421; *De sensu,* 443]. The first and last items on this list—sweet and bitter—he believed to be primary; the other four, derivative. It is difficult to decide, however, just what Aristotle meant when he said that smell and taste correspond in this way. Did he mean the sensory qualities themselves are analogous? Or the objects that produce them? If it is the former, we are dealing properly with a type of cross-modality matching between qualities of sensation on different modalities; but if it is the latter, we are dealing with cross-modal transmission of stimulus information.

Sometimes these two types of matching can be the same, for instance, when a person matches visual to tactile size. Both visual and tactile sensations display extensiveness, and this spatial attribute of sensory experience usually bears a close relation to the actual size of the object that produces it. Large objects appear large both to the eye and to the hand. Other times, however, the two types of matching are rather different. Brightness to the eye and hardness to the touch are both quantitative, intensive characteristics of sensation, but high brightness and great hardness need not imply anything common about their stimuli. This dichotomy between features of objects and attributes of sensation is difficult to apply to Aristotelian doctrine because Aristotle did not make a clear distinction between sensation and the physical dimensions of stimuli that produce sensation. To the extent that he did not separate the phenomenal from the physical, his proposal that taste and smell are similar pertains more properly to equivalence of stimulus information than to analogous attributes.

The most extensive empirical literature concerning analogies among sense qualities deals with synesthesia. Because this is a complex

and important subject deserving special scrutiny, I will defer consideration of synesthesia to a special section later in the chapter. Aside from
these studies, however, data on direct cross-modal comparison of sensory quality are scanty. This is not to deny that qualitative analogies
have been considered. Indeed, significant research, especially early
research on sensory processes, was stimulated, in large measure, by the
notion that qualities of sense in different modalities exhibit important
parallels. An example is the way that some research on taste mixtures
was patterned after experiments and concepts with color mixtures (e.g.,
von Skramlik, 1926).

In this connection, it is constructive to take each individual sense
and look at the dimensions along which its sensations can vary. Because
sensations generally vary along several dimensions, characterizing a
sensation requires specifying values on all of them. If these dimensions
are represented geometrically, as axes in space, then the dimensional
values that denote any given sensation also correspond to a particular
point in the space. Points near each other in the space represent similar
sensations; points far from each other represent dissimilar ones. Attempts have been made to construct geometrical models representing
the multidimensional nature of sensory variations. An interesting question is whether the psychological structure of multidimensional sensory
spaces bears any resemblance from one modality to another.

The qualities of visual experience have been represented in the
well–known color solid, which is a three-dimensional space presumed
to hold all tints, shades, and lightnesses of surfaces. The color solid has
as its simplest representation a spindle: The color spindle contains an
elongated white–black dimension and a circular hue dimension (see
Figure 3.6). On the surface lie the most deeply saturated colors; paler
(grayer) ones fall closer and closer to the center. By way of analogy,
three-dimensional structures have been proposed to describe gustatory
and olfactory qualities (Henning, 1916a,b). The four taste qualities
presumed to be primary appear as the points of a tetrahedron, the six
odor qualities presumed to be primary as the points of a triangular
prism (Figure 3.7). Both geometrical representations have regular
forms, that is, in Henning's theory the primaries lie equally distant
from each other.

The basic features of Henning's (1916b) taste tetrahedron—at least,
the primacy of salty, sweet, sour, and bitter as groupings that are
fundamental, though not necessarily equidistant from one another—
appear in results obtained by Gregson (1965) and by Schiffman and
Erickson (1971). Primary odor qualities, if they exist, have been elu-
sive. Schiffman (1974) reanalyzed several of the empirical attempts to

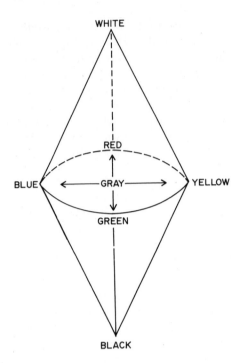

Figure 3.6. The color spindle, a three-dimensional representation of the colors of objects. Pure hues inhabit the circular rim, with psychologically opposed hues (red vs. green, blue vs. yellow) directly opposite one another. The colors become less and less saturated (more and more like neutral gray) closer and closer to the spindle's center. The vertical dimension gives the lightness of the color experience.

determine the multidimensional psychological properties of odors. Schiffman's analysis produced a two-dimensional scheme (a scheme that, incidentally, differs markedly from Henning's [1916a] odor prism), in which one dimension appears to portray pleasantness and unpleasantness, while the other can be interpreted as sharpness, and perhaps corresponds to odor brightness. One cannot help wondering, though,

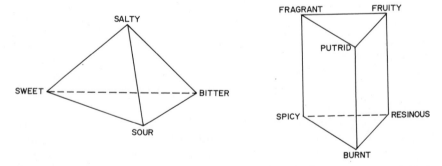

Figure 3.7. Henning's (1916a,b) taste and smell solids. Each of the four primary taste qualities sits at a corner of the tetrahedron on the left. Each of the six presumed primary odor qualities sits at a corner of the triangular solid on the right.

to what extent these spatial representations of qualitative similarity actually reflect the psychological structure of sensory quality, to what extent the representations reflect the conceptual structures of psychologists.

A small number of experimental studies have sought to learn whether certain sensory qualities show any cross-modal similarities. Békésy (1957a, 1959b, 1961) pointed to a marked phenomenal resemblance among the sensory qualities produced by stimuli that arouse various senses: He pointed in particular to the qualities of tones produced by acoustic vibration of the ear, and of touch produced by mechanical vibration and by electrical stimulation of the skin. Indeed, some sensory scientists use the term "pitch" to describe all three perceptual qualities. As a stimulus's vibratory frequency increases, tactile as well as auditory pitch increases.

Simpson, Quinn, and Ausubel (1956) tried to determine the relation, if any, between visual hue and auditory pitch. The subjects were 1096 schoolchildren (grades 3 to 6), who listened through earphones to pure tones. The tones ranged in frequency from 125 to 12,000 Hz, and all were played at sound pressure levels between 40 and 50 dB. The children's task was merely to name the hue that seemed to "go with" each sound—a task much less formidable and demanding than is the quantitatively more precise method of cross-modality matching. The colors that were named bore some regular relation to pitch (sound frequency). Violet and blue were predominantly associated with the lowest sound frequencies, orange and red with intermediate frequencies, green and yellow with high frequencies.

One of the most interesting of the experimental studies is that of Wicker (1968). He asked subjects to judge the similarity of pure tones to one another, of patches of colored papers to one another, and of pure tones to patches of colored papers. From the judgments, Wicker discovered that all of the stimuli—both colors and tones—could be embedded in a single spatial representation, to be more precise, in a bisensory, two-dimensional, Euclidean space. In Euclidean space, the perceived dissimilarity between any two stimuli—here, between tone and tone, between color and color, or between color and tone—is given as the simple distance between the stimuli in the space. In Wicker's study, the multimodal space was a single flat plane. Visual sensations usually need a three-dimensional space like the color solid of Figure 3.6; Wicker's results showed no simple visual dimension related to hue, presumably because there was no simple auditory analogue to hue. The main problem posed by the results was how to uncover the meaning of the space's two orthogonal dimensions.

Sensations of pure tones display two salient characteristics—loudness and pitch. This suggests organizing tonal similarity in a two-dimensional space, as shown in Figure 3.8. Loudness and pitch are represented here as being orthogonal to each other. Shown also in the figure are the dimensions of tonal volume and tonal brightness, which were considered earlier in this chapter. Loud, low pitched sounds are most voluminous; loud, high pitched sounds are most bright. So volume and brightness too are orthogonal to one another. Thus the two dimensions of auditory space could conceivably be taken to be either pitch and loudness or to be volume and brightness. Wicker came to the same conclusion; furthermore, he noted that if pitch and loudness were selected to describe the auditory dimensions of his bisensory space, then the corresponding visual dimensions were brightness and contrast. If auditory volume and brightness were taken, the visual analogues were brightness and "vividness."

A secondary experiment by Wicker (1968) tested the way relations transfer cross-modally from sound to color; its results implied that the primary auditory dimensions were, in fact, pitch and loudness. It follows that the analogous visual dimensions were brightness and contrast. The correlation between auditory pitch and visual brightness is the same one already encountered in the work of Hornbostel (1931). On the basis of psychophysical studies of auditory brightness (Figures 3.3–3.5), though, we might have expected that auditory brightness itself, not just pitch would correlate most strongly with visual brightness. Why didn't it?

Probably what mattered most was that Wicker presented his colored samples against neutral gray backgrounds of medium lightness. Both very dark and very light samples contrasted strongly with their backgrounds. Perhaps it should not be surprising, then, to find that loud tones were judged similar both to color samples that were much more luminous and to samples that were much less luminous than the background. A similar relationship is seen in Figure 3.9, which displays

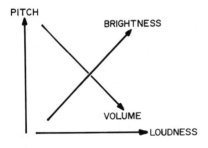

Figure 3.8. A two-dimensional representation of the relationships among four perceptual dimensions of pure tones. Brightness comprises high pitch and high loudness; volume comprises low pitch and high loudness.

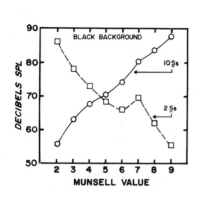
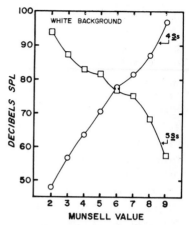

Figure 3.9. Sound pressure levels of a 1000-Hz tone matched to gray surfaces that differ in lightness. The grays appeared against either black backgrounds (Munsell value of 1) or white backgrounds (Munsell value of 9.5). On the scale of Munsell value, equal steps should correspond to equal changes in perceived lightness; increasing value means increasing lightness. From Lawrence E. Marks, On associations of light and sound: The mediation of brightness, pitch, and loudness, *American Journal of Psychology,* 1974, *87,* 173–188. Reprinted by permission.

some data that I collected. Plotted are sound pressure levels of a 1000-Hz tone judged to match gray surfaces presented against black and white backgrounds (Marks, 1974a). Clearly, some people find that increasing loudness goes with increasing surface brightness, regardless of the backgound. For other people, however, increasing loudness goes with increasing surface brightness when the background is black, but with decreasing brightness when the background is white; in other words, for these people, increasing loudness goes with increasing difference between figure and background. Perhaps under conditions where loudness associates with brightness contrast, it is pitch that associates with visual lightness per se.

HARTSHORNE'S THEORY
OF FUNDAMENTAL QUALITIES

One of the strongest theoretical claims for cross-modal analogy among sensory qualities is that of Charles Hartshorne (1934). His remarkable theory is unique not only in that it posits specific equivalences amongst qualities of virtually all sensory modalities, but also in that it attempts to provide an explanation, in terms of adaptive evolution, to account for the phenomenology of different qualities. According to Hartshorne's theory, three fundamental dimensions, in addition to time and space, dominate all of our sensory experiences. These dimensions are bipolar, and they are designated as activity–passivity, joy–sorrow, and intensity–faintness. In vision, the corresponding colors are said by Hartshorne to be red–green, yellow–violet, and white–black, respectively. Thus redness is given as the visual manifestation of activity, yellowness as the visual manifestation of joy, white as the visual manifestation of intensity. Red is often acknowledged as a "vibrant" or "stimulating" color: G. D. Wilson (1966) discovered that subjects do describe red as a more "lively" and "exciting" color than green; in fact, red was more effective than green in eliciting a galvanic skin response (sweating on the palm of the hand). Bornstein (1975) found that infants attended longer to red light than to any other equally bright spectral color.

In hearing, the dichotomy between high pitched and low pitched sounds is assumed to correspond to the opposition between joy and sorrow. In Hartshorne's scheme, high pitched sounds are analogous to yellow, low pitched sounds to violet. The reader may recall that this postulated correlation between pitch and hue is exactly like that demonstrated empirically by Simpson *et al.* (1956). To children, at least, the colors blue and violet do appear to correspond to low pitched sounds, the color yellow to high ones. Even Wicker's (1968) data, obtained from adults, show a tendency for yellows to associate more closely with high frequency sounds, blues with low frequency sounds.

In the somesthetic senses, Hartshorne's theory relies on the famous dichotomy between warm and cool colors—his analogies are between warmth and orange–red on the one hand and between cool and pale blue–green on the other. "Part of the difference between blue and red," wrote Hayek (1952), "[is] that blue is associated with coolness and red with warmness [p. 20]." The correspondences between yellowness and gaiety, between redness and activity, between blueness and coolness were anticipated more than a century earlier by Goethe (1810).

A flavor for Hartshorne's approach is perhaps best conveyed by the following passage, in which he examined taste quality both from the point of view of his own system and from that of Pikler (1922), to whose work Hartshorne was strongly indebted.

On the whole, the best working hypothesis is that proposed by Pikler, according to which the following order obtains:

SWEET

BITTER   SOUR

SALTY

This corresponds formally with the order of colors, with saturated intermediates, analogous to orange, etc., in sweet–sour, sour–salt, salt–bitter, bitter–sweet, while sweet–salt and sour–bitter correspond to the complementary pairs of primary colors. Pikler considers the analogy as material as well as formal, and regards salt as a sort of gustatory yellow (on the ground of its sharpness or brightness), sour as gustatory green, sweet as blue-like (because of its mildness and dullness), red as akin to bitter (both being duller than yellow or salt, but "rougher" than green or sour). One objection to this is that bitter seems distinctly darker than sweet, whereas red is brighter than blue. On the other hand, I at least have always felt something sweetlike in blue, something mild and caressing. Starting from the color, I could arrive at no other taste as its analogue, and the same is no less true of the green affinity of sour. For red and yellow only bitter and salt would remain; the brightness of salt would suggest yellow while the darkness of bitter would absolutely exclude this color [From *The philosophy and psychology of sensation* by Charles Hartshorne, pp. 237–238. Copyright 1934 by the University of Chicago. Reprinted by permission.].

Hartshorne concluded his discussion of the chemical senses with the Aristotelian deduction that the same (here four) basic qualities (and the same analogies) apply to smell as well as to taste.

The theory of Hartshorne is foremost an affective one. It presumes the various sensory qualities to be modes of affect; thus the theory purports to explain why as well as how, to show not only in what ways qualities are similar or different, but also why they are as they are—why red looks red, why sour tastes sour, why warm feels warm. According to Hartshorne, the sensory qualities evolved and developed in essential correspondence to the objects that produce them. Yellowness came to be yellowness because it holds the pleasure of warmth from sun; greenness came to be greenness because it captures the cool relief that foliage provides from activity; and so on. Hence yellowness expresses brightness and intensity, greenness expresses passivity. The taste qualities sweet and bitter reflect, respectively, the nutritive and life-threatening aspects of stimuli, such as foods and poisons, that produce them. "The actual correlation of stimulus and response is in a broad way in accordance with adaptive requirements. The exposure to warmth which falls short of heat is incomparably more advantageous than that to cold of a degree to be felt (through the fur or other protective covering) as cold. The feeling tones of these two sensations are the faithful conscious expressions of these facts [Hartshorne, 1934, p. 260]." And it is interesting to note, in conjunction with this example, that Jeddi (1970) found cross-cultural evidence to support the view that the sensation of warmth is intrinsically more positive in affect than is the sensation of cold.

To argue, as Hartshorne did, that sensory qualities are faithful psychological expressions of the physical stimuli that cause them is to take a stance akin to that of Stern (1938) quoted earlier. It is to blur the border between perception of primary and secondary qualities of objects. It is to assert that experiences can resemble on more than one level, on the affective as well as the denotative.

A study by Wright and Rainwater (1962) bears some relevance to the cross-modal analogies that Hartshorne postulated. They had subjects evaluate 50 color samples on a variety of semantic scales. In line with Hartshorne's scheme, red identified with warmth and white with intensity. Other of Hartshorne's correspondences, however, were notably absent. Happiness, for instance, which should have closely identified with yellow, turned out not to be related to hue at all, but rather to high brightness and saturation. The fact that yellow is perceptually the least saturated of the phenomenally unique colors scarcely helps improve the situation.

At the beginning of the present discussion, I described Hartshorne's theory as "remarkable." That designation stemmed largely from subsequent empirical evidence, which accords with the idea that three common, bipolar dimensions underlie all sensory experience. For it turns out that the same three dimensions that Hartshorne derived have been established, it appears totally independently, from studies on the connotative meanings of verbal concepts.

Osgood, Suci, and Tannenbaum (1957) set out to index the linguistic meanings of concepts. A goal of this research was to obtain a limited set of verbal responses that can be elicited from people, responses that map all of the important dimensions of meaning. The technique they developed goes by the name *semantic differentiation*. One of their basic experiments went as follows. First, the experimenters constructed a set of 50 bipolar dimensions, selected so as to cover a wide conceptual gamut; and most important for present purposes, the set included many pairs of sensory opposites (white–black, bitter–sweet, red–green, loud–soft, among others). Next, 100 subjects rated graphically each of 20 verbal concepts with respect to all 50 dimensions. To the matrix of data that resulted, Osgood *et al.* applied centroid factor analysis, from which they distilled three major factors: These they called *evaluation, potency,* and *activity.* Other experiments, employing somewhat different techniques, also yielded the same three basic factors.

The three factors derived through the semantic differentiation of concepts correspond exactly, or almost exactly, to the bipolar dimensions that Hartshorne (1934) proposed to underlie sensory quality. The clearest agreement is in the dimension of activity. Since that dimension was the same in both cases, little else need be said right now. A second factor derived through semantic differentiation is potency, exemplified by such contrasts as large versus small and loud versus soft. Potency corresponds to Hartshorne's dimension of intensity–faintness. This second factor of both Hartshorne and Osgood *et al.* has to do with strength, magnitude, intensity. Evaluation is the third semantic factor. Its essence blooms in the contrast between good and bad; but it also crops up in the dimensions beautiful–ugly and pleasant–unpleasant. Thus this factor is thoroughly affective or hedonic. Hartshorne's corresponding third dimension is joy–sorrow, which may reasonably be allied to its cousin, evaluation.

As I have already mentioned, Osgood *et al.* (1957) included many pairs of opposing sensory qualities among the 50 bipolar scales that they employed. This makes it possible to select sensory qualities that display opposition and compare the factor loadings obtained on evaluation, potency, and activity on the one hand to the dimensional assignments given by Hartshorne on the other. By doing this, we can go beyond the superficial equivalence between the two sets of dimensions, to ask whether people's semantic evaluations of sensory adjectives agree with the specific affective representations that Hartshorne proposed.

First, recall that Hartshorne postulated the white–black dimension to be the visual representation of intense–faint (potency, in the terms of Osgood *et al.*), the red–green dimension to be active–passive (activity), and the yellow–blue dimension to be joy–sorrow (evaluation). Results of semantic differentiation indicate that white distinguishes itself from black on evaluation as well as on potency. This result is probably not surprising, since the semantic associations and connotative implications of these colors (for instance, white signifying purity, black degradation) far transcend the simple sensory qualities and properties.

Closer in line with Hartshorne's hypothesis, the opposition of red and green correlates well with activity versus passivity, but again there is, in addition, some evaluative connection (green as good, red as bad). Contrary to the hypothesis, the dichotomy between yellow and blue fails to correlate well with differences along the dimension of evaluation; as a matter of fact, yellow failed to distinguish itself from blue on any of the three semantic factors. To the slight extent that there was some evaluative connotation, its direction was opposite to that predicted by Hartshorne.

In the domain of hearing, Hartshorne made the interesting argument that pitch is the auditory manifestation of sensory intensity. And equally interesting is the parallel finding that the connotative difference between bass (low pitch) and treble (high pitch) can be accounted largely by the semantic-differential factor of potency. Hence agreement here seems good. Note, however, that pitch also exhibits an evaluative factor, and, in one study by Osgood *et al.*, a large activity factor. Moreover, a similar result obtained with loud–soft. That is, loudness primarily connotes potency, but it also exhibits an evaluative compo-

nent. Thus semantic differentiation discloses similar connotative meanings to both the dimensions of loudness and pitch.

Most of the remaining bipolar sensory dimensions that appear in
the study by Osgood *et al.* expressed themselves, perhaps not surprisingly, as evaluative. These included the pairs sweet versus sour, sweet
versus bitter, fragrant versus foul, smooth versus rough, and bland
versus pungent. The dimension heavy–light emerged mainly as potency, and sharp–dull and hot–cold mainly as activity.

It is disappointing to find so little support for Hartshorne's theory
in the specific experimental results of semantic differentiation, especially given the high expectations aroused by the strong similarity
between the two triads of dimensions. Somewhat to Hartshorne's de-
fense, it should be pointed out that these later, semantic studies
required people to assess verbal names of sensory qualities, the *concep-
tions* of the qualities, hence not necessarily the sensory qualities themselves. Operationally considered, semantic differentiation deals with
the connotations of words. Color words and colors can produce different evaluations (Osgood, 1960). Even so, it is probably true that
Hartshorne's theory is inadequate. Sensory qualities just do not seem to
distribute themselves in so simple a manner as he thought. It may be
that red is somewhat more active than is green, but there is also a
difference between their evaluative connotations (good–bad). Redness
is not just the visual manifestation of activity. It is much more.

Is the correlation between the dimensions proposed in
Hartshorne's theory and those derived from semantic differentiation
only fortuitous? Perhaps. But even if Hartshorne's theory is only partially correct, it stands as an historically significant portent, given the
generality and usefulness of semantic differentiation and of the three
factors that its methods yield. For there is good indication that evaluation, potency, and activity *are* fundamental properties of cognition.
And since cognition leans so heavily on sensation, it is not surprising to
find these same three dimensions prominent also in the affective
makeup of sensory qualities. The three dimensions probably do make
up an important part of the differences among sensory qualities, even if
dimensions and qualities do not line up in the direct and one-to-one
manner that Hartshorne supposed.

Setting aside for now the questions of how correct is Hartshorne's
theory, how apt are the analogies he gives among specific sensory
qualities, one point of the theory is worth noting. An important way
that sensations of different modalities resemble each other is through
their hedonic value and tone. The dimension of evaluation stands
prominent among the three factors of connotative meaning. A century
ago, Wilhelm Wundt (1874) formulated a psychophysical function that

he believed applicable to the hedonics of many different senses. According to Wundt's function, stimulation at low intensities (just above threshold) is pleasant, and, as stimulus intensity increases pleasantness tags along for a while and increases to a maximum. Further increase in stimulus intensity, however, causes pleasantness to decrease until a point of hedonic indifference is reached, after which the sensation turns unpleasant and grows more so as stimulation further increases. Unfortunately, the scheme does not always apply. The failure of the scheme to account for hedonics in all of the senses has been documented elsewhere (Marks, 1974b). Suffice it to say here that even very mild stimulation, as by electric shock, may be unpleasant, while very strong stimulation, as by sugar, may not be unpleasant. Still, despite the evidence against the generality of Wundt's psychophysical formulation, the senses surely are vehicles for pleasure and pain. Sight and taste, hearing and smell, all reveal affective components: Swinburne's "Birthday Ode" alludes to

> *Sounds lovelier than the light,*
> *And light more sweet than song from night's own bird.*

The sweet taste, mild warmth, certain colors and sounds appear intrinsically pleasant, whereas the bitter taste, electric shock, and intense stimulation in general appear intrinsically unpleasant; it is not difficult to imagine an experimental paradigm in which subjects are asked to set the pleasantness or unpleasantness of one stimulus to equal that of another. In fact, a study of this sort compared how rats responded to aversive stimulation in different modalities (Woods & Campbell, 1967). It just might be that the affective or hedonic dimension of sensation forms, in part, a basis for qualitative similarities among the senses. To the extent that this may be so, Hartshorne's theory deserves further attention. The hypothesis brings to mind a couplet from an Egyptian love poem translated by Foster (1971); the poem is a hieroglyph from the New Kingdom, XIX–XX Dynasties, about 1300–1100 B.C., whose lines express sensory analogy by means of strong emotional link:

> *The sound of your voice is sweet,*
> *full like the taste of dark wine.*

Sound Symbolism

Analogies among the senses are not just bloodless, abstract symbols entered on a scientific ledger, but vital phenomena of mental life.

Lest the reader feel unconvinced of this point, it is imperative to make the argument more compelling. Where does the unity of the senses play a vivid role in thinking and behavior? In particular, where can one find virile embodiments of cross-modal translations among sensory qualities?

For one, in the phenomenon known variously as phonetic symbolism or as sound symbolism in speech: Elemental speech sounds, both individually and in combination, sometimes serve in and by themselves to evoke meanings—as if the sounds that constitute a word form part of the semantic content. Sound symbolism transcends the relatively simple process of onomatopoesis. In onomatopoesis, consonants and vowels of speech actually mimic some naturally occurring, nonspeech sound; well-known examples of the latter are onomatopoeic words like "buzz," "crackle," "swish," and "meow." Sound symbolism proper enters the scene when sounds and referents differ, when sounds express some nonacoustical property of nature. In his extensive review of sound symbolism in English words, Marchland (1958) claimed, for example, that / r / symbolizes vibration, that / p / at the end of verbs of motion symbolizes quickness, that long vowels in verbs of motion symbolize slowness.

The present concern is not with the entire province of sound symbolism, but with a subset of the counties that it comprises, namely, with the ways that speech sounds can convey sensory meanings, whether visual, tactile, gustatory, or olfactory. This is, of course, a question of cross-modal translation; what I wish to propose is an account of one aspect of sound symbolism—that vowels and consonants suggest referents in other sensory modalities by dint of certain psychoacoustic characteristics of speech, to wit, through the operation of suprasensory attributes.

Language and speech are amenable to analysis at a number of different levels. At one level, language presents itself as an abstract system of symbols, together with sets of rules that define structural and sequential relations among the units (morphemes, words) and that define relations between units and their referents. At this level, meanings are denotative, and the relationship between sound and meaning is wholly arbitrary. It does not matter, for instance, whether the class of physical structures that serve as domiciles is designated by the word "house" or by the word "flix." As long as the appropriate linguistic rules are obeyed in a consistent fashion, the denotative representation is served equally well by both words. And it does not matter if the words are spoken, printed, or displayed in Morse code.

But at another linguistic level, the relationship between language and meaning is not always wholly arbitrary. Language comes fundamentally through the vocal and auditory systems; the basic mode is speech, and speech is processed by complex psychoacoustic mechanisms that transform acoustical waveforms into perceptual responses. At this level, it is important to bear in mind, speech sounds arouse perceptions that, in some ways, behave like perceptions aroused by nonspeech sounds. Here may be found the power of sound *qua* sound, the power to evoke or suggest meanings in ways that are not arbitrary. Wolfgang Köhler (1947), the eminent Gestalt psychologist, quoted with obvious approval the poet Morgenstern's observation that "All seagulls look like their name is Emma." Köhler's own contribution to the intimacy of sound and meaning consisted of an experiment in which subjects were asked to match the pseudowords "maluma" and "takete" to the visual forms depicted in the upper part of Figure 3.10. Most subjects did not hesitate in matching the sibilant "maluma," with its long duration, low pitched vowels, to the softly rounded figure on the upper left; and in matching the sharper "takete," with its short duration, high pitched vowels, to the angular figure on the upper right. Köhler's

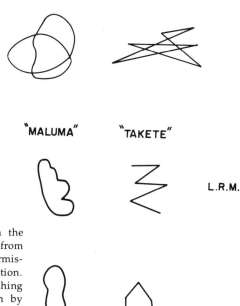

"MALUMA"   "TAKETE"

L.R.M.

L.J.M.

Figure 3.10. Top: "Maluma" is on the left, "takete" on the right. Reprinted from W. Köhler, *Gestalt psychology*. By permission of Liveright Publishing Corporation. Copyright 1947 by Liveright Publishing Corporation. Bottom: Figures drawn by two children, 9-year-old L.J.M. and 12-year-old L.R.M., to correspond to the words "maluma" and "takete."

experiment can also be turned around. The lower part of Figure 3.10 gives my two daughters' visual representations of the pseudowords "maluma" and "takete."

Köhler's finding of consistent matches between nonsense words and visual figures was confirmed by Holland and Wertheimer (1964), who, in addition, had subjects evaluate the implicit meanings of the two sets of stimuli. Both words and forms were perceived to differ along the same semantic dimensions, including angularity, strength, and size. R. Davis (1961) found that English and Tanganyikan children agreed about associations between spoken words and drawings.

Sound not only can serve as a medium for conveying meanings, but the medium itself can serve to express meanings. And these expressed meanings, or at least some of them, represent the relative values of suprasensory attributes like size and brightness. The vowel sound / a / seems to refer to a larger object than does the vowel / i /. Children as well as adults, and native speakers of Chinese as well as native speakers of English, agreed that "mal" suggests a larger table than does "mil" (Sapir, 1929). Sapir (1929) constructed nonsense syllables containing different vowels and asked subjects about the size of the objects they refer to. Newman (1933) reanalyzed Sapir's data and repeated the experiment. The results, shown in Table 3.1, confirm Sapir's finding that words with the vowel / a / suggest larger referents than do words with

Table 3.1

Rank orders of the sizes and brightnesses suggested by different vowel sounds in nonsense syllables and of the pitches of the vowels [a,b]

Vowel	Size		Brightness	Pitch
	Sapir	Newman	Newman	
/i/ (meet)	7	5	1	1
/e/ (French é)	6	—	—	2
/I/ (mitt)	—	6	2	3
/ɛ/ (met)	5	—	—	4
/æ/ (mat)	4	4	4	5
/a/ (mop)	3	—	—	6
/ɑ/ (mar)	—	2	3	7
/o/ (moat)	2	—	—	9
/ɔ/ (maul)	1	1	5	8
/u/ (moot)	—	3	6	10

Source: Based on data of Sapir (1929) and Newman (1933).

[a] Sound frequencies of the second format.

[b] Highest rank is number 1.

the vowel / i / . What is most striking about these results is their relationship to vowel pitch. The pitch of a vowel is closely associated with the sound frequency of the second formant (Delattre, Liberman, Cooper, & Gerstman, 1952). A formant is a packet of energy in the sound spectrum, that is, energy concentrated in a small frequency band; the frequency band that constitutes the second formant lies above the band that constitutes the first formant. As Table 3.1 shows, there is an orderly relation between the size of the object suggested by each vowel sound and the frequency of the vowel's second formant. The higher the frequency, the smaller is the implied size.

This relationship between connoted size of referent and sound frequency reflects the operation of the attribute of auditory size or volume discussed earlier in this chapter: As the frequency of a sound increases, the sound's phenomenal size—its appearance of spatial extent—diminishes (see Figure 3.1, p. 54). This leads us to hypothesize that vowel sounds can express largeness or smallness in objects to the degree that the vowels themselves appear phenomenally to be large or small. A similar hypothesis recommends itself in the case of the expression of brightness: Vowel sounds express brightness or darkness, sharpness or dullness to the degree that the vowels themselves display these attributes. Newman also investigated the symbolism of brightness by vowels, and those results too are given in Table 3.1. As the table shows, brightness is directly related to frequency of second formant. High pitched vowels suggest brightness, low pitched vowels suggest darkness. Werner (1940) wrote, "A four-year-old girl says: 'Father talks just like Santa Claus . . . boom, boom, boom! As dark as night . . . ! But we talk light, like the daytime . . . bim, bim, bim!' [p. 262]." Here, as is most often the case, the symbolic connotations of sound reinforce the denotations. Occasionally, however, language plays perverse, creating conflicts between denotation and connotation, as Stéphane Mallarmé (1935) noted:

> . . . mon sens regrette que le discours défaille à exprimer les objets par des touches y répondant en coloris ou en allure, lesquelles existent dans l'instrument de la voix, parmi les langages et quelquefois chez un. A côté d'*ombre*, opaque, *ténèbres* se fonce peu; quelle déception devant la perversité conférant à *jour* comme à *nuit*, contradictoirement, des timbres obscur ici, là clair [p. 242].[4]

Sometimes it takes a poet's ear to notice a discrepancy between what a word's sound implies it should mean and what it does.

[4] "My poetic sense laments the fact that discourse fails to express things with those touches of color and charm that exist in the instrument of voice, and among languages, sometimes in one language. Compared to *ombre's* [shade's] opacity, *ténèbres* [obscurity] is hardly dark; how deceptive it is, that perverseness that, in contradiction, gives to *jour* [day] a dark tone, to *nuit* [night] a bright tone."

Although this last point is not worth belaboring, it does have the incidental virtue of helping to establish the validity of sound symbolism itself. For one might rightly raise the objection that some, perhaps many, examples of so-called sound symbolism—where individual sounds, sound sequences, stresses, rhythms, and cadences purportedly indicate meanings in and by themselves—are really nothing of the sort, but instead occurrences of the reverse, in that denotative meanings of words or phrases have become attached to sounds and hence seems to be conveyed by them. Thus Samuel Johnson's (1778) famous critique of Alexander Pope's precept notes that

> our language having little flexibility, our verses can differ very little in their cadence. The fancied resemblances, I fear, arise sometimes merely from the ambiguity of words; there is supposed to be some relation between a *soft* line and a *soft* couch, or between *hard* syllables and *hard* fortune.
>
> Motion, however, may be in some sort exemplified; and yet it may be suspected that even in such resemblances the mind often governs the ear, and the sounds are estimated by their meaning [p. 182].

No doubt this is sometimes so. But, if I may extend Mallarmé's observation in Johnson's terms, to perceive that mind and ear conflict is to grant that they may act independently.

Among these independent purveyors of meaning are the expressions of dimensions common to the experience of different sense modalities. Correspondences between vowel pitch on the one hand and size, brightness, sharpness on the other can be observed in several studies on sound symbolism (e.g., Bentley & Varon, 1933; Czurda, 1953; Tsuru & Fries, 1933). Although many investigators of sound symbolism tested artificial verbal materials (nonsense words), some, like Tsuru and Fries (1933), employed real words taken from foreign languages that their subjects were not familiar with. Tsuru and Fries's study showed a greater than chance matching of pairs of English to Japanese antonyms. Positive findings like this, with materials from natural languages, imply that sound symbolism is not just the construct of a psychological laboratory, but forms an undercurrent running through real, spoken language.

Brown, Black, and Horowitz (1955) asked subjects who were unfamiliar with Chinese, Czech, and Hindi to select pairs of antonyms from those languages that they believed to match pairs of English antonyms. Successful translations occurred at a rate much greater than could be expected by chance. Subsequently, McMurray (1960) selected those pairs of antonyms from the three foreign languages that had been translated successfully in the study by Brown *et al.* and asked a group of subjects to evaluate these words on several descriptive scales. The results evidenced two major factors—one a factor of high vowel pitch, which was described as small, sharp, bright, quick, and active; the other, of low vowel pitch, was described as large, dull, dark, slow, and passive.

A prominent feature of sound symbolism is the way that a single, low level property of sounds—here the vowel pitch, or more properly formant frequency—can express so many different qualities. Sounds embody many potential referents; sounds are, to use H. Werner and Kaplan's (1963) terminology, *plurisignificant.* Any search for universals in sound symbolism must take plurisignificance into account, lest the domain of reference wander from one word to another or from one person to another. Brown and Nuttall (1959) pointed out a reason why certain studies failed to show sound symbolism. These were studies in which subjects were asked to match words from two languages both of which were unfamiliar. Such an open-ended task lacks any indicated sensible dimension to guide the process of translation. If sounds have the potential to specify meanings along several dimensions, one may first have to specify the appropriate dimension of significance before one can ask whether people agree.

Sound symbolism in speech, or phonetic symbolism as it is sometimes called, has generated considerable interest among linguists, philosophers, and estheticians, as well as among psychologists. The existence of suprasensory dimensions of experience provides one mode for the expression of meaning through speech sounds, but it may not be the only mode. In some instances, the cross-modal translations may not even depend on sound. Meaning may be mediated through proprioception, by dint of the position of the mouth and tongue, or through kinesthesis, by dint of movements of the lips and tongue (cf. Grammont, 1930). The consonantal combination "sp" found at the beginning of many words that refer to emission or expulsion (e.g., spit, spew, sputter) might signify the action of the tongue and lips pronouncing it. Vladimir Nabokov remarked that in his own synesthesia

I present a fine case of "colored hearing." Perhaps hearing is not quite accurate, since the color sensation seems to be produced by the physiological act of my orally forming a given letter while I imagine its outline [1949, p. 33].

Given their proprioceptive rather than psychoacoustic basis, it is not surprising to discover that Nabokov's colored vowels and consonants fail to evidence any simple relation between brightness and sound.

In this context, we should note R. C. Johnson, Suzuki, and Olds's (1964) finding that sound symbolism was present among hearing but not among deaf individuals. This was true even though the deaf had learned to speak, and thus had had the opportunity to learn associations between meanings and kinesthetic and proprioceptive cues. Sound itself matters.

Before concluding this section, it is only proper to consider the question, How important a role does sound symbolism play in verbal communication? True, there is a small, but measurable ability on the part of individuals to translate words from unfamiliar natural languages; some words utter their meanings loudly enough to be heard and comprehended, while others murmur in a muted undertone that is often indistinct. On the other hand, there is little point in attempting to deprecate the predominant role played by abstract, formal symbolism in the relation of words vis-à-vis their referents. For the most part, meanings are denoted, and denotations are arbitrary. Sound symbolism functions only to a limited degree under normal circumstances, serving to modulate a system that is primarily abstract. Words are more important to meaning than are the sounds that constitute the words. To be sure, the way words are spoken is important. The sequence of sounds that forms the utterance "I am certain" can be declared in a forceful fashion that bespeaks certainty, or whined in a plaintive fashion that belies it. But this is a different matter from the subject of sound symbolism that is being considered here.

Somehow, through the process of learning and using a language, the sound structure of a word can become closely connected to its meaning. Such an intimate relation is often readily observed when a person attempts to remember a word that is at "the tip of his tongue," when the endeavor to remember a target word first brings to mind words that sound like the target; this suggests that the target word's sound and meaning are at least partially stored together or associated in memory (Brown & McNeill, 1966). Again, though, this is not sound symbolism.

That sound symbolism proper exists in natural languages, albeit to a small degree, is evidenced by positive success found in matching meanings of words cross-linguistically. But, I would venture to say, the symbolic arousal of meaning by sound plays only a minor role in business conversations, weather broadcasts, and marital squabbles. Sound symbolism becomes more significant, however, in one very special circumstance—in that liaison of sound with sensible content commonly known as poetry.

One prominent feature that distinguishes poetry from other forms of verbal expression is the central role played by the words themselves—not merely the precision of diction, the judicious use of the mot juste, the subtlety and nuance of connotation, but moreover the close relation between the sound of a word and its meaning in the context of the poem. The reading, enjoyment, and comprehension of poetry is a complex of behaviors that calls into play and blends perceptual, affective, and cognitive responses. The total apprehension of a poem requires sensitivity to several linguistic levels that operate concurrently—not just to the formal representations of meanings by words, but also to the simultaneous, complementary evocation of meaning by sound. As Alexander Pope said, and despite Dr. Johnson's reservations,

> 'Tis not enough no harshness gives offence,
> The sound must seem an echo to the sense.[5]

Northrop Frye (1957, p. 262) noted the way the alliterative rhythms in

> Swarte smekyd smethes smateryd wyth smoke
> Dryue me to deth wyth den of here dyntes

serve to strengthen by imitation the simple repetitive tempo of the hammering in the fourteenth-century poem "The Blacksmiths." Sound symbolism is a medium through which the poet can display his command of "the *vestigia communia* of the senses . . . the excitement of vision by sound and the exponents of sound." A fuller treatment of sound symbolism in poetry awaits Chapter 7.

Synesthesia

Without any doubt, cross-modality equivalences express themselves most forcefully and vibrantly in the variegated phenomena known as synesthesia. A small minority of people experience a curious sensory blending, where stimulation of a single sense arouses a mélange of sensory images. Stimulation evokes not just those sensations that are normally considered proper to that modality, but also evokes sensations or images that are normally considered proper to other modalities. To a synesthetic individual, a voice may take on colors and tastes as well as sound. Most frequently encountered in synesthesia is the form known as *colored hearing;* to people so endowed, sounds—especially speech

[5]"Essay on Criticism." Pope likely borrowed from Vida's "The Art of Poetry": "'Tis not enough his verses to complete, / In measures, numbers, or determined feet; / . . . / To all, proportioned terms he must dispense / And make the sound a picture to the sense."

and music—produce both auditory perceptions and colored visual images.

To those of us who are not ourselves synesthetic, the very phenomenon may seem strange, perhaps even dubious. Yet is is difficult not to be impressed by the seriousness that it provokes and by the impact that it generates in those who are synesthetic. Curiously enough, this may be evidenced in rather different ways. Some synesthetic individuals—even adults—express unfeigned surprise to discover that their way of perceiving is not universal; they had assumed that everyone perceives the colors and tastes of names, voices, music. Others, by contrast, are too acutely aware of the distinction between synesthetic and non-synesthetic perception; some people have commented to me how they learned to suppress any hint of synesthesia, occasionally hiding it even from friends and relatives, and, in a few instances, seeking medical help. To synesthetes, their mode of perceiving is real enough.

One of the first, if not the first, reported cases of synesthesia appeared at the beginning of the eighteenth century: From Louis-Bertrand Castel (1735) we learn that the English ophthalmologist Thomas Woolhouse knew of a blind person for whom sounds were said to arouse visual sensations. Castel, who was a friend of Woolhouse, was himself the inventor of the first color organ—the instrument whose multimodal music Castel believed could express the fundamental unity of light and sound. Its music was a colored music, which could be comprehended by the blind or deaf, as well as by the sighted and hearing.

The concepts of synesthesia and synesthetic relationships were clearly in the air from the late seventeenth through the nineteenth centuries. John Locke (1690) was affected by the *Zeitgeist*, when he raised a closely related issue. Locke wrote of "a studious blind man, who . . . bragged one day, that he now understood what *scarlet* signified. Upon which, his friend demanding what scarlet was? the blind man answered, it was like the sound of a trumpet [Locke, 1690/1894, Vol. 2, p. 38]." Locke's query, soon after reiterated by Gottfried von Leibniz (1704), is reminiscent of the passage, cited at the beginning of this chapter, in which a blind woman essayed to teach a congenitally blind girl visual meanings through cross-modal analogies. Are there actual relations between qualities of sight and sound? Does the color scarlet in some way resemble the sound of a trumpet? Are there some properties of auditory and visual sensation that are shared by these two perceptual events? The poet Swinburne evidently thought so, for he wrote

Like fire are the notes of the trumpets
that flash through the darkness of sound.[6]

Interestingly, there are several records of synesthetic associations between colors and the sounds of musical instruments. The composer Joachim Raff did perceive the color of the trumpet's sound to be scarlet (Krohn, 1892). Synesthetic individuals—synesthetes, as they are called—described by L. Hoffmann (see Krohn, 1892) and by Ortmann (1933) called it bright red. But not all do. Other synesthetes found the sound of the trumpet to be yellow–red (Lomer, 1905), yellow (Anschütz, 1926; de Rochas, 1885), and blue–green (Anschütz, 1926).

Although synesthetic phenomena attracted sporadic attention in the eighteenth century, it was not until the nineteenth century that synesthesia began to impel significant and serious study, both scientific and otherwise. Indeed, as that century progressed, the reports of synesthesia, particularly of colored hearing, increased rapidly in number—so rapidly in fact that several volumes devoted solely to the subject appeared before the century closed (e.g., Bleuler & Lehmann, 1881; Flournoy, 1893; Suarez de Mendoza, 1890). All of these works emphasized the predominant form of synesthesia—colored hearing.

This explosion of interest continued on into the early years of the twentieth century. As an indicant of the scientific interest in synesthetic phenomena, let us consider the number of papers published. What we find is a peak reached in the 1930s. My tabulation from *Psychological Abstracts* shows 44 references appearing between 1927—when that publication began—and 1940, but only 14 appearing between 1941 and 1970 (and only 3 of these between 1961 and 1970).

Let me back up to the nineteenth century. In that period, interest began to focus on synesthesia from several quarters. Not only did physicians and scientists become concerned with synesthetic perception and what it implies about abnormal and normal mental functioning, but, moreover, synesthetic expressions of sensory unity appeared with regularity, occasionally even as doctrine, in literature and in music. As evidence, witness the production of multimodal concerts—music with light, sometimes with odor. These concerts often employed color organs, keyboards on which each key, when struck, produced a colored light as well as a musical note. As I mentioned earlier, the first color organ thus far documented was built in the early eighteenth century by Woolhouse's friend Louis-Bertrand Castel (1735); many others were built over the next century and a half. One culmination of

[6]"Erechtheus."

this particular tradition is found in the multisensory music of Alexander Scriabin, whose *Prometheus* was written for piano, chorus, and color organ.

In literature, too, expressions of synesthetic correspondence among the senses virtually abounded in the nineteenth century. Chapter 8 will examine some of these expressions in greater detail. For present purposes, it is sufficient to point out two notable and relevant examples. One is Charles Baudelaire's "Correspondences," a poem that served as a focus for the subsequent literary movement known as Symbolism. The symbolic relationship between phenomenal appearance and underlying reality is mirrored, in the poem, by the way

> *Perfumes, colors and sounds intertwine*

and in particular by the

> *perfumes fresh as children's flesh*
> *Sweet as oboes, green as prairies.*

Here we see a statement of correspondences among three, even four, different senses.

The second example is Arthur Rimbaud's "Sonnet of the Vowels," which begins

> *A black, E white, I red, U green, O blue; vowels,*
> *One day will I tell of your latent birth.*

Rimbaud's lines are of special interest because of the central role that speech—particularly vowels—plays in synesthesia. Vowel sounds have a peculiarly great potency in arousing visual images synesthetically. To see just how, it is encumbent to inquire more deeply into the nature of colored hearing synesthesia.

COLORED HEARING SYNESTHESIA

An obvious question with which to begin is to ask whether colored hearing synesthesia obeys the same rules of cross-modal translation as the nonsynesthetic analogies that were elucidated earlier in this chapter. In order to answer the question, let us start by examining the most prevalent form of colored hearing, namely, colored vowels.

It is both curious and intriguing to discover so enormous a disproportion in the types of synesthesia that are reported. If we work with a scheme of five external sense modalities—for example, sight, hearing, touch, smell, and taste—then there are 10 possible pairs that may be conjoined synesthetically, that is, sight with hearing, sight with touch, smell with taste, and so forth. Moreover, synesthetic relationships typically are not symmetrical. To a synesthete, sight may arouse taste, or taste may arouse sight, but synesthesia usually operates in only one direction, not both. Synesthesia tends to be a one-way street. If we take the direction of the synesthetic association into account, there become 20 possible pairwise combinations.

Given this large set, it is remarkable to find that most cases of synesthesia involve only one type, namely colored hearing, the arousal of colored visual images through sound. Moreover, of all the sorts of sounds in the environment, speech sounds turn out far and away to be the most powerful stimuli in arousing these visual images. And finally, within the domain of speech sounds, it is the sounds of vowels that tend to dominate. Thus, words that contain the same vowels, but different consonants, typically produce similar or identical secondary visual images.

Colors of vowels. An enormous number of reports on vowel-color synesthesia exist, a sizeable portion of which are summarized in Table 3.2. This summary represents the associations between vowels and colors obtained from over 400 people, as culled from many different studies. Most of these synesthetic individuals spoke either French or German as their native language, but a few spoke English, and others spoke Italian, Czech, or Serbo-Croatian.

Listed in each section of the table are the numbers of synesthetic individuals who reported each of the major vowels to arouse images that were colored yellow, red, green, blue, violet, white, gray, black, and brown. In cases where a vowel produced an image of mixed color (such as blue–green), each component color (in this instance blue and green) was given the value of one-half.

It requires only a casual perusal of Table 3.2 to convince one that there are several regular and systematic relations between vowels and synesthetically induced colors. The vowel *a* most often induces images of red and blue, *e* most often induces yellow and white, *i* induces yellow, red, and white, *o* induces red and black, and *u* and *ou* induce blue, brown, and black. Actually, in order to specify the relations between vowel and color with any precision, it is necessary to denote the appropriate phonetic description of the vowels. Synesthetic colors of vowels depend on how the vowels sound. Hence Table 3.3 presents these same data, pooled across all studies, with the color responses assigned to categories in accord with the best assessment of the way each vowel was pronounced.

Table 3.2

Frequencies of synesthetic associations between colors and vowels

Vowel	Yellow	Red	Green	Blue	Violet	White	Gray	Black	Brown
			Summary of results from 32 studies[a]						
a	4.5	34.5	1	18.5	0	20.5	5	20.5	6.5
e	29.25	9.75	9.5	10	1	25.5	23	0	2
i	19	21	5	11	0	22	5	22	1
o	11.5	25	1.5	5.5	1	12.5	4	16	23
u	5.5	9	11	15.5	5	7	5	20.5	9.5
ou	3	1.5	3.5	4.5	0	1	4	6	9.5
			From data of Fechner (1876)						
a	0	15	1	10	0	26	0	1	0
e	21	2	13	11.5	0	7.5	4	0	1
i	28	10	12	2	0	6	1	0	0
o	2	16	5	14	0	0	4	7	5
u	0	1	3	11	6.5	0	1	24	13.5
			From data of Bleuler and Lehmann (1881)						
a	7	13	1	10	0	6	0	15	3
e	28	3	5	5	0	4	3	0	2
i	7	3	4	2	0	36	0	0	0
o	13	12	0	7	1	0	1	7	9
u	4	11	4	4	2	0	8	10	7
			From data of Flournoy (1892, 1893)						
a	11	50	3	26	3	52	4	45	6
e	38	14	17	36	2	29	27	11	6
i	28	49	19	19	2	43	6	16	2
o	42	38	12	6	6	16	6	26	17
u	15	12	53	24	21	1	7	13	21
ou	9	18	11	12	12	1	17	10	34

[a] Data compiled from Sachs, Perroud, Mayerhausen, Lauret, and Raymond (as compiled by Suarez de Mendoza, 1890), and by Galton (1883), de Rochas (1885), Baratoux (1887), Lauret and Duchaussoy (1887), Klinckowström (1890), Quincke (1890), Beaunis and Binet (1892), Binet and Philippe (1892), Philippe (1893), Grafé (1898), Laignel-Lavastine (1901), Claparède (1903), Stelzner (1903), Ulrich (1903) Lemaitre (1904), Lomer (1905), Gruber (reported by Marinesco, 1912), Schultze (1912), Hug-Hellmuth (1912), Langenbeck (1913), Ginsberg (1923), Henning (1923), Anschütz (1926), Argelander (1927), Collins (1929), Reichard, Jakobson, and Werth (1949), and Masson (1952).

Table 3.3

Data on vowel–color synesthesia from Table 3.2, assigned to specific phonetic representations

Vowel		Yellow	Red	Green	Blue	Violet	White	Gray	Black	Brown
/a/	(mop)	22.5	112.5	6	64.5	3	104.5	9	81.5	15.5
/e/	(mate)	116.25	28.75	44.5	62.5	3	66	57	11	11
/i/	(meat)	82	83	40	34	2	107	12	38	3
/o/	(moat)	68.5	91	18.5	32.5	8	28.5	15	56	54
/U/	(mush)	7.5	22	10	21.5	9.5	3	11	37	24.5
/u/	(moot)	14	21.5	22.5	22.5	12	5	21	20	47.5

Brightness. A noteworthy feature of Table 3.3 is the way the synesthetic colors progress regularly from lighter to darker as vowel pitch descends from high to low: /e/ and /i/ are high pitched, bright sounding vowels, and they produce the whitest colors—or, at least, they produce white colors most often; /o/, /U/, and /u/, on the other hand, are low pitched, dark sounding vowels, and they produce the darkest colors. Bleuler and Lehmann (1881) and Flournoy (1892, 1893) were among the first to note this simple relationship, and they suggested that colored hearing synesthesia obeys a *law of brightness:* Bright vowel sounds produce bright visual colors. This is, of course, the embodiment of Hornbostel's theory of universal brightness described earlier in the chapter.

The law of brightness rears what should now be quite a familiar head. Brightness's role in visual–auditory synesthesia bears a strong resemblance to its role in sound symbolism. If one compares the data on synesthesia (Table 3.3) to those on sound symbolism (Table 3.1), one cannot help being struck by the similarities. Words like "beat" and "bait," with their bright sounding vowels, suggest relatively bright referents, whereas "boat" and "book," with their darker sounding vowels, accordingly suggest darker referents. In a similar vein, synesthetes report that words like "beat" and "bait" arouse brightly colored images, while "boat" and "book" arouse darker ones.

In sound symbolism, the brightness of the referent reflects the brightness of the vowel. So too in synesthesia: The brightness of the secondary visual image mirrors the brightness of the inducing vowel sound.

As I mentioned earlier, the brightness of a vowel sound itself depends on the distribution of frequency and energy in the vowel's sound spectrum. Vowels are like other sounds in this respect: Brightness is greatest when sounds are high both in frequency and in energy.

As might be expected, there is a perfect ordinal relation between the lightness (whiteness–blackness) of the visual images that the vowels arouse and the auditory brightness of the vowels themselves. The relation is depicted in Figure 3.11; here, a score on a dimension of whiteness–blackness was calculated for each vowel and plotted against the sound frequency that typically characterizes or matches that vowel's pitch.

The relation between auditory pitch or brightness and visual lightness or brightness is undoubtedly the most salient feature of colored hearing synesthesia. The same relationship pops up even when sounds other than speech induce the visual images. Music yields a similar correspondence (e.g., Mudge, 1920). Among synesthetes for whom musical notes produce visual images, it is rare to find much regularity or agreement about the relation between color and note. Everybody tends to have his own scheme for ascribing colors. Nevertheless, one point where virtually all synesthetes agree is on brightness. Regardless of the hue, the higher the note's pitch, the brighter the visual image. If middle C evokes red, high C evokes a brighter red; if middle C evokes green, high C evokes a brighter green.

As has already been indicated, we should more properly speak of this relationship as one between auditory and visual brightness, rather than between pitch and brightness. For it turns out that visual brightness that is produced synesthetically often varies directly with the loudness of the inducing sound (e.g., Pedrono, 1882; Wheeler, 1920), as

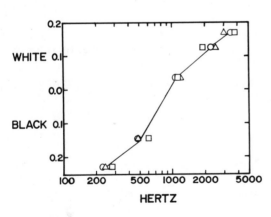

Figure 3.11. A measure of the relative frequency that vowel sounds produce white and black sensory images in synesthetic individuals. The vowels are, in increasing order of brightness, /u/, /o/, /a/, /e/, and /i/. Scores are based on the data in Table 3.3 and they are plotted against three measures of the sound frequency that characterizes the pitch of the vowel. From L. E. Marks, On colored-hearing synesthesia: Cross-modal translations of sensory dimensions. *Psychological Bulletin*, 1975, *82*, 303–331. Copyright 1975 by the American Psychological Association. Reprinted by permission.

well as with its pitch. This is as it should be if the visual brightness expresses auditory brightness, for, ceteris paribus, loud sounds are brighter than soft ones. The brightness of a visual image produced by a sound is a direct function of both sound frequency and sound intensity, and therefore it parallels the attribute of auditory brightness (see Figures 3.3 and 3.4).

What this means, of course, is that in colored hearing synesthesia—and, more generally, in visual–auditory synesthesia—the brightness of secondary visual images varies in a simple and direct way with the brightness of the primary auditory sensations. Translations from sound to sight, so to speak, take place by means of at least one common sensory attribute, namely brightness.

Hue. It would be most rewarding to be able to discover similarly simple relationships between acoustic properties of vowels and the hues aroused synesthetically, so that it would be possible to account for all of the data summarized in Tables 3.2 and 3.3—for instance, to explain why the / a / of "hot" and the / o / of "boat" so often induce the color red. The data suggest that a vowel's potency in eliciting synesthetically a red image depends on its formant structure. The vowels / a / and / o / are called compact, in that the sound frequencies of the first and second formants fall close together, and these vowels tend most often to yield images colored red. With diffuse vowels like / i / and / e /, the frequencies of the first and second formants lie far apart, and, correspondingly, diffuse vowels tend more often to arouse green, or at least less often to arouse red (see Marks, 1975). Still, it must be confessed that the relationship between red–green on the one hand and vowel compactness–diffuseness on the other seems much less powerful a cross-modal association than that between white–black and high pitch–low pitch.

Size. Perceived size is another attribute that is common to both visual and auditory sensations and that plays a leading role in sound symbolism. The deep, low pitched vowels / u /, / o /, and / a / conjure up a sense of large and spacious objects, whereas the thinner, high pitched vowels / i / and / I / hint at delicate and smaller ones. There is no surprise, at this point, in discovering that perceived size, like brightness, provides a medium also for cross-modal transfer in visual–auditory synesthesia.

Many reports of synesthesia note that the sizes of secondary visual images vary according to the nature of the inducing sound (Anschütz, 1925; Bleuler & Lehmann, 1881; Dudycha & Dudycha, 1935; Karwoski & Odbert, 1938; Riggs & Karwoski, 1934; Vernon, 1930; Voss, 1929; Zigler, 1930), and, in particular, the observation has repeatedly been made that visual size increases systematically as auditory pitch diminishes. High pitched sounds produce synesthetic visual images that are small in size; low pitched sounds produce images that are larger. The synesthesia of the subject described by Riggs and Karwoski (1934), a 7½-year-old girl, is typical:

> . . . the size of the colours was related to the pitch of the tones. Tones of the middle range of the piano were reported between one and three inches in diameter. The high tone of a Galton whistle was reported as "small as a pea" [p. 31].

Size bears an interesting parallel to brightness, for, it turns out, visual size depends not only on auditory pitch, but also on auditory loudness: The louder the sound, the larger the induced visual image (e.g., Bleuler & Lehmann, 1881; Karwoski & Odbert, 1938; Voss, 1929). The apparent size or voluminousness of a sound follows the same rule—increasing with increasing loudness, but decreasing with increasing pitch. Just as the brightness of secondary synesthetic visual images appears to reflect directly the auditory brightness of the inducing sounds, so too the perceived size of secondary synesthetic visual images appears to reflect directly the auditory size of the sounds. There exist, then, at least two common or supramodal attributes through which visual–auditory synesthesia operates: brightness and size.

Synesthesia from music. Speech and music are the most potent of all sound stimuli in their capacity to evoke visual images. And these two types of auditory stimulus play by many of the same rules. For instance, when a musical sound synesthetically stirs sight, both brightness and size are conveyed phenomenally from one sensory domain to the other. Musical synesthesia exhibits its idiosyncrasies, to be sure; but it exhibits its invariances and consistencies as well. To some individuals, as I already noted, the sounds of musical instruments can produce specific colors. The philosophers Locke and Leibniz, among others, suggested that the sound of a trumpet is akin to the color scarlet. To both the painter Kandinsky (1912) and the poet Tieck (1828) the music of the flute was blue, "bright blue" to Kandinsky, "sky blue" to Tieck. But the colors of instruments are capricious. More salient, or at least more reliable, than instrumental hues are their brightnesses, especially as related through musical register or pitch. A systematic investigation by Mudge (1920) of the visual impressions from musical instruments found that, in general, the sounds of a flute and of a clarinet suggest bright colors, those of a trombone, dark ones.

Any given synesthetic individual typically finds the visual expressions of music to be regular, consistent, and reliable. Disagreement and inconsistency more often characterize comparisons from one synesthete to another. For instance, some musical synesthetes claim that particular musical notes regularly and repeatedly arouse specific colors—this is the principle that underlies the color organ. Unfortunately, it is hard to find two synesthetes who agree with each other as to which colors go with which notes. Diversity marked the results of a survey that Gruber conducted and Marinesco (1912) reported.

Newton (1704), Castel (1725), and others maintained that there is a real analogy between elementary colors and the notes of the musical scale. Newton, for example, named seven supposedly primary colors of the spectrum—red, orange, yellow, green, blue, indigo, and violet— one to parallel each note on the musical scale. Castel incorporated his own scheme into his color organ: blue for do, green for re, yellow for mi, red for sol, etc. Castel's version was in turn criticized by Field (1820), who proposed still another organization. And so it went. Sadly, one finds that synesthetic associations between colors and musical notes fail to favor any particular scheme over the others.

Music is a complex form of art, so it is not surprising that visual images aroused by music often show a complexity that can itself be related to many features of the music. So we find that when synesthetes listen to music, their visual responses—color, form, movement—may shift, surge, and ebb according to musical key, to musical pattern, to musical progression. But here too results are divergent, with little specific agreement on the images reported by different individuals. There are, however, a few notable exceptions. Karwoski and Odbert (1938) discovered a systematic relation between the shapes of synesthetic visual forms and the tempo of the music: The faster the music, the sharper and more angular the visual image.

This outcome is in line with findings of Willmann (1944), who asked composers and students of musical composition to write music for each of several visual themes. These themes comprised a set of line drawings: a square; a rounded, sailboat-like shape; a squat, multipointed form; and an elongated shape that resembled a bolt of lightning. As might be expected, each line drawing elicited a host of different musical compositions; but the compositions written for each visual theme also contained certain common features. The angular and irregular drawings yielded louder sounds, faster tempos, and syncopated rhythms.

SYNESTHESIA OF TASTE, TEMPERATURE, AND PAIN

Although colored hearing constitutes the bulk of reports on synesthesia, from time to time other types crop up. Sensory qualities of smell, of taste, or of touch may appear in synesthetic conjunction with stimulation of hearing, of sight, or of both. This was true in a study by Martin (1909), who presented art reproductions as visual stimuli and asked for verbal reports of sensory images. Kinesthetic, thermal, tactile, gustatory, and olfactory images, as well as auditory images, appeared. Synesthesia involving the so-called lower senses can also go the other way, in that stimulation of a lower sense may arouse visual or auditory images.

Sometimes these minor forms of synesthesia occur together with colored hearing, but in other instances they are isolated phenomena. The relatively small number of cases of synesthesia involving the lower senses makes it difficult, if not impossible, to systematize the cross-modal relationships and uncover general rules—if any exist. Some of the results, though, are suggestive. The present section serves primarily to give the flavor of what these other, minor forms of synesthesia are like.

Taste. In J.-K. Huysmans's novel *A rebours* (1884), the synesthetic "hero" Jean des Esseintes admires the close connection between taste and music, a connection that he experiences by playing melodies of liqueurs on his taste organ. Each liquor has its instrument: curaçao a clarinet, mint a flute, kirsch a trumpet.

> The similarity carried even farther; tonal *relations* existed in the music of liqueurs. Thus, to give one example, benedictine represents, so to speak, the minor key of that major key of the alcohols that merchants designate by the symbol of green chartreuse.
>
> These principles once admitted, he established by erudite experiments how to play silent melodies on his tongue, mute funeral marches in full dress; how to hear in his mouth crème de menthe solos and rum and vespetro duets [p. 63].

Believe it or not, there once was a serious proposal to build what may have been a progenitor to des Esseintes's taste organ—a first cousin, it would seem, to the color organ. The Abbé Poncelet (1755) offered the following scheme of associations between musical notes and flavors: A—sour, B—insipid, C—sweet, D—bitter, E—harsh, F—austere, and G—piquant. Seven musical notes demand seven taste qualities! Poncelet's assumption was that, under this system, consonant combinations of musical notes would correspond to consonant combinations of tastes, dissonant notes to dissonant tastes.

Wheeler (1920) reported the synesthesia of a blind subject, for whom tastes and smells, as well as sounds, produced colors. Whereas the colored hearing synesthesia was systematic and regular, in that colors increased in brightness as the sounds increased in pitch, the colored tastes and colored smells showed no such regularity. Schultze (1912) recounted the responses of a synesthete who associated tastes as well as colors with vowel sounds. The vowel /e/ yielded a yellow, sugary image, /o/ a brown chocolate, and /u/ a black coffee. It seems quite feasible here to interpret the connections between hues and tastes in terms of learned associations.

Sometimes so-called taste responses can be complex, seemingly an amalgam of taste, smell, and touch images. Thus we find Pierce's (1907) report of a young woman who found spoken names produced a multitude of savors. To give some examples, "Francis" evoked a flavor image of baked beans, "French" evoked charlotte russe, and "Italy" evoked "very small, white pickled onions."

A case of pure gustatory synesthesia was described by Downey (1911). Here the synesthesia worked in the opposite direction, in that the tastes acted as stimuli and produced different colors. Sweet yielded black, bitter was orange–red, sour gave green, and salt was clear. It is interesting that two of the four pairs (bitter and orange–red, sour and green) agree with Hartshorne's (1934) and Pikler's (1922) theory, described earlier, which says that these qualities are cross-modal analogues. Even the association between salty and clearness might be considered analogous to Hartshorne and Pikler's salty–brightness.

Charles Féré (1892) described the case of a woman who suffered from *anorexia nervosa*, the condition of extreme loss of appetite; whenever she tasted vinegar, the woman said her visual field first turned red, then later green. Ginsberg (1923), in the course of discussing his own synesthesia, described taste–colors. For Ginsberg, the correspondences were sweet as orange–red, salty as blue, sour as green, and bitter as black. Note again the association between sourness and green. This same pairing also appeared in the taste synesthesia reported by Collins (1929); whereas all of the other three primary taste qualities induced reddish visual images, acid (sour) induced green ones. A close affinity between sour and green was also mentioned by Suarez de Mendoza (1890).

The most extensive collection of reports on synesthesia involving taste is that of Bleuler and Lehmann (1881). Eugen Bleuler was a psychiatrist, an early promotor of the psychoanalytic theory of Sigmund Freud, and himself a synesthete. Ten of Bleuler and Lehmann's 77 subjects reported tastes to have colors. Unfortunately, these subjects agreed with one another only slightly in the way they linked taste qualities and hues. Consider first the sour taste: Just 3 of 9 subjects reported sour to be green (though, it may be noted, no other color was named even that many times). Furthermore, 2 of 5 named green as the color aroused by salty tastes. The sweet taste produced a wide range of responses (two blues, two greens, one each of red, yellow, gray, white, and clear). Only the bitter taste showed any semblance of interindividual constancy: Five of 9 subjects reported bitter to be brown, another reported it to be black, while the remaining 3 said yellow. Taken as a whole, these results—even to the extent that they demonstrated some very slight consistency—appear at variance with most of the predictions made by Hartshorne and Pikler.

To conclude this section, I will mention the subject (S.) studied extensively by Alexander Luria (1968); Luria's interest in this subject stemmed not primarily from his synesthesia, but rather from his remarkable memory. The mnemonist S. was perhaps only incidentally multiply synesthetic. Aside from the commonly observed colored hearing, S. also displayed a robust gustatory hearing:

> Presented with a tone pitched at 50 cycles per second and having an amplitude of 100 decibels, S. saw a brown strip against a dark background that had red, tongue-like edges. The sense of taste he experienced was like that of sweet and sour borscht, a sensation that gripped his entire tongue . . . .
> Presented with a tone pitched at 2,000 cycles per second and having an amplitude of 113 decibels, S. said "It looks something like fireworks tinged with a pink–red hue. The strip of color feels rough and unpleasant, and it has an ugly taste—rather like that of a briny pickle [pp. 45–46].

Temperature. Aldous Huxley wrote in his novel *Point counter point* (1928),

> Like the warmth of a body transposed into another sensuous key, the scent of her gardenias enveloped him. There are hot perfumes and cold, stifling and fresh. Lucy's gardenias seemed to fill his throat and lungs with a tropical and sultry sweetness [p. 170].

Ginsberg (1923) noted that colors arose in himself not only from tastes, but also from thermal sensations: Mild cold was white, whereas extreme heat and cold were red. Collins's (1929) subject reported cold as white and heat as red; the identical relationships were reported by Suarez de Mendoza (1890).

Three of Bleuler and Lehmann's subjects reported that thermal stimulation induced colors. In contrast to reports by Ginsberg, Collins, and Suarez, two of Bleuler and Lehmann's subjects reported cold as black; the third reported it as only slightly tinted. Hot stimuli were said by the three to be red–brown, yellow, and white. Again, as in the case of colored tastes, there seems to be little agreement from one synesthete to another. At the risk of providing an ad hoc explanation, I would suggest that the differences in these correspondences between temperature and hue are most likely due to selected associations: Thus cold may be associated with black because both sensations can be thought of, in one manner, as the result of "low-level" stimulation; on the other hand, cold may be associated with white because of the more direct, empirical connection with ice and snow.

Temperature, like taste, is sometimes on the receiving end. That is, stimulation of other senses can arouse thermal images. To give one example, Coriat (1913a, b) reported a case of synesthesia where a woman perceived the vowel sounds / e / and / i / as cool.

Actually, certain associations between temperature and color are a matter of common experience, and seem to be widespread, even in everyday language. Colors produced by light of long wavelengths (red and yellow) are typically perceived as warm, whereas colors produced by shorter wavelengths (blue and green) are typically perceived as cool. According to Sully (1879), the coolest colors—blue and green—fall in the middle of the spectrum, with yellow and red very warm and violet slightly warm. More about warm and cool colors, and their origin, will be discussed in Chapter 8.

Pain.

> A pain, of another musical tone than intercostal neuralgia or that strange ache which a great cardiologist had told her came from a "shadow behind the heart," entered into excruciating concords with the orchestra [p. 207].

So, at least, wrote Vladimir Nabokov in his novel, *King, queen, knave* (1968).

As far as I have been able to discover, only a few scientific reports of synesthesia involving pain exist. Bleuler and Lehmann's (1881) survey included four cases of colored pain: a woman who reported pains to be yellow; a young woman and a girl, both of whom reported toothaches to be red; and a man who reported toothaches to be yellow. It is of some incidental interest to note that Bleuler, himself a synesthete, had not only colored hearing and colored taste, but also colored pain. Bleuler experienced most strong pains as white; the exception, headache, was black.

An extensive description of pain synesthesia was given by Dudycha and Dudycha (1935). In that study, the cross-modal correspondences between pain and sight appeared to travel along a path of brightness: The subject found dull pain to produce dark colors, sharp pain to produce bright ones. Again, we have evidence of the existence of an underlying dimension of brightness that determines the course of synesthetic associations.

Synesthesias of the minor senses are idiosyncratic. Synesthesias that involve the so-called minor or lower senses of taste, smell, touch, temperature, and pain stand in marked contrast to synesthesias of sight and sound. Whereas colored hearing synesthesia is dominated by regular and systematic correlations between visual and auditory dimensions of sensory experience, other forms of synesthesia are generally much more erratic and idiosyncratic, in that they rarely reveal common patterns or dimensions. The only significant exceptions to this generalization appear to be (*a*) the widespread, if not universal, perception of blue and green as cool colors, red and yellow as warm colors, and (*b*) the less manifest, but nevertheless reliable perception of darker and more saturated colors as heavy (Alexander & Shansky, 1976; Bullough, 1907). Other than these, there seem to be no other analogues in touch, taste, or smell to the simple and powerful cross-modal translations that take place between sight and sound, as in auditory and visual brightness and in auditory and visual size. This is not to deny either the reality of other types of synesthesia or the meaningfulness of these cross-sensory correspondences to synesthetic individuals. On the other hand, the lack of generality suggests that, aside from possibly color and temperature, and color and weight, there may be little in the way of *intrinsic* equivalence between the sensory qualities of sight and sound on the one hand, and of taste, smell, and the somesthetic senses on the other.

Synesthetic and Nonsynesthetic Correspondences

Despite the fact that synesthesia involving the minor senses fails to reveal much in the way of systematic relationships, we should not lose sight of the significant nomothetic principles, discussed previously, that are revealed in colored hearing. If there is one main conclusion to be drawn from findings on visual–auditory synesthesia, it is that synesthesia is not wholly idiosyncratic. For the most part, cross-modal relations are more than just the result of experiencing associations between randomly or accidentally conjoined sensations. Sometimes this may be so, but usually not. Synesthesia emanates ultimately from a more primitive and intrinsic unity of the senses.

We are left with these major questions that need inquiry: What makes synesthesia, synesthetic correspondences, different from nonsynesthetic analogy? What, if any, is the functional role of synesthesia?

GENERAL PRINCIPLES

Before attempting to answer directly either of these questions, let me review and summarize the major points. First and foremost, synesthesia consists of the correlation between sensory dimensions. Colored hearing, in its plethora of manifestations, embodies dimensional correlations: When speech or music has that peculiar capacity to conjure up visual images and qualities, the lightness or brightness of the visual image relates directly to the auditory brightness of the galvanizing sound, the size of the image to the auditory volume of the sound. Although it is these two sets of auditory–visual correlates—brightness and size—that are most readily evidenced in synesthesia, other suprasensory equivalences do appear. When visual imagery is awakened by music, for instance, the faster the music, the sharper and more angular the associated photisms.

A second general principle is that dimensions that are linked cross-modally in synesthesia tend also to be linked in nonsynesthetic forms of analogy. Nonsynesthetic individuals perceive weak, high frequency sounds through hearing to be small, and in synesthetes these same sounds produce small visual images. Nonsynesthetic individuals perceive intense, high frequency sounds to be bright, and in synesthetes these same sounds produce bright visual images. Synesthetic visual responses to music resemble semantic judgments made by nonsynesthetes. Karwoski, Odbert, and Osgood (1942) obtained, from nonsynesthetic subjects, verbal judgments of meanings suggested by music. Verbal dimensions of meaning were similar to qualities embodied in visual responses obtained from synesthetes; Lehman (1972) reported a similar finding. Phenomena that fall under the rubric of sound symbolism also exemplify the general principle. The sounds of a word can supply implicit meanings to it, and these meanings are born out of the phenomenal qualities of the sounds. Again, the dimensions of brightness and size are salient.

SYNESTHESIA INDUCED BY DRUGS

It is hard to talk about sensory correspondences in synesthetic perception and nonsynesthetic analogy without pointing out one way that even nonsynesthetic individuals can sometimes experience synesthesia. Several of the consciousness-altering drugs, especially hashish, mescaline, and LSD (lysergic acid diethylamide), are known to evoke synesthesia, at least on occasion. That this happens has one clear implication, namely that a capacity for true synesthetic perception lies latent and dormant within most if not all people, ready to come forth when properly catalyzed. The potential to experience synesthesia is probably universal.

Marijuana is sometimes reported to produce synesthesia. Tart's (1971) survey of 150 marijuana smokers revealed that 56% of them often or occasionally experienced colored hearing synesthesia. This percent-age seems rather large. One should take into consideration the fact that 105 of the 150 respondants admitted to prior or simultaneous use of stronger psychedelic drugs, like LSD. Perhaps there is some additive or synergistic action between drugs in inducing synesthesia.

Strong forms of cannabis—for example, hashish—are well known to provoke colored hearing, and sometimes other forms of synesthesia as well. Théophile Gautier and Charles Baudelaire observed the effects of eating hashish at meetings of the Hashish Club. Gautier (1846), at least, participated. Both writers described their experiences with the drug, including vivid depictions of how, under hashish's influence, they experienced a synesthetic unity of sound and sight. Baudelaire, with particular acumen, abstracted out the essential feature of drug-induced synesthesia, which he related in *Les paradis artificiels* (1860/1923). Drugs, he wrote, add nothing new, but instead energize analogies that normally are latent in the mind:

> Sounds clothe themselves in colors, and colors contain music. That, one will say, is quite natural, and every poetic brain, in its healthy and normal state, readily com-prehends these analogies [p. 218].

Baudelaire's conclusion finds support in observations on the synes-thesia brought about by mescaline, where colored hearing displays the general law of brightness (Beringer, cited by H. Werner, 1940).

SYNESTHESIA IN THOUGHT AND LANGUAGE

What are the differences between synesthetic and nonsynesthetic correspondences—between the dramatic, but sometimes puzzling cross-modal associations described by synesthetic individuals and the similarities and analogies noted by individuals not endowed with synesthetic perception? One difference is in vividness. To a synesthetic person, speech or music not only suggests analogies of colors and forms, but the auditory experience actually results in vibrant visual images or in a blending of visual characteristics with the vocal or musical sounds.

The strength of imagery is, of course, a relative matter. The issue of imagery brings to mind what was several decades ago a major con-troversy in psychology. The controversy centered on the question of whether thinking must involve sensory images of one sort or another. On one side of the debate stood E. B. Titchener (1909), stalwart defender of the opinion that sensory elements form the core of thought; on the other side stood members of the Würzburg school—Külpe, Ach, Watt—who emphasized nonsensory cognitive processes like set and determining tendency, which may activate thought processes without the need for images as intermediaries. Eventually, the controversy cooled. If the only difference between synesthesia and cross-modal analogy is the vividness of secondary images, then the difference should perhaps be treated as one of quantity rather than of quality.

There is, however, a second difference. Synesthetic translations from one modality to another tend to be rigid and inflexible, from which we may deduce that these translations derive, in part, from some basic, intrinsic similarity in the underlying structures and mechanisms. To the extent that the cross-modal analogies perceived by nonsynesthetic individuals follow the same rules (dimensional alignments) as those found in synesthesia, these analogies most likely stem from the same underlying sensory unity.

But nonsynesthetic individuals do not always perceive the cross-modal equivalences in an automatic way, certainly not always in a rigid or inflexible way. Instead, some individuals at least, perhaps all individuals at one time or another, can and do shift the way that they associate heteromodal sensory qualities or align stimulus dimensions on different modalities (Marks, 1974a). For instance, on one occasion a person may match increasing auditory loudness to increasing visual brightness, but on another may tergiversate and match loudness to darkness. Though some basic, intrinsic, and, we might say, natural alignments exist between senses, superimposed on these intrinsic correspondences is the perhaps peculiarly human ability to alter alignments, to manipulate the ways that dimensions on different modalities can parallel each other. There is, then, a creative aspect to nonsynesthetic analogy that is generally lacking in synesthesia proper.

The ability to transcend fixed, synesthetic relations, the power to manipulate cross-modal correspondences, and to express these correspondences verbally, takes us from the domain of sensation to what is more generally considered to be that of cognitive processes (though this is not to deny that the topic of sensation falls properly under cognition's rubric). More will be said about this subject in Chapter 8, which examines the manifestations of cross-modal analogy and correspondence at the verbal level.

True synesthesia forms a universal, sensory–perceptual basis for cross-modal equivalence: Certain properties or features of sensory experience are shared by several sense modalities, and perception expresses these shared properties, in their most vivid form, as synesthetic transfer. Heinz Werner (1940) claimed that synesthesia is an important and integral part of children's thought. Synesthesia is common in children, a fact that contrasts markedly with synesthesia's relatively infrequent occurrence in adulthood. Because the relevant longitudinal studies do not seem to have been conducted, it is not possible to document directly the deduction that synesthetic perception is often lost with age; nevertheless, given the drop in frequency from about 40–50% in childhood (e.g., Hall, 1883; Révész, 1923) to at most 10–20% in adulthood (e.g., Bleuler & Lehmann, 1881; Ulich, 1957), it seems eminently reasonable to conclude that synesthesia often diminishes or disappears when child grows into adult.

But to say that synesthesia disappears is only to mean that primary sensory stimuli no longer contain the power of automatic or Pavlovian-like arousal of images on a secondary modality. It is not, however, to say that the analogies between modalities disappear. Just the opposite: Cross-modal relations between analogous attributes remain very much alive.

As I have argued (Marks, 1975), synesthesia is a direct and economical, a salient and compact mode of childhood cognition, laden with the physiognomic characteristics of perception. As such, synesthesia may play an important transitional role in the sharpening of modes of information processing. It is transitional because it may be superseded by the more abstract representations embodied in the linguistic mode of cognition.

The unity of the senses, which expresses itself through attributes common to different senses, transcends the synesthesia of childhood, burrowing deeper into the mind, remaining viable in adulthood, even when only latent. But although these correspondences remain viable in their original, primal form, their sensory–perceptual representation is subdued, and the correspondences accordingly come to be released through the dominant mechanism of adult cognition, namely language.

For this reason, we find that what I have called nonsynesthetic correspondences between the senses—analogies, equivalences, translations of sensory qualities—that these often take place without the mediation of imagery, that these often express themselves, and are themselves revealed, through language. At the verbal level, however, cross-modal analogies need not remain solely the rigid, synesthetic manifestations of a primitive unity of the senses. The richness of thought and language provides the opportunity for permutation and even reversal in dimensional association.

In other words, the verbal expression of cross-modal equivalence can take either of two forms: the representation of some primitive synesthetic unity, that is, the revelation of an *intrinsic* correspondence;

or the assimilation of a new intermodal relationship, that is, the construction of an *extrinsic* correspondence. To disclose an intrinsic relationship, such as that between visual and auditory brightness, it is necessary only to state or exemplify the relevant categories. Indeed, were it not for the existence of multiple significances—like the symbolization of smallness as well as brightness by high pitch—it would be necessary to give only one side of the expression, since the intrinsic property of the relationship would suffice to convey the appropriate concept.

When Edgar Allan Poe wrote, for example, of "the sound of coming darkness,"[7] he implied, intrinsically, one type of sound, a sound like "the murmur of the gray twilight."[8] The imposition of extrinsic correspondence, on the other hand, must perforce be less subtle, for by their very nature extrinsic correspondences require the creation of newly converging properties of sense, ones that may even run counter to intrinsic correspondences. Twilight, as W. S. Merwin apprehended, need not whisper, but can come in a different form, stronger and more powerful, like

> *the blackness . . . growing as it came down*
> *Whirring and beating, cold and like thunder.*[9]

Metaphoric expressions of the unity of the senses evolved in part from fundamental synesthetic relationships, but owe their creative impulse to the mind's ability to transcend these intrinsic correspondences and forge new multisensory meanings. Intrinsic, synesthetic relations express the correspondences that are, extrinsic relations assert the correspondences that can be.

---

[7] "Tamerlane."
[8] "Al Aaraaf."
[9] From "The Annunciation" by W. S. Merwin. In W. S. Merwin *The first four books of poems*. Copyright © 1955, 1956, 1975 by W. S. Merwin. Reprinted by permission of Atheneum.

4

The Doctrine of Common Psychophysical Properties

The scientific study of sensation starts with psychophysics. Psychophysics can be defined broadly as the science that deals with the dependence of the psychological on the physical—with the relationship between sensations or sensory responses on the one hand and characteristics of physical stimuli on the other. Psychophysics deals, therefore, with functional relations between output and input, between sensation and stimulus, between certain classes of behaviors and the environmental conditions that elicit those behaviors.

Studying the senses can excite and reward. It is especially gratifying to a student of the senses to fathom that some unity lays behind seeming diversity: to discover that general principles apply to the input–output relations of more than one sensory system, to realize that the multiplicity of separate and distinct senses only partially disguises an underlying kinship. The senses are, to be sure, distinct entities, though their exact number has, through history, been a matter of controversy: Aristotle supposed them to number 5; Galen stepped the number slightly to 6; Erasmus Darwin later jumped the value to 12 before von Frey reduced it to 8. The very process of numbering the senses means looking at how they differ, while the goal of this work is to see how they are alike. Aristotle himself indicated several similarities among the senses. And as sensory scientists learn increasingly more about their subject, the examples of universal sensory principles become more and more numerous, and the principles themselves become more and more general in their applicability. Notable in this respect is the emergence of general psychophysical principles from the works of Georg von Békésy (1959a, 1967b) and S. S. Stevens (1957, 1958).

This doctrine of general psychophysical properties is most agreeable to one of the basic aims of science: to condense our knowledge, to discover generic laws of nature, to reveal the seeds that contain the potential tree of knowledge. In psychophysics, one goal is an understanding of the senses that is not only complete, but also, whenever possible, simplified. Surely it becomes more convenient, more simple to deal with sensory systems when one comprehends that they operate in ways that are at least somewhat uniform. A single psychophysical law, applicable to many senses, is more powerful, more elegant, more beautiful, than 5, 6, 8, or 12 individual laws. The esthetic appeal of such a scientific doctrine challenges that of literature and art.

We might place the origin of the notion of common psychophysical properties with the Greek thinkers Empedocles, Democritus, and Leucippus, who viewed all sensation as dependent on, and therefore as forms of, touch. According to their view, sensations are aroused when the sense organs come in contact with streams of atoms. Right at the start of philosophic if not scientific inquiry, therefore, one sees the quest for a unifying theme. It is to Empedocles that we owe the idea that the sense organs contain passages into which the appropriate stimulating particles enter. But it was Democritus who, to the best of my knowledge, first tried to establish explicit and definite psychophysical relations. As Theophrastus reported in *De sensibus,* Democritus believed that qualities of sensation depend on the shapes, the "figures" of atoms. Democritus paid special regard to the senses of taste and vision: Each of the six gustatory qualities, sour, sweet, astringent, bitter, salty, and pungent, and each of the four visual qualities, white, black, red, and green, was presumed to arise from the particular size, angularity, regularity, and roundness of the stimulating atoms.

Closely allied doctrines were later espoused by Plato and by Aristotle. For example, Plato, in the *Timaeus,* proposed that large particles cause contraction of the sensorium, small particles cause dilation: Contraction produces the sensation of blackness in vision, of cold in temperature sensation, whereas dilation produces sensations of whiteness and of warmth.

The same sorts of ideas appeared in subsequent speculations, for example, in Hobbes's (1651) mechanistic view that all sensation results from pressures, or, as he wrote, "divers motions," and in Newton's (1704) view that both color and sound depend on physical motion. But it has taken modern empirical, psychophysical research to extend these pre-empirical doctrines and to uncover the extent to which the input–output relations of different sensory systems really do show qualitative and quantitative similarities.

The search for common psychophysical processes embraces the topics of both the previous chapters—both the Doctrine of Equivalent Information and the Doctrine of Analogous Attributes. That is to say, the psychological half of psychophysics refers to all sensory traits and attributes, to the perceptions of primary as well as secondary qualities. In considering common psychophysical properties, the specific sensory or perceptual variable of concern may be either an attribute that resembles stimuli or a purely phenomenal quality. We may be searching, therefore, for a single set of psychophysical processes governing perception of size and form, of duration and spatial location; or we may be searching for a single set of processes governing perception of sensory intensity and of sensory quality.

It takes only a moment's reflection to uncover some rules that must govern the psychophysics of equivalent sensory information. First of all, to the extent that perception is veridical, and accurately reflects traits of properties, the psychophysics must consist of simple linear relations. This is the property of structural identity discussed in Chapter 2. Moreover, when two or more senses provide equivalent, veridical information, the same linear psychophysical function must apply to the several senses. We have already encountered examples of this sort—for instance, Figure 2.1 (p. 16), which shows that distance or extent, whether perceived visually or kinesthetically, is directly proportional to physical length.

The present chapter will deal almost exclusively with the psychophysics that pertains to analogous sensory qualities. As a reminder that this is only part of the story, I will take a moment now to consider briefly one example of a psychophysical approach to cross-modal perception of equivalent forms, a study reported by Owen and Brown (1970a). Random geometrical shapes, differing in number of sides, provided the stimuli that were judged by two groups of subjects. One group received visual versions, the other group tactile equivalents; subjects in both groups had the task of rating each form's complexity. Rated complexity grew as the number of sides increased, and in an identical fashion for the two groups. Both visual and tactile complexity were, for these stimuli, strongly related to a factor that Owen and

Brown called "jaggedness," a stimulus trait that, in turn, seemed to depend on the number of sides, perimeter, and distribution of angles. It is possible that there are several component perceptual dimensions to perceived complexity, and that these same components also provide one basis for the integration of information among several senses and for the transfer of information from one modality to another.

The main business at hand is the psychophysics of phenomenal sensory attributes. Again, note that we have already encountered a few examples of psychophysical relations applicable to several modalities. One is the way the perceived sizes of sounds, vibrations, and shocks all diminish when the frequency of the stimulating sinusoid increases (Figure 3.1 p. 54). Békésy's (1957a) results imply that every time the frequency doubles, the apparent size of the sensory impression drops by one-half. Similarities among the senses are readily apparent when one considers the ways that the senses restrict their sensitivity to select ranges of stimulus energy, the ways that the senses discriminate stimuli that differ in intensity, and the ways that the subjective magnitude of sensation depends on stimulus variables like intensity, duration, and spatial distribution of stimulation over the sensory surface.

Sensitivity

How readily a sense organ reacts to a stimulus is the property known as sensitivity. Sensitivity is defined as the inverse of the amount of stimulation that is needed to evoke some given level of behavior. Usually, the task is to detect the stimulus, and the measure is the amount of stimulation needed for a person to perceive the stimulus 50% of the time. (This measure of sensitivity is known as absolute threshold; other measures, though, like the stimulus magnitude required to produce a given sensation magnitude, can be and often are used.) Hence sensitivity is not a direct measure of a sensor's vigor, for it is a measure not of the output, but of the input. To be twice as sensitive to one sound as another, for instance, means that it takes half as much sound energy to yield the same level of detection or the same sensation of loudness.

BAND-PASS CHARACTERISTIC

Every sensory system restricts itself to a relatively small set of physical stimuli to which it is especially sensitive, and it restricts itself in two ways. First, each sense—with the possible exclusion of pain— has only one appropriate type of stimulation, be it electromagnetic, mechanical, or chemical. The eye, for instance, is adapted to respond to electromagnetic energy; despite the fact that a blow to the head may arouse a visual sensation, the proper stimulus for vision is light energy, not mechanical energy. Second, each sense responds best to a narrow range of stimuli within its domain. Sensitivity is selective.

The visual system responds efficiently to a narrow band of electromagnetic energy: The human eye responds most vigorously to wavelengths around either 500 or 560 nanometers (nm). The peak in sensitivity depends basically on whether the eye is adapted to the dark (peak at about 500 nm) or to bright light (peak at about 560 nm), a duality that reflects the presence on the surface of the retina of two classes of neural receptor: rods and cones. Sensitivity falls off rapidly at wavelengths greater and smaller than the peaks, as Figure 4.1 shows. One frequently encounters the statement that the visible spectrum runs from 400 to 700 nm, and that these two values constitute, respectively, the lower and upper limits on visual sensitivity. This is a convenient

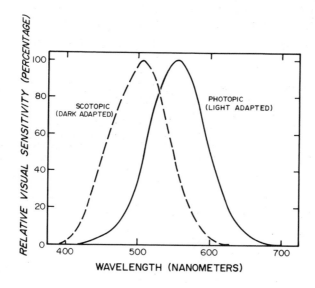

Figure 4.1. The visual system's relative sensitivity to lights of various wavelengths throughout the visible spectrum. Relative sensitivity is inversely proportional to the intensity of the stimulus needed to produce a fixed perceptual response. For instance, on the photopic curve, relative sensitivity at 500 nm is about 35%; thus three times as much light energy is needed at 500 as at 560 nm to produce the same sensation of brightness. The photopic curve represents cone sensitivity, measured in the light-adapted eye or in the all-cone fovea. The scotopic curve represents rod sensitivity, measured in the dark-adapted peripheral retina.

rule of thumb. Even though it is true that the visual system can respond to radiation in the ultraviolet (wavelengths smaller than 400 nm) and in the infrared (wavelengths greater than 700 nm)—given sufficiently high levels of energy—this qualification does not detract from the basic principle, namely that only a narrow range of stimulus wavelengths produces vision. Sensitivity is extremely poor outside the range of wavelengths 400–700 nm, and the natural environment rarely provides enough energy for us to see with ultraviolet or infrared radiation. In a nutshell, the visual system, like other sensory systems, displays what is called band-pass sensitivity.

An analogous narrow band of wavelengths mediates the sense of hearing (Figure 4.2). The mechanical waves that the ear responds to are much larger than the electromagnetic waves of vision. The human auditory system is most sensitive to sounds with wavelengths of about 11 centimeters (cm). It is more common—though confusing for the present purpose of comparison—for acousticians and psycho-acousticians to speak of sound frequency than wavelength: A wavelength in air of 11 cm corresponds to a sound frequency of 3000 hertz (Hz, cycles per second). The often-quoted lower and upper limits of hearing are 20 and 20,000 Hz, respectively, though, as in

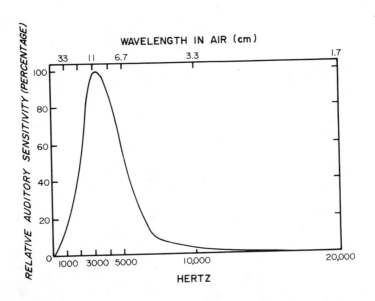

Figure 4.2. The auditory system's relative sensitivity to sounds of various frequencies (lower ordinate) or wavelengths (upper ordinate) throughout the audible spectrum.

vision, when energy is sufficient, human beings can hear sounds at lower and at higher frequencies. Nevertheless, the ear responds best to frequencies between the narrow limits of several hundred and several thousand hertz.

The so-called lower senses also show restricted ranges of sensitivity. The capacity of the tactile system to respond to vibratory stimulation of the skin in some ways resembles the capacity of the auditory system to respond to vibratory stimulation of the ear. Tactile sensitivity depends strongly on vibration frequency; sensitivity is maximal to frequencies around 250 Hz, as Figure 4.3 shows.

With other senses—taste and smell—it is clear from everyday experience that only certain substances are capable of eliciting sensory responses. A modern hypothesis is an update of Democritus's theory that the sensory receptors in the tongue and in the nose are specialized to accept molecules that have certain shapes or configurations. The better the shape of an impinging molecule "fits" the receptors, the more likely we are to sense the substance, or the stronger the sensation will be (e.g., Amoore, 1974). However, when it comes to asking specifically what properties of the stimulus are crucial to determining how readily stimuli can be perceived, answers get hard to come by. It is not unfair to make the general statement that we know much less about the chemical senses than we do about vision and hearing.

This overview serves primarily to earmark some salient characteristics about sensitivity—how each sense is specialized not only with respect to the class of physical stimuli that excite it, but also with respect to the relatively small number or range of stimuli within that class. In fact, the concept of sensitivity is complex. Many other properties of stimuli besides their intensity and composition help determine

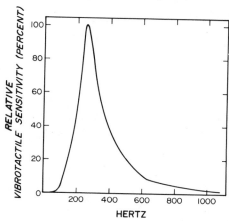

Figure 4.3. The touch system's relative sensitivity to sinusoidal vibrations of the skin at various frequencies. Note that the tactile sensitivity curve is virtually identical to the auditory sensitivity curve, except that the touch system responds to frequencies one-tenth as great.

how readily they will be perceived. In this context, it is worth mentioning that even the band-pass nature of sensitivity, or the width of the band, can be influenced by other stimulus variables. For instance, tactile sensitivity to vibratory stimuli shows a much broader band-pass characteristic when the vibrator is very small in size than when it is large (Verrillo, 1966). That is, sensitivity is much more uniform over the frequency range 20–500 Hz when the energy is delivered through a small stimulator on the skin. Verrillo has taken this as evidence that the touch sense is mediated by at least two different types of receptor.

MINIMUM ENERGY

A second feature of sensitivity common to at least two modalities is their minimal sensible energy. As J. D. Harris (1950) and S. S. Stevens (1958) have pointed out, the visual and auditory systems can, under ideal circumstances, detect quite similar—and incredibly small—amounts of energy. In a study of absolute visual sensitivity that is now classic, Hecht, Schlaer, and Pirenne (1942) determined how many photons—quanta of light—are needed in order to arouse a barely perceptible visual sensation in the peripheral retina, under conditions aimed at eliciting the best possible sensitivity. Their measurements showed that in order to detect a brief flash of light 60% of the time, between 5 and 14 quanta of light at wavelength 510 nm must be absorbed by visual photopigment. In terms of energy at the retina of the eye, this range corresponds to 2.1–5.7 × 10⁻¹⁰ erg (2.1–5.7 × 10⁻¹⁷ W-sec); in terms of energy estimated to have actually been absorbed by the retinal receptors (rods), the range corresponds to 1.92–5.3 × 10⁻¹⁷ W-sec. Other investigations (e.g., Bouman & van der Velden, 1947) suggest that only 2 quanta need be absorbed; if this is so, the corresponding absorbed energy is 7.7 × 10⁻¹⁸ W-sec.

Similar values characterize the sense of hearing. Psychoacoustic experiments (see H. Davis & Kranz, 1964; Sivian & White, 1933) suggest that maximal sensitivity in audition (lowest absolute threshold) corresponds to a sound pressure of about 7.5 dB SPL[1] (5 × 10⁻⁵ N/m²); from this value I calculated the acoustical power of the stimulus at threshold to equal 3.0 × 10⁻¹⁶ W.[2] Given that the auditory system integrates acoustic power over a time period equal to .2 sec (Garner, 1947), the threshold energy comes to 6.0 × 10⁻¹⁷ W-sec. Needless to say,

---

[1] Decibels (dB) SPL = $20 \log(P/2 \times 10^{-5})$, where P is pressure in newtons per square meter.

[2] The computation is based on the equation $P^2 = J\rho c/a$ where $\rho = 1.2$ kg/m³, $c = 3.44 \times 10^2$ m/sec, and $a = 5.5 \times 10^{-5}$ m² as the area of the tympanic membrane (from Békésy, 1960). The energy flux $J = 3.0 \times 10^{-16}$ watt when the sound pressure $P = 7.5$ dB SPL or 5×10^{-5} N/m².

the minimal energies for vision and for hearing, besides being strikingly similar are also extremely small.

It would be interesting to know whether any other sensory systems show comparably high absolute sensitivities. Touch does not. Touch is good, but not that good. At its best, the sense of touch is acute enough to detect sinusoidal displacements (vibrations) of the skin that are smaller than the wavelength of visible or even ultraviolet light—displacements of one ten-thousandth of a millimeter (.1 μm) and less (Wilska, 1954). Yet even this tiny amplitude is 10,000 times as great as the estimated movement of the eardrum at the lowest threshold of hearing (Wilska, 1935).

Visual studies conducted by Hecht et al. (1942) and by others indicate that an individual sensory receptor in the human eye responds when it absorbs a single quantum of light. In animal species such as the silk moth, an individual olfactory receptor responds when it absorbs a single molecule (Schneider, 1974). Perhaps the human olfactory system is similarly acute. De Vries and Stuiver (1961) deduced from measurements of human absolute sensitivity to the compound mercaptan (skunk odor) that a single human olfactory cell probably responds to the presence of one molecule, certainly requires no more than eight molecules. The nose, like the eye and the ear, performs at its best about as well as laws of the physical world permit.

Discrimination

The sensitivity of a sensory system, its capacity to detect stimulus energy, is a measure of the sense's ability to discriminate stimulation from no stimulation. Let us consider the processes involved in the arousal of a just detectable, or as it is called a threshold sensation of light, as in the study by Hecht et al. (1942) described earlier. Visual sensation is one of the end-products of a sequence of events that begins with the absorption of light energy at the retina. More specifically, the light energy activates photochemicals that reside in retinal receptor cells. Hecht et al. assumed that the excitation of a minimal visual response is the result of the absorption of a fixed number of light quanta by the retinal photopigment. This assumption implies an abrupt transition between visibility (when enough quanta are absorbed) and invisibility. But the definition of a threshold—of any sensory threshold—is fundamentally a probabilistic one: The threshold is defined as a level of stimulation that produces a response on a certain fraction of presentations.

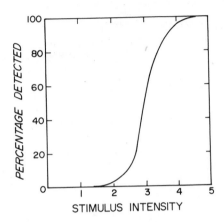

Figure 4.4. A psychometric function, showing how the probability that a subject will detect the presentation of a stimulus depends on the stimulus intensity. The ogival curve is the integral of a normal probability distribution.

The probabilistic nature of threshold is shown by Figure 4.4, which plots the likelihood of detection—the fraction of stimulus presentations that a subject reports as detected—against the intensity of the stimulus. There is no abrupt jump from never detected to always detected, but instead a continuous increase in the percentage of positive responses with increasing magnitude of the stimulus. For this reason, the threshold must be defined as the stimulus level that yields positive responses on some fixed fraction of presentations. The fraction selected—.50, .75, or whatever—is itself a matter of definition and convention. Most often, .50 is used, but recall that Hecht *et al.* used .60. What is important is the notion that the threshold is *not* a level of stimulation that suffices *always* to produce a response. Central to the concept of threshold is *variability of response*.

If light is seen whenever a fixed number of quanta is absorbed by receptors, why is the threshold a variable quantity? Hecht *et al.* made a second assumption—that most of the variation encountered in measuring the visual threshold was due to quantal fluctuations in the stimulus itself. Light is absorbed in little packages or quanta, and, according to laws of quantum physics, a nominally constant stimulus cannot lead to an invariant response. Given a constant stimulus, some fluctuation must take place, from time to time, in the number of absorbed quanta. Hecht *et al.* argued that these fluctuations suffice to account for the probabilistic nature of visual sensitivity: Not every stimulus presentation is detected because not every presentation, even of a nominally constant stimulus, results in the absorption of a sufficient number of quanta. This interpretation puts most or all of the variability in the stimulus, not in the sensory system.

The existence of this physical source of fluctuation cannot be denied. There is, however, an alternative view, namely that sizeable statistical fluctuations can also take place inside the organism; these fluctuations have a biological basis, and they too can influence the measured threshold. Barlow (1956), for example, proposed that light is reported as seen when a fixed number of events (quanta-like absorptions) occur, and that these events can also arise both from absorption triggered by external light and from spontaneous breakdown of photopigment in the retina.

No sensory system is without "noise," that is, spontaneous fluctuations in sensitivity, spontaneous activity in its neural chain. Many nerve cells found in sensory pathways discharge occasionally even when no external stimulus is applied to the sense organ. Stimulation of a sense organ usually produces an increased rate of discharge, but in many significant cases stimulation actually produces a suppression of ongoing spontaneous discharge. More importantly in the present context, both the rate of spontaneous firing and the rate of activated firing induced by a nominally constant stimulus can fluctuate from moment to moment.

Taking this view as a new starting point, we can see the outline of a unitary theme in sensory discrimination: The senses function similarly in their capacity to detect stimuli because the process of detection consists of discriminating signals (stimuli) from noise (nonstimuli or comparison stimuli). In the work of Crozier and Holway (1937) we find an early statement of the general relation between discriminability and variability in sensory systems:

> The really significant and characteristic properties of [discrimination] data are essentially nonspecific with reference to their receptor-organs. . . . The properties of . . . ΔI . . . [the change that must be made in the intensity of a stimulus in order for the change to be detected] are determined by probability considerations which are completely independent of specific structural or other properties of the receptor field [p. 23].

What is perhaps the most extensive theory in psychophysics—the theory of signal detectability—makes this the core assumption (Swets, Tanner, & Birdsall, 1961).

THEORY OF SIGNAL DETECTABILITY

Measurements of absolute sensitivity, such as those considered in the last section, boil down to measurements of a person's ability to discriminate presentations of stimulus from presentations of no stimulus. The theory of signal detectability starts with the postulate that there is spontaneous activity in the sensory system even when no stimulus is presented; the core of the theory states that fluctuations in the level of this spontaneous activity can be confused with changes brought about by the action of an external stimulus.

Absolute sensitivity, then, becomes a special case of differential sensitivity. Differential sensitivity refers to the ability to differentiate between two nominally different stimuli, for example, between a background stimulus and a background plus superimposed test stimulus, or between a standard, reference stimulus and a slightly different, test stimulus. When signal-detection theorists interpret measurements of differential sensitivity, they assume that the background or comparison stimulus produces sensory acitivity whose magnitude fluctuates from one moment to the next or from one presentation to another. Thus, these theorists assume that the experimental subject confuses intrinsic changes—here fluctuations in the sensory effect of the background or reference stimulus—with changes that are produced by increments added to the background stimulus or by the greater effectiveness of a stronger test stimulus.

This potential for confusing the fluctuations in the effect of a reference stimulus with the presentation of a more intense test stimulus is depicted by the two curves in Figure 4.5. Both curves give hypothetical distributions of the probabilities of various levels of sensory activity. The curve on the left shows the distribution of activity produced by the background, the reference, or the noise stimulus; the curve on the right gives the distribution produced by the background plus increment or the test stimulus. Under any particular set of instructions, the subject will have certain expectations that lead him to set a given criterion; the criterion—a point along the abscissa—is a value of sensory activity that the subject uses as a cutoff to decide whether any particular trial contained a test stimulus. According to the theory, the subject responds "yes" when, but only when, the level of sensory activity on a given trial surpasses the criterion. Assume that the criterion is set at the point where the two curves cross; the subject will respond "yes" to about 84% of the presentations of the test stimulus, since about 84% of the area of the right-hand curve falls above the criterion; but the subject will also respond "yes" to about 16% of the presentations of the comparison stimulus, the area of the left-hand curve that falls above the criterion. The theory, then, deals with probabilities, not with "thresholds."

Several predictions follow from this theoretical approach. One is that the probability of a subject responding "yes" when a stimulus is presented [$p(Y \mid S)$] is not independent of the probability of saying "yes" when no stimulus is presented [$p(Y \mid N)$]. In fact, each of these two

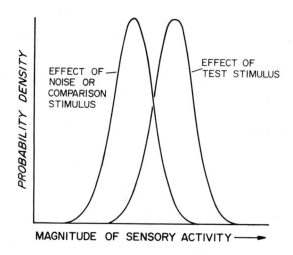

Figure 4.5. The theory of signal detectability hypothesizes two distributions of sensory events. According to the theory, a nominally constant stimulus produces a sensory effect whose magnitude is not invariant, but fluctuates from moment to moment or from trial to trial. In a detection experiment, one distribution (on the left) describes the sensory responses to no stimulus, while the other (on the right) describes the sensory responses to the stimulus. In a discrimination experiment, the two distributions describe the sensory responses to the standard and comparison stimuli. In both experimental paradigms, the subject's task is to decide from which distribution a given observation comes. Where the curves overlap there is ambiguity, and the subject has no way to know which stimulus condition produced the sensory event.

probabilities corresponds to the area of the corresponding curve that falls above the criterion. From the curves in Figure 4.5, p (Y $\mid$ S) will equal .84 when p (Y $\mid$ N) equals .16. Another prediction from the theory is that in a multiple-choice task some information remains even when a subject's initial response (first choice) is erroneous. Consider an experiment where a stimulus appears during one of four intervals, and the subject's task is to decide which one. Even if the subject's first response is incorrect, the probability of a correct identification on a "second guess" should, according to theory, be better than one in three. And it is (Swets *et al.*, 1961).

The most extensive application of the theory of signal detectability has been to the sense of hearing, and in particular to the detection of pure tones embedded in a background of noise. But the theory has also been applied successfully to the detection of visual (Nachmias & Steinman, 1963), gustatory (Linker, Moore, & Galanter, 1964), olfactory

(Semb, 1968), and thermal stimuli (Vendrik, 1970). Detection considered as discrimination of signal from noise is a general psychophysical feature of sensory systems.[3]

DISCRIMINATION OF SENSORY INTENSITY AND WEBER'S LAW

A concern of sensory psychophysics for over 100 years has been the way that our capacity to discriminate one stimulus from another depends on the intensities of the stimuli. How much must a stimulus be changed—increased or decreased in intensity—for the change to be perceptible? How does the size of the change depend on the starting intensity?

Early in the history of psychophysics, Ernst Heinrich Weber (1834) discovered the quantitative rule that now bears his name as law. Weber's law says that a change in intensity, in order to be detected, must be a constant percentage of the initial value. If we begin with stimulus intensity φ and augment or diminish it by $\Delta\varphi$, the $\Delta\varphi$ will be just barely noticeable, regardless of the initial intensity φ, as long as the ratio $\Delta\varphi/\varphi$ is constant. If a change of 1 unit from 10 can be noticed, then so can a change of 10 from 100, of 100 from 1000. In other words, in order to discriminate a minimal sensory change, the signal-to-noise ratio must remain constant. A fixed proportional change in stimulation is just detectable. The solid line in Figure 4.6 shows this relation.

Although it receives criticism from time to time, Weber's law turns out to serve rather well as a general law of discrimination, albeit with some modification and restriction. Even in the nineteenth century, it was known that the law breaks down over low stimulus intensities (near the absolute threshold). Fechner (1860) proposed that Weber's law be modified to state that the difference threshold, $\Delta\varphi$, is proportional not simply to φ, but to $(\varphi + \varphi_0)$, where φ_0 corresponds to a hypothetical level of spontaneous activity in the sensory system, activity that is present even when external stimulation is absent. Such a modification makes sense; without it, Weber's law predicts that the difference threshold $\Delta\varphi$ gets infinitesimally small as φ approaches zero. By adding a constant to Weber's law, the absolute threshold becomes a limiting case of the differential threshold: The absolute threshold is the stimulus

---

[3] I shall just mention a rather different theory of discrimination, one that may hold when noise and variability are minimized. This is the *neural–quantum theory*, and it hypothesizes discrete units of sensory activity (thresholds) in discrimination. S. S. Stevens (1972) argued in favor of this as a general theory, applicable to several modalities.

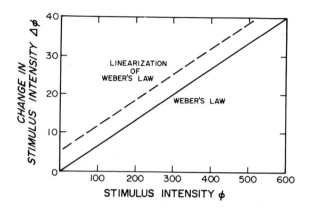

Figure 4.6. The magnitude of the change in stimulus intensity $\Delta\varphi$ from its baseline φ needed for the change to be detected. $\Delta\varphi$ is plotted as a function of the baseline stimulus intensity φ. Weber's law (solid line) states that $\Delta\varphi$ is fully proportional to φ. The linear generalization (dashed line) says that $\Delta\varphi$ is proportional to φ + constant. The value of the Weber fraction $(\Delta\varphi/\varphi) = .067$ is only illustrative.

intensity that must be added in order to detect a change in the level of the background of intrinsic noise (φ_0). This modification is sometimes termed the "linear generalization of Weber's law," and it is shown as the dashed line in Figure 4.6. The generality of Weber's law is illustrated in Figure 4.7, which characterizes intensity discrimination in five sense modalities. This is a double logarithmic plot, so the simple form of Weber's law shows as a straight line with unit slope; with the linear generalization, the line is not straight throughout, but tails off at low values of stimulus intensity and becomes horizontal in the vicinity of the absolute threshold.

Miller (1947) showed that the linear generalization could be used to describe well the discrimination of increments in the intensity of white noise: The size of the Weber fraction $\Delta\varphi/(\varphi + \varphi_0)$ equaled about .1. Results of many studies on discrimination of visual stimuli (e.g., Graham & Kemp, 1938; Mueller, 1951) can also be described by the linear generalization. (A few others cannot. The linear generalization often fails when there is significant spatial contrast between standard and comparison fields [e.g., Steinhardt, 1936].) The Weber fraction for brightness varies in size from .01 when visual test and comparison fields border one another (Steinhardt, 1936) to .1 when they do not (Graham & Kemp, 1938). The linear generalization has also been verified for olfaction (Stone & Bosley, 1965), where the Weber fraction

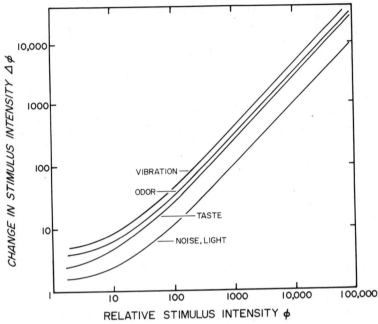

Figure 4.7. Intensity discrimination in five sense modalities. Note that the spacing of stimulus values along both axes is logarithmic. The touch system is least sensitive to changes in physical intensity; the visual and auditory systems are most sensitive. The linear generalization of Weber's law provides a good, approximate description of sensory discrimination.

approximated .25–.3;[4] for taste (Bujas, 1937), where the fraction varied from less than .2 to more than .3, depending on the compound; and for touch (Craig, 1972), where the Weber fraction for vibratory intensity was about .4.

One curious departure from the ubiquitousness of Weber's law arises in the auditory discrimination of pure tones. Although, as I just mentioned, discrimination of noise follows the law, discrimination of tones does not—at least not quite. In a log–log graph like that of Figure 4.7, the discrimination function for tones does plot as a straight line. The line's slope is not unity, however, but slightly smaller—typically about .9 (McGill & Goldberg, 1968; Schacknow & Raab, 1973). The reasons for this lack of proportionality between $\Delta\varphi$ and φ, a "near-miss to Weber's law," as it is called, remain unclear.

[4]Recent data of Cain (1977) suggest that olfaction is a much more precise sense than has heretofore been recognized. When variability in the stimulus is minimized, the Weber fraction for smell can be .1 and smaller.

The size of each Weber fraction reported here should be considered to be only indicative of the way that stimuli are distinguished from one another by any particular sense. Weber fractions are not invariant. Discriminability depends on other stimulus variables besides intensity, variables like frequency or wavelength, duration, size, and so forth. Often, the discriminability of small or brief stimuli is proportional to stimulus size and duration; that is, small, brief stimuli may be harder to tell apart than large, long ones, at the same intensities. Thus the values listed above are more suggestive than definitive. More important than the exact values is the generality of the Weber relation itself, that is, the generality of the principle that discrimination is relative.

At the same time, I think it worth pointing out that Weber's law may not apply in a simple fashion under all stimulus conditions. For example, our ability to discern the difference between one sound and another may be adversely affected by the presence of a third, extraneous sound that masks both of the first two. An extraneous vibratory stimulus disrupts vibrotactile discrimination. Nevertheless, it is interesting to find yet another similarity between these two sense modalities: In both, one may salvage Weber's law by assuming that a fraction of the intensity of the extraneous, masking stimulus adds to the intensities of the comparison and test stimuli (Craig, 1974; Sherrick, 1959).

Weber's law fails more seriously in certain visual paradigms, especially when visual test stimuli consist of very small and very brief increments added to larger, steady backgrounds. Here, $\Delta\varphi$ is found to be proportional to the square root of φ rather than to φ itself (Bouman, 1950), a law first proposed by Cattell (1893). This is the psychophysical relation one would predict from the assumption that discriminability is governed primarily by the statistical fluctuations in the stimulus. Treisman (1964) has proposed a signal-detection model that incorporates variability from several sources—background stimulus and neural pathways. The model predicts both Cattell's law and Weber's law, each under appropriate conditions. Thus Treisman's model assumes that stimulus variability underlies Cattell's law, whereas neural variability underlies Weber's law. It is possible, of course, that similar relationships hold, under comparable conditions, in other sense modalities; hence both laws may apply to all or at least most of the senses.

DISCRIMINATION OF QUALITATIVE, SPATIAL, AND TEMPORAL FEATURES

The topic of discrimination covers much more than just the detection of differences in intensity. Questions about the processes and properties by which people tell one stimulus from another may be asked about any or all of the attributes of sense perception. We just found, when we inquired into the perception of intensity, that there is a simple relationship that seems widely applicable to most if not all modalities—a linear relation between differential threshold and stimulus intensity. Similar inquiry can be made into the rules that govern our ability to discern small differences in other sensory attributes and perceptual features, such as quality, shape, size, number, and duration.

Quality. Again let us consider quality, that thorn in the doctrine of sensory unity. Not surprisingly, it is hard to find profound commonalities in the ways that people differentiate colors, pitches, touch, taste, and smell qualities. After all, if few of these qualities themselves seem phenomenally similar, why should the psychophysics display universal principles? Color is not very much like pitch, so why should hue discrimination resemble pitch discrimination? To be sure, they are similar in that all mechanisms of discrimination may ultimately be limited by variability in sensory processes, and the same theory of signal detectability may apply to discrimination of quality as well as discrimination of intensity in all modalities.

Beyond this, however, lies a vast and treacherous terrain. I say treacherous because resemblances between different senses always carry the danger of inducing one to clasp onto indirect, dubious, or false analogies, or to extend correct ones too far. An example that comes to mind is the analogy between the auditory pitch of a sound and the tactile pitch of a vibration. Touch the plucked string of a violin or guitar and feel the pitch. It surprisingly resembles sound. Is, then, the psychophysics of pitch discrimination by the skin like the psychophysics of pitch discrimination by the ear?

Maybe. But first ask, Is this the proper comparison? Békésy (1955) emphasized a rather different analogy: He noted that sounds of different frequency are represented by different sites of maximal stimulation along the basilar membrane of the inner ear. That is, the sense organ of hearing is extended in space, and sound frequency maps spatially onto it: Békésy suggested that an appropriate model for hearing is a mechanical wave that travels along the sensory surface, reaching its maximal amplitude at a particular locus that depends on the stimulus frequency. Given this model, one might suppose it most appropriate to compare pitch discrimination in hearing not to pitch discrimination on the skin, but to space discrimination on the skin.

Should we eschew the analogy based on phenomenological resemblance and embrace the one based on similar mechanisms? And if we do, how can space discrimination by the skin be compared to frequency (pitch) discrimination by the ear? One complication is that different senses may utilize similar mechanisms in the periphery, but different mechanisms more centrally. In processing pitch, the auditory system might employ a spatial representation on the basilar membrane, but some other representation in the brain (perhaps one similar to that for vibrotactile pitch). The question remains, Which analogy is best for discrimination?

Shape and size. Owen and Brown (1970b) compared visual and tactile discrimination of randomly articulated geometrical shapes. An important physical property of the stimuli they used was the number of sides, which ranged from 4 to 20. One question is, How discriminable are different shapes that have a given number of sides? If discriminability were to follow a relationship of the type codified in Weber's law, then we might expect that a person's ability to distinguish one shape from another should decrease in direct proportion to the number of sides: The more sides, the harder it should be to tell shapes apart. But this was not the result. Instead, discriminability first increased, then decreased with increasing number of sides. Random shapes with 8 sides were more readily distinguished from one another than were shapes with greater or smaller numbers of sides. What is perhaps even more interesting is that this relationship between discrimination and number of sides was the same in both modalities, vision and touch. It is tempting to conclude that the processes underlying shape discrimination are similar in the two modalities—or that a single set of processes operates in both.

There is an intriguing addendum to this finding. The way that rhesus monkeys learn to distinguish random shapes appears to provide a possible corollary to Owen and Brown's (1970b) finding—at least if we are willing to treat number of trials to learn as analogous to difficulty in discrimination. For it turns out that monkeys needed the smallest number of trials to learn when the shapes had eight sides (Carlson & Eibergen, 1974). Perhaps similar, curious processes of shape discrimination operate in monkey and man.

Let us turn now briefly to the question of simple discrimination of size. Kelvin (1954) found discrimination between aluminum disks to be roughly the same for the tactual and the visual modalities. In fact, cross-modal discrimination, where the task was to decide whether a tactile test stimulus was larger or smaller than a visual standard, was about as good as intramodal discrimination in men, though not quite as good in women.

Time. The remainder of this section will be devoted to consider the discrimination of time and temporal order in different senses. One of the earliest of such studies was conducted a century ago by Exner (1875), who determined the interval of time that had to separate two stimulus events in order for a person to perceive the events as successive rather than simultaneous. The ear may justifiably brag of its superiority to the eye at this task. Exner found a much smaller interval was required to resolve two auditory clicks than to resolve two flashes of light—the values were 2 and 40 msec, respectively.

In a more modern experiment, Gescheider (1967) compared the temporal acuity of hearing and touch in their capacity to resolve pairs of clicks; again, the experiment determined the time interval (Δt) between two sensory events that was necessary to perceive them as dual instead of unitary. On an absolute scale, auditory temporal acuity turned out to be 10 times as great as tactile acuity, in that a pair of tactile pulses had to be separated by an empty interval 10 times as long. Nevertheless, there is a remarkable similarity between the processes operating in these two senses. Our discriminative capacity is not invariant in either modality, but depends in a systematic manner on the stimulus intensities of the two pulses or clicks. As Figure 4.8 shows, the way intensity influences acuity is strikingly alike in hearing and touch. If the intensity of the first stimulus is held constant, temporal acuity increases (Δt decreases) with increasing intensity of the second stimulus. If the intensity of the second stimulus is held constant, acuity is maximal when the first stimulus has a magnitude 15 dB above threshold.

Hirsh and Sherrick (1961) asked a related, but slightly different question about temporal discrimination: How much time must separate two stimuli in order to perceive which came first? To test the ability of the visual system to distinguish temporal order, they presented flashes of light that were separated spatially; that is, the two flashes illuminated different portions of the retina. To make the appropriate comparison in the auditory system, they presented pulses of sound that either differed in frequency, that stimulated separate ears, or that both differed in frequency and stimulated different ears. To make the appropriate comparison in the tactile system, they applied vibratory stimuli to different fingers. The findings were remarkable in that the thresholds of successiveness were identical in all three modalities—equal to about 20 msec. The threshold remained at 20 msec even when the pair of stimuli was multimodal, that is, when the first pulse was delivered to one sense and the second pulse to another. It is tempting to speculate that the perception of temporal order of sensory events is processed not separately in each system, but in a single nonspecific center, that is, in the *sensus communis*.

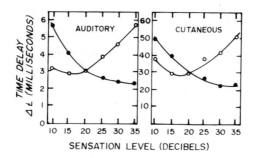

Figure 4.8. The temporal acuity of hearing and touch compared. Plotted are the time intervals needed between two pulses in order for subjects to perceive two pulses instead of one. Filled symbols: The intensity of the first stimulus is held constant at a level 20 dB above threshold; as the intensity of the delayed stimulus increases, temporal acuity improves (the needed time delay diminishes). Open symbols: The intensity of the delayed stimulus is held constant at a level 20 dB above threshold; temporal acuity is best when the first stimulus is about 15 dB above its threshold. The shapes of the curves are nearly identical in the two sense modalities, but the touch system requires time delays about 10 times as great. From G. A. Gescheider, Auditory and cutaneous temporal resolution of successive brief stimuli. *Journal of Experimental Psychology*, 1967, 75, 570–572. Copyright 1967 by the American Psychological Association. Reprinted by permission.

Some interesting perceptual phenomena can emerge when stimuli are presented in rapid succession; just what does emerge will depend on whether the two stimuli strike the same or different portions of the sense organ. When two qualitatively different stimuli are applied to the *same* locus on the sensory surface very rapidly, rapidly enough so that the two stimuli are perceived as a single event, the perceptual qualities of the two merge. Curiously, though, under such a condition the sequence of the events X followed by Y can still be distinguished from the sequence Y followed by X (Efron, 1973), apparently because whichever stimulus in the pair comes second tends to dominate the percept. A 1000-Hz pulse followed immediately by a 2000-Hz pulse sounds higher in pitch—more like the 2000-Hz pulse heard alone—than does the reverse sequence. This is true also in vision, when the pair of stimuli comprises different wavelengths, and in touch, when the pair of stimuli comprises different vibratory frequencies. In all three modalities—hearing, vision, and touch—stimuli that are delivered in such rapid succession that their temporal order cannot be perceived directly are nonetheless perceptually distinct. Such stimuli can be discriminated from one another by dint of perceived quality (pitch, hue). As Efron pointed out, temporal information is transformed, if you will, into qualitative variation.

Other sorts of perceptual events result when stimuli are delivered one after the other to *different* spatial regions of the sensory surface. Geldard and Sherrick (1972) encountered in the sense of touch a new and striking illusion, which they dubbed the cutaneous "rabbit." They delivered a series of brief taps to a spot on the arm just above the wrist, followed immediately by a series of taps to the mid-forearm, followed immediately by a series of taps to a spot near the elbow. What was perceived was not a sequence of events at three points on the skin, but "a smooth progression of jumps up the arm, as if a tiny rabbit were hopping from wrist to elbow [Geldard & Sherrick, 1972, p. 178]." Rabbits also run across the auditory and visual fields (see Geldard, 1976)—a fact that perhaps should not be surprising, given the rabbit's proverbial fertility.

The rabbits jump, hopping from spot to spot. But a sequence of stimuli can also yield the perception of smooth movement between two discretely stimulated points (as Exner, 1875, noted in vision). Whether *apparent movement*, as it is called, materializes, and how like real movement it is, depends critically on the interval of time that separates the stimuli.

Apparent movement is a phenomenon well studied in vision, where it is known to depend on several stimulus variables, such as intensity, duration, time interval between stimuli, and spatial separation. Apparent movement occurs in the tactile sense as well. Sherrick and Rogers (1966) studied the apparent movement that takes place when two 150-Hz vibratory stimuli are applied to the skin of the thigh; they found that optimal movement depends on both the duration of the two stimuli and on the time interval between them, as Figure 4.9 shows. For comparison, Figure 4.9 also gives results of similar studies conducted with visual stimulation and with electrical stimulation of the skin. The absolute correspondence is striking: "The conditions for good apparent movement are not modality-bound [Sherrick & Rogers, 1966, p. 179]." We should, however, inject a dram of caution. Another study (Kirman, 1974) found the absolute sizes of the interstimulus intervals in touch to be about 20% smaller than those reported by Sherrick and Rogers. To find differences in absolute values is not surprising, when one considers that Kirman stimulated the fingertip rather than the thigh, used a square wave rather than a sinusoid, and employed a

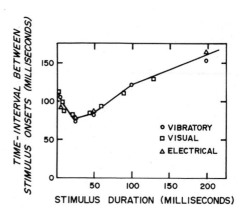

Figure 4.9. Apparent movement in vision and touch. In both senses, optimal movement depends on both the time interval between the onsets of successively presented stimuli and on their durations. From C. E. Sherrick and R. Rogers, apparent haptic movement. *Perception & Psychophysics*, 1966, *1*, 175–180. Reprinted by permission.

stimulator of .025 in. diameter instead of .25 in. It is precisely because parametric differences in stimulating conditions can so influence the exact values that we must exercise a little caution in drawing conclusions about results obtained in different sense modalities. Yet despite this caveat, it is important to indicate that the shape of the function that Kirman obtained parallels very closely that of Sherrick and Rogers. There seems little doubt that the fundamental nature of the processes underlying apparent movement are similar in the eye and on the skin.

Psychophysics of Sensory Intensity

SENSORY SCALES AND STEVENS'S LAW

For centuries a major quest of philosophers and scientists has been to understand the relation between mind and body; over the last two centuries this quest has been channeled partly into the inquiry of how sensation intensity—the psychological magnitudes of brightness, loudness, warmth, and so on—depend on the energy level of the corresponding physical stimulus. In 1860, when experimental psychology was still in its crib, Gustav Theodor Fechner proposed to quantify mental events (sensations) and thereby to state mathematically the rule of translation between the mental and physical realms. Ever since, psychophysics has been fraught with relentless controversy over whether and how mental quantities are to be measured. Are sensations quantities? Can they be added together like lines strung out end to end? And if sensations are quantities, how can their sizes be determined?

I wish to argue that sensory experience is quantitative—that one thing can look brighter or smell stronger than another, and that this psychological attribute of intensity can be specified in mathematical form. One of the ways devised to measure sensations—and one of the most simple and forthright at that—is known as magnitude estimation (S. S. Stevens, 1957). This method calls on people to tag numbers in proportion to the size of each sensation. If one light looks twice as bright as another, or one tone sounds twice as loud, the person gives a number twice as great. Results averaged across a group of 10 or more subjects are generally stable and reliable.

Using the numerical estimates that people apply to their sensations in order to "measure" sensation seems straightforward enough, but the method has had its critics, who question the validity of treating such numerical responses as mathematical entities. How, a skeptic may ask, can we justify taking a subject's numbers at face value? When a person says one sound is twice as loud as another, how do we know it is *really* twice as loud? The criticism hinges on what the skeptic means by "really twice as loud." Some criteria may be applied. One of the most interesting harks back to a commonly accepted and well established notion that many types of measurement—measurements of physical as well as psychological quantities—use the primitive operation of addition (Marks, 1978). Perhaps sensations can, in some instances, be added to one another, like line segments strung out end to end, so that two sensations added together give a sensation equal to the simple sum of the parts.

A few examples from hearing offer themselves. A pair of pure sine waves, widely separated in sound frequency, will, when played together, have a total loudness that is the sum of the individual loudnesses of the two tones. Analogously, when tones of the same sound frequency are played simultaneously to the two ears, we hear a unitary sound whose loudness equals the sum of the loudnesses of the two individual components presented separately. Figure 4.10 gives an example: The graph shows the way people judge the loudness of a 1000-Hz tone played at various intensities to the two ears. Each curve represents what happens to loudness when the intensity presented to the left ear is kept constant, while the intensity to the right ear increases. A fixed intensity to either ear adds a constant amount of loudness, regardless of the intensity to the other ear. It follows that the loudness of each binaural stimulus, as judged by numerical estimations, equals the loudness of the component presented to the right ear plus that of the component presented to the left ear. Evidence like this suggests that these numerical judgments do tap directly the magnitudes

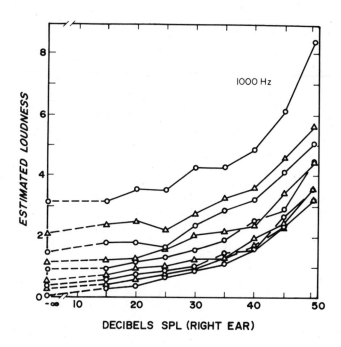

Figure 4.10. Magnitude estimates of the loudness of a 1000-Hz tone. Nine intensity levels to the right ear were combined in all possible ways with the same nine levels to the left ear, making a total of 81 different stimuli in all. The magnitude estimates are plotted as a function of the sound pressure level (SPL) in decibels presented to the right ear; each curve represents a constant SPL presented to the left ear. The fact that the curves are approximately parallel (equally spaced vertically) suggests that overall loudness is a linear sum of left-ear loudness plus right-ear loudness.

of sensory experience, and that the overall sensation of loudness is the linear sum of its two parts.

What is the relation between sensation magnitude and stimulus? Data from many studies on virtually all sense modalities point to a general psychophysical law relating sensation to stimulus: If the theory of signal detectability is the best theory in sensory psychophysics, then S. S. Stevens's (1957) power law of sensory intensity is its best law. Applicable, virtually without exception, to sensory attributes that are quantitative in their nature (or "prothetic," as Stevens [1961] called them), Stevens's law states that the subjective strength or intensity of a stimulus is proportional to its physical intensity raised to some power. Another way of expressing the law is to say that equal ratios of stimulus intensity produce equal ratios of sensation intensity. Two sounds whose acoustical energies bear a ratio of 8-to-1 may give loudnesses in the ratio of 2-to-1, whereas the same 8-to-1 ratio of electrical currents may give perceived shocks in the ratio of 25-to-1. In mathematical terms, Stevens's law can be written

$$\psi = k\varphi\beta.$$

ψ represents perceived intensity; φ represents stimulus intensity; k is a constant of proportionality; and β, the exponent, describes the rule of ratios for the modality (and stimulus conditions).

The way that stimulus ratios couple to sensory ratios in any sense department expresses itself in the size of the exponent β of the power equation, which is the mathematical statement of Stevens's law. Loudness grows about in proportion to the one-third power (cube root) of sound energy, shock about in proportion to the three-halves power of electrical energy (see Figure 4.11).

The value of the exponent in a power equation mirrors sensation's rate of growth, as Figure 4.11 shows. Large exponents—exponents greater than 1—mean that sensation magnitude increases more and more rapidly as physical intensity increases, whereas small exponents—exponents less than 1—mean that sensation magnitude increases less and less rapidly. To some extent, such differences in rate of

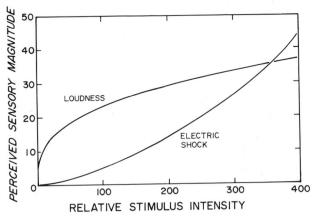

Figure 4.11. Psychophysical functions for loudness and electric shock. Loudness increases here as the .33 power of acoustical energy, perceived shock as the 1.5 power of electrical energy.

growth are likely to be reflected also in the ease with which one stimulus can be discriminated from another, for example, in the size of the Weber fraction. In order to double a sound's perceived loudness, the acoustical energy must be multiplied by a factor of 8–10; to double perceived electrical shock, the electrical energy must be multiplied by a factor of only 1.6. Given this, it seems eminently likely that, in order to detect a minimal change in sensation magnitude, it will take a much larger proportional change in acoustical energy than electrical energy.

This notion was formalized by R. Teghtsoonian (1971), who collated data on sensory magnitude and discrimination in nine perceptual continua. On the basis of these data, he suggested a mathematical formulation to relate the exponent of the psychophysical power function for intensity to the Weber fraction for discrimination. Teghtsoonian's hypothesis states that, in general, we are able to notice the change in sensation magnitude, on any modality, when that change, in psychological units, equals about 3%. According to the hypothesis, differences in discriminability (Weber fraction) from one modality to another come about because it takes different increases in physical intensity to augment sensation by this same 3%.

Examined in detail, this proposal does not always quite work (Marks, 1974b), probably because discriminability does not depend solely on the rate of change in sensation magnitude; discriminability also depends on the degree of variability in the sensory system. For example, the rate of growth of loudness of a 1-msec burst of noise is the same as that of a 1-sec burst. Yet discriminability of the short burst will be poorer because noise is by its nature variable, and a brief sample must perforce lead to greater statistical fluctuations. A more conservative statement of the relation between sensory magnitude and discrimination would turn the order around and say: When the same constant, proportional change in sensory magnitude yields a constant level of discriminability, then it is appropriate to conclude that the variability in the different sensory systems is also the same.

Stevens's power law appears to hold up as a general principle not only across all of the senses, but also under many of the conditions under which any given sensory system may be stimulated. The perceived intensity of a sensory event depends on a host of variables—variables of the stimulus, such as wavelength or frequency, duration, size, and presence of inhibitory stimuli; and variables of the sense organ, such as its state of adaptation. Indeed, the study of sensory processes concerns itself to a significant degree with elucidating just how sensation depends on all aspects of the stimulus and the sense organ. Too brief an exposure to the eye, as to the camera, may render a light or an object invisible. When one first enters from outside, objects in the dark movie theater are indiscernible, but gradually they appear to brighten; and, conversely, when one leaves the theater the outside world dazzles at first, but gradually its brightness is muted.

Variables like adaptation not only modify the magnitude of sensation; they also may influence the size of the exponent in the power equation. But when they do, they typically leave unaltered the form of the power equation itself. For this reason, it is an oversimplification, though admittedly a convenient one, to imply, as I did earlier, that an 8-to-1 ratio of acoustical energies always yields a 2-to-1 ratio of loudnesses. Under restricted conditions of stimulation, such as listening in the quiet to pure tones of frequencies greater than 300 Hz, the rule is correct; under other conditions, such as listening to speech, to pure tones of frequencies less than 300 Hz, or to any sound in a noisy environment, somewhat different rules apply. But they all remain ratio rules. Similarly with electric shock: Under some conditions, the exponent of the power function ranges from 1.5–2, but under other conditions may be as great as 3.5. A full account of the ways that parameters of stimulation influence sensory magnitude and some mathematical formulations of these psychophysical relationships can be found elsewhere (Marks, 1974b).

What is most significant here for the Doctrine of the Unity of the Senses is the generality of the rule "Equal stimulus ratios produce equal sensation ratios." It suggests a kind of matching up of the psychological to the physical domains, of "the veil" with its "sensible content, the inner dynamic arrangement of the *object*." Yilmaz (1967) interpreted Stevens's law in terms of a Principle of Perceptual Invariance. His core assumption is that there are relations among sensory values (such as ratios of sensations) that remain invariant when the environment changes in a systematic manner. For instance, if one changes the overall illumination of a room, say by adding an additional light, the luminances of surfaces change in approximate proportion. Only if sensation relates to stimulus by a power law will the brightness *ratios* be left unchanged under different illuminations. Sensations, therefore, contain some of the same structural relationships that exist in the external world; this property is of epistemological import (see pp. 43–48). Invariant sensory ratios may provide a basis for the extraction in perception of invariant features of the environment.

CROSS-MODALITY MATCHING

Given that there is a rule for relating the strength of a sensation to the intensity of the stimulus that evokes it, and given that the rule can be applied to all sensory domains, then it should be possible to make quantitative predictions as to which sensations, taken from different modalities, match in their subjective strength. That is, once we have an equation that describes the growth of sensation magnitude on Continuum A, another that describes growth on Continuum B, the matching equation follows. Consider the following experiment. We find a level of acoustical energy whose loudness matches the subjective strength of a particular intensity of electric shock. With suitably selected stimulus parameters, loudness will double when the acoustical energy increases by 700%, but perceived shock will double when electrical energy increases by only 60%. Thus if the sound level is multiplied by a factor of 8, and the electrical level is multiplied by a factor of 1.6, the two new stimulus intensities should still match. And they do. Cross-modality matching relationships, like those evidenced in Figure 3.2 (p. 55), attest to the internal consistency of Stevens's power law.

Cross-modality matches do more than just this. They also attest to the very universality of intensity as an attribute of sensation. The simple experimental paradigm of allowing people to select from different modalities those stimuli whose perceived magnitudes are equal crystallizes and quantifies some of those same intersensory relationships that are captured in the metaphorical and poetic analogies of sense. With the help of cross-modality matches between loudness of sounds and brightness of lights (Marks & Stevens, 1966; J. C. Stevens & Marks, 1965), sensory scales and literary metaphors illustrate one another:

Luminance (candelas/meter^2)		Sound pressure (newtons/meter^2)
10,000	*the dawn comes up like thunder* —RUDYARD KIPLING	3.5
1000	*sunlight above roars like a vast invisible sea* —CONRAD AIKEN	1.1
100	*music bright as the soul of light* —ALGERNON CHARLES SWINBURNE	.35
10	*the music . . . suddenly opened, like a luminous book* —CONRAD AIKEN	.11
1	*sunset hovers like the sound of golden horns* —EDWIN ARLINGTON ROBINSON	.035
.1	*a soft yet glowing light . . . like lulled music* —PERCY BYSSHE SHELLEY	.011

Luminance (candelas/meter²)		Sound pressure (newtons/meter²)
.01	*the murmur of the gray twilight* —EDGAR ALLAN POE	.0035
.001	*the quiet-coloured end of evening* —ROBERT BROWNING	.0011
[.000001	best absolute sensitivity	.00005]

STIMULUS VARIABLES THAT DETERMINE SENSORY INTENSITY

I have already alluded to a number of variables besides intensity—variables of the stimulus, like duration and size; variables of the sense organ, like state of adaptation—that help determine the subjective strength of our sensations. Sensory psychophysicists devote themselves largely to unraveling all of these effects in a systematic fashion. One outcome of this effort has been to reveal several instances of general principles, instances where variables like stimulus duration behave in the same manner in different sense departments. The present section can aim only to sample a few of the general laws governing sensory functioning. More information about the material presented in this section appears in Marks (1974b).

How responsive a sensory system is to stimulation depends not just on how intense the stimulus is, but also on how long it lasts and how much of the receptor surface it activates. A short click may be inaudible, a longer lasting noise readily heard; the heat from a flame may be imperceptible to a solitary finger, yet warm to the entire hand. Sensory systems integrate energy over time and over space. These processes are commonly termed *temporal* and *spatial summation.* And not only are temporal and spatial summation virtually universal as sensory phenomena, but moreover the quantitative rules that govern summation are themselves analogous from one sense to another. What follows is a brief sketch of the ways that temporal and spatial summation operate.

Over short periods of time, the duration of a stimulus will deeply influence the sensory responses, in that it will determine both the likelihood that a weak stimulus is perceived and the apparent intensity that a stronger stimulus will have. A short sound pulse lasting a few thousandths of a second may be imperceptible or very soft, but the same sound intensity extended through time to several tenths of a second may be quite distinct, even moderately loud. The exact length of time over which sensation continues to increase in magnitude itself changes from modality to modality, but the general principle of increase remains always the same. Analogous relationships hold with regard to extension through space. A tiny dot of light that is barely visible may, when enlarged, but kept at the same physical intensity, be distinct and bright. Figure 4.12 characterizes both temporal and spatial summation.

One of the direct routes to assessing temporal and spatial summation is to study how the magnitude of sensation grows with time and with size. Recent years have seen several attempts at such direct assessment. But the more traditional route has been somewhat different, and, unfortunately, more indirect. Instead of charting the course of sensation as it grows or diminishes, the older procedures ask the subject to make stimuli of different durations or sizes appear equally intense; subjects do this by making suitable adjustments in the physical intensity of the stimuli. If, for instance, two stimuli have the same physical intensity, but one is larger in size or longer-lasting, it consequently will appear stronger than the other. But the two stimuli can be made to appear equally strong subjectively by making either an appropriate decrease in the physical intensity of the one or an increase in the physical intensity of the other.

Within certain limits, there are equivalences between stimulus intensity and stimulus duration, and between stimulus intensity and stimulus size. To the extent that sensation depends on all three variables—intensity, duration, size—any one can be traded for another and the sensation left invariant: Decrease intensity, but increase duration or size appropriately, and the sensation magnitude is unchanged.

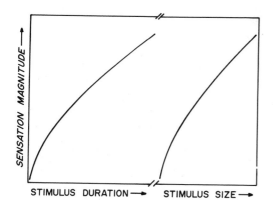

Figure 4.12. Curves characterizing temporal summation and spatial summation: The magnitude of a sensory experience increases with increases in both the duration and the size of the stimulus.

Most important in the present context, the rules of temporal and spatial reciprocity are, in many sense modalities, mathematically similar, in that they are hyperbolic in form:

$$\varphi t^a = \text{constant}$$
$$\varphi A^a = \text{constant}$$

where φ represents physical intensity; t represents duration; and A represents area. In order to keep the magnitude of sensation constant when stimulus duration or size changes, stimulus intensity must change in just the opposite way. A hyperbolic relation means, mathematically, that a given, constant proportional change in duration or size can be offset by some constant proportional change in intensity. When the proportions are equal, as they are in the case of temporal summation of light energy, the reciprocity is perfect: The exponent a equals unity. Doubling the duration has an effect identical to that of doubling the intensity. This relation is known as Bloch's law, and it implies that the visual system completely integrates luminous energy over time. Auditory temporal integration is nearly perfect, though perhaps not always quite so. Actually, suprathreshold temporal summation of the loudness of noise may be somewhat greater than perfect (J. C. Stevens & Hall, 1966), in that doubling a noise's duration seems more effective in increasing loudness than does doubling its acoustical intensity.

Figures 4.13 and 4.14 illustrate temporal and spatial summation in various sense departments. Each line shows the way that stimulus intensity and duration, or stimulus intensity and size, can trade one for the other in order to maintain a constant sensory experience. Let me preface this discussion by pointing out that these functions are meant only as examples. The rules of summation can vary with stimulus conditions, even within a single sense modality. For instance, some evidence (e.g., Watson & Gengel, 1969) suggests that temporal summation in hearing changes systematically when sound frequency changes. Figures 4.13 and 4.14, then, do not tell the whole story. But they are representative.

Because both coordinates in each figure are logarithmic, a hyperbolic relationship plots as a straight line, and the slope of the line indicates the degree of temporal or spatial summation. In the case of a simple reciprocity—for example, Bloch's law in vision—the slope equals -1.0. Slopes with absolute values greater than 1.0 mean that a given percentage change in duration requires an even larger percentage change in intensity to offset it; hence summation is impressively great.

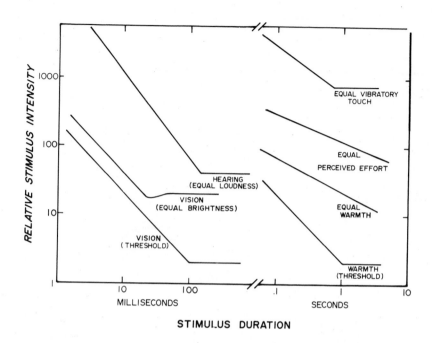

Figure 4.13. Temporal summation in vision, hearing, warmth, proprioception, and touch: The effectiveness of a stimulus in arousing a sensory experience depends on the stimulus's duration. These idealized curves show how the intensity of a stimulus must decrease when its duration increases, in order to give a constant sensory response. The temporal limit on summation is known as the *critical duration;* critical durations are shown as the abrupt transitions between summation and no summation.

In audition, the slope (for noise) equals −1.25. Slopes with absolute values smaller than 1.0 mean that a given percentage change in duration requires a smaller percentage change in intensity to offset it; hence summation is less impressive. Temporal summation is less than perfect in touch (slope of −.7), warmth (slope of −.5 to −1.0), and perceived muscular effort (slope of −.4).

Bloch's law has a spatial analogue, namely Ricco's law. Riccò's law states that the visual system completely integrates luminous energy over space, and, by analogy with temporal summation, it plots in double-logarithmic coordinates as a straight line with slope of −1.0 (Figure 4.14). Perfect spatial summation takes place also in hearing and in touch. In hearing, sound frequencies enjoy a spatial representation on the basilar membrane of the inner ear's cochlea; the reason they do is

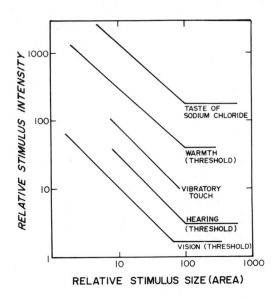

RELATIVE STIMULUS SIZE (AREA)

Figure 4.14. Spatial summation in vision, hearing, touch, warmth, and taste: The effectiveness of a stimulus in arousing a sensory experience depends on the stimulus's size. These idealized curves show how the intensity of a stimulus must decrease when its size increases, in order to give a constant sensory response. The spatial limit on summation is known as the *critical area*; critical areas are shown as the abrupt transitions between summation and no summation.

because the locus of maximal displacement of the basilar membrane changes systematically with frequency. Furthermore, energy is summed across limited ranges of sound frequency and therefore is summed spatially over the basilar membrane. The range of frequencies over which energy sums is called a critical band (Zwicker, Flottorp, & Stevens, 1957); critical bands appear, therefore, to reflect roughly equal areas of the basilar membrane. In touch, spatial summation of vibratory energy is perfect (shows simple reciprocity) when the skin is stimulated with several vibrators (Craig, 1966). Figure 4.14 illustrates spatial summation in vision, hearing, and touch, and gives typical functions for warmth and for taste.

In most sense modalities, summation over time is a short-term affair, lasting a few tenths of a second or at most a few seconds. But when stimuli are delivered for long periods of time, the resulting sensations—of light, taste, smell, temperature, and perhaps sound— adapt; that is, the sensations wane in magnitude and occasionally even

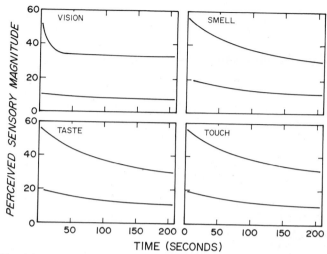

Figure 4.15. Adaptation in vision, taste, smell, and touch: These curves show how sensation decays over time when stimulus duration becomes very long. Note that in vision, the rate of adaptation is relatively much more rapid at high stimulus intensity. In all of the idealized curves drawn here, sensation magnitude ψ decays as an exponential function of time t, according to the formula $\psi = be^{-t/\tau}$.

disappear. Phenomena of *adaptation* were described long ago by Aristotle, who wrote in *De insomniis* [459] of the temporal changes in sensitivity and of the aftereffects of stimulation (afterimages). Contemporary psychophysical research has revealed how different senses display similar patterns of adaptation. In general, once sensations are fully aroused, they next begin to decrease, rapidly at first, then more slowly until an asymptotic value is attained. In mathematical terms, this time course is expressed by saying that sensory magnitude declines in approximately an exponential manner. These exponential curves in vision, smell, taste, and touch appear in Figure 4.15. Though the rate of brightness adaptation itself depends on the light's physical intensity, the rates of olfactory, gustatory, and tactile adaptation are constant, and, indeed, most similar to each other.

PSYCHOPHYSICS OF SENSORY INHIBITION

Strong stimulation tends, in general, to weaken, inhibit, or suppress the sensory effects of weak stimulation, as Aristotle long ago noted [*De sensu*, 447]. It is a common observation, and as well a consternation, that bright headlights of oncoming cars decrease visibility on the road, that low-flying jet planes make conversation virtually impossible. S. S. Stevens (1966), following a model first proposed by J. C. Stevens (1957), argued that the psychophysical processes of brightness contrast in vision and of masking in hearing are similar, and Békésy (1969) sought to demonstrate that the principles underlying spatial and temporal inhibition are common to most if not all of the senses.

The presence of an inhibitory light or sound stimulus not only can alter the perceived quality or depress the perceived intensity of other stimuli, but actually can transmute the sense's input–output function. This is so because masking stimuli exert a more potent suppressing effect on stimuli weaker than on stimuli stronger than themselves. Dim lights and whispers are knocked way down, while bright lights and shouts remain relatively untouched. Such asymmetries imply that the subjective ratio between two brightnesses or between two loudnesses itself changes when an inhibitory stimulus enters the scene. With inhibition, the subjective ratio increases, because the weaker of two sensations will be depressed more than will be the stronger. In terms of the psychophysical power law, then, inhibition acts to increase the size of the exponent (S. S. Stevens, 1966).

There are two fundamental rules about inhibition, surely applicable to vision and hearing, and probably applicable to many or all other sensory systems: First, the stronger is the inhibiting stimulus, the greater is the inhibitory effect; and second, the greater is the difference between the stronger and weaker stimuli, the greater is the inhibitory effect. According to Stevens's (1966) model, inhibition is unidirectional. For example, bright lights inhibit dimmer ones, but dim lights leave bright ones unaffected. This means that inhibition is a nonlinear sensory and physiological process.

An extensive and brilliant series of studies, which compare inhibition in all of the senses, was conducted by Georg von Békésy and is summarized in his book *Sensory inhibition* (1967b). The philosophical framework behind these studies is similar enough to that of the present work to warrant quotation:

> If we look at any handbook of physiology or psychology, it is surprising how neatly the different sense organs are separated into different chapters and each one is treated, in general, by a different author. Unfortunately, I find this disturbing because it creates an artificial separation barrier between different parts of physiology where we would expect some cross-correlations [Békésy, 1969, p. 711].

One of the best-known examples of an effect of sensory inhibition is the perception of Mach bands in vision. Ernst Mach (1868) discovered that sudden changes in the spatial distribution of light intensity over a surface can give rise to the perception of bright and dark bands. If a surface is illuminated evenly over one side, say the right, then abruptly begins to increase steadily in illumination, a dark band is seen at the point of transition. If the illumination abruptly stops increasing and becomes constant again, here over the left side, a bright band is seen at the second transition. Figure 4.16 sketches the spatial distribution of light intensity and the resulting perception of brightness.

A similar perceptual pattern emerges when an analogous spatial distribution of stimulation is applied to the skin. Békésy (1958) found that a vibratory stimulus whose amplitude of displacement followed the stimulus pattern of Figure 4.16 produced a vibrotactile sensation with distinct weak and strong bands. Similar results were reported with sensations of static pressure (Békésy, 1969), heat (Békésy, 1962), warmth, cold, and taste (Békésy, 1967a).

Actually, these phenomenal Mach bands demonstrate more than merely inhibition. Because "overshoot" occurs as well as "depression," the model that Békésy formulated to account for the perceptual events had to incorporate spatial summation as well as inhibition. As I just noted, spatial summation occurs in most or all of the senses. Presumably, the positive and negative Mach bands represent the outcome of spatial summation of both the excitatory and inhibitory effects of stimulation. Békésy's model, unlike Stevens's, contains no nonlinear process in the mechanisms of inhibition. Inhibition is assumed to be proportional to the level of excitation produced by the inhibiting stimulus, and excitation and inhibition are assumed to combine their effects in a linear manner. Békésy (1958) used the term *funneling* to identify situations where summation and inhibition take place simultaneously.

Funneling can also take place when two stimuli, which are ex-

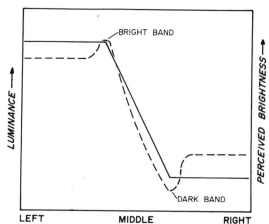

Figure 4.16. Mach bands. Abrupt changes in the spatial distribution of light produce bright and dark bands in perception.

LEFT   MIDDLE   RIGHT

tended or separated in space, are also separated in time. When two pulses of sound, equal in physical intensity, are presented in sequence one to each ear, both the loudness and the perceived location depend on the time interval between them (Békésy, 1957b). With relatively long intervals separating the two pulses, that is, several milliseconds, what is heard is a sequence of two equally loud clicks. As the interval between the pulses is decreased, the second click is progressively inhibited by the first until, with a separation of about 1 msec, only a single click is heard, and it is localized at the ear that received the first click. Precisely the same pattern of events emerges in the localization of two brief vibratory stimuli applied seriatim to different spots on the skin. Again, complete lateralization (inhibition of the second stimulus) occurs when the onset of the second stimulus is delayed about 1 msec (Békésy, 1957b). When the conditions are selected so that lateralization is complete, the loudness of a lateralized click is greater than the loudness heard when only a single click is played (that is, a click to one ear). In the process of laterlization, the second of two clicks may lose its identity, but not its influence: The "inhibited" stimulus does not manifest itself as a separate phenomenal event, but funnels into the first click, to whose loudness it adds (Békésy, 1959a).

Lateralization takes place in the olfactory sense, when stimuli are presented to the two nostrils, and again a difference between onsets of only 1 msec suffices to displace the perceived location (Békésy, 1964a). The same result obtains with sensations of taste produced by sequential stimulation of two regions of the tongue (Békésy, 1964b) and with sensations of shock produced by sequential electrical stimulation of two sites on the skin (Békésy, 1963). Lateralization even takes place when two points on the skin are heated in sequence (Békésy, 1962), but here a time delay of 1 msec is not sufficient. The interval needed for complete lateralization of heat sensation was 140 msec, that is, it had to be 2 orders of magnitude greater than the interval needed with any other sense modality.

The phenomena just considered only scratch the surface of the study of inhibition. Békésy (1971) identified four types of inhibition in hearing, most or all of which have analogues in the other senses. Two of these have received attention here: simultaneous and forward inhibition. I shall conclude this section—and this chapter—by mentioning a third, namely backward inhibition. As we just saw, in forward inhibition the first of two stimuli may be perceived intact, even heightened in strength, while the second is phenomenally suppressed. In backward inhibition or backward masking the reverse happens, in that the second of two successive stimuli may be perceived while the first one is weakened or even completely erased (Raab, 1963). Vision, hearing, and touch all show inhibitory effects of this type. Again, the pivotal variable is the time interval between stimuli. Time intervals must, in general, be somewhat less than 100 msec. Békésy (1971) reported the optimal interval to be 60 msec in both vision and hearing.

Hence we see again, as so many times before, parallel psychophysical processes operating in different sense modalities. One seems to be led almost inexorably to the next topic, which deals with evidence concerning parallel and common physiological mechanisms in different senses. All of the similarities among the senses—but most of all the analogous psychophysical processes just considered—point to, and may in some instances demand, the existence of analogies in the anatomical structures and physiological mechanisms that must mediate sensory perception in different modalities.

5

The Doctrine of
Neural Correspondences

In the first four chapters, I focused attention on the psychological side of the issues—on the side of perception, phenomenology, and psychophysics. Now, however, I want to cross through the looking glass, to inspect some of the same issues from another side, where all of the principles and theories, all of the questions and problems, translate from the realm of psychology to that of neurophysiology. Sense perception, like thought, emotion, and phenomena of mind in general, may at times seem impalpable and evanescent—to be what William Butler Yeats called "disembodied powers," seemingly unlike the material stuff of the external world. But mental events do have their palpable physical and chemical counterparts. And though psychologists and physiologists, philosophers and physicists have held diverse views on whether and how mind depends on brain, just about everyone concurs with the tenet that *some* sort of relation exists; moreover, most acknowledge that this relation, whatever it may be, is especially intimate.

What physiological processes embody sensory experience?

What neural events correlate with analogies and equivalences among the senses?

It is not feasible to try to delve into all of the topics considered in the previous chapters.[1] Instead, a better strategy is to sample a few high points. How does the nervous system pull together information about spatial and temporal characteristics of objects and events? What makes space or number a common sensible? Does the nervous system use a single code to represent the brightness of lights, the loudness of sounds, and the intensities of smells and of tastes? What makes intensity a suprasensory attribute?

Searching for correspondences between domains as different as perception and physiology is much like wending through Baudelaire's "forest of symbols," where, like leaves, ambiguous hints flutter about. Which should be picked up, which followed, which explored? The search for correspondences requires first and foremost a base of principles, a set of rules for relating the psychological to the physiological. Usually, these rules remain implicit or obscure. My goal in this chapter's first section is to give a broad overview of the search for physiological correspondences—to make explicit the rules that guide the search, to provide what is in essence a prolegomenon to the possible theories of psychophysiology that may eventually come forth. Part of this includes pointing out some of the difficulties in evaluating the empirical evidence. Following this, I will delve into the substantive questions: What neural mechanisms underlie the integration in perception of inputs coming from different senses? And what neural mechanisms underlie similarities among the psychological attributes of sensations of different modalities?

---

[1] There are several ways to cut up the pie. Because this chapter is so selective and does not try to evaluate the physiological underpinnings to all qualitative dimensions of sensory experience, I take this opportunity to indicate another direction. Hartshorne's (1934) theoretical analysis of sensation and Osgood, Suci, and Tannenbaum's (1957) empirical analysis of meanings in sensory words indicate that three fundamental dimensions—good–bad, strong–weak, active–passive—pervade sensory qualities. Osgood, May, and Miron (1974) suggested that these dimensions may have their neural counterpart in activity of diffuse systems such as the reticular formation. (The reticular formation is a relatively nonspecific system, receiving inputs from many if not all senses, that runs through the central spinal cord into the bulb (medulla and pons), mid-brain, and thalamus [Magoun, 1963].)

Let me indicate a particularly interesting possibility. Börnstein (1936, 1970) hypothesized that there is a universal sensory attribute of brightness and that brightness's universality rests on the arousal of common muscular tonus. This hypothesis, which finds its most elaborate expression in H. Werner and Wapner's (1949) sensori-tonic field theory of perception, states that one end result of sensory stimulation is the production of a general muscular (tonic) response, the magnitude of which correlates with the "brightness" of the associated sensation. On the physiological side of the coin, one of the first important studies of the reticular formation (Allen, 1932) pointed to a possible relation between reticular function and tonicity. Subsequent research showed that reticular formation plays an important role in the inhibition and facilitation of motor performance (Magoun, 1963). Also of interest: Buser and Imbert (1961) discovered multisensory cells in the motor areas of the cerebral cortex of cats that respond to light, sound, and touch.

Two Faces of Sensation

The search for a neural basis to sensory experience demands no commitment to a particular philosophy about the relation between mind and brain. A materialist will maintain that the mental aspects of all sensory events merely reflect, in a fixed, regular, and systematic fashion, the particular array of physical acts in the nervous system that underlie them; the materialist's eye sees matter and its physicochemical activity as the basic stuff of the universe. Physical activity is primary, mental activity secondary, in that mental events emerge as more or less accidental by-products of physical processes. But, as I said, faith in the intimate association between mental and bodily events is not limited to partisans of a single philosophy; it can be embraced by the idealist as well as the materialist, by the dualist as well as the monist. For a relation may be close even if it is only a co-relation—if, for example, the mental and physical universes are condemned, as Leibniz (1705) believed, to run perpetually like two perfectly synchronized clocks, wholly parallel but nonetheless independent of each other.

To one way of thinking, it really does not matter whether what we call mental activity has—in and by itself—an ontological footing equal with what we call physical, or whether it is a mere will-o'-the-wisp. In either case, meaningful problems await scrutiny and investigation. Questions that can be asked about the phenomenal characteristics of sensory events—about sensations—can also be asked of the neurophysical processes that parallel them. And often they are. Physiologists frequently seek out correlates to psychophysical findings, in the hope of discovering the neurological basis to sensation. Some consider the quest for neurophysiological underpinnings to be the most significant endeavor in understanding perceptual behavior.

BRAIN AND MIND: THREE HEURISTIC PRINCIPLES

For every nuance of color vision or of taste perception, for every discernible smell or musical pitch there must be a corresponding, unique neural process. The present chapter's safari into the nervous system is predicated on the assumption that there is a basic correspondence between the brain and the mind, specifically, on the assumption that there is a basic correspondence between neural activity and perception. Resting on what used to be called psychophysical parallelism, this *Principle of Nomination*, as I will name it, is propaedeutic to all that follows, and it declares that for every change in the state of the mind there is a change in the state of the nervous system.

The principle places little restriction on the possible ways that mental activity can relate to neural activity. Virtually any systematic set of rules can govern the relationship. All that the Principle of Nomination demands is the ability to classify mental and neural events as different or as the same, as varying or invariant. What the principle eliminates is the possibility that identical physical processes give rise to different psychological events; but this is all it eliminates. For the principle only says: Whenever the nerve activity is the same, perception must also be the same.

Is the converse also true? When perception is the same, must nerve activity be the same? Some believe so. When, for instance, G. E. Müller (1896) postulated his five so-called "psychophysical" axioms—five principles by which mental events purportedly relate to physiological processes—he stated them in a symmetrical, reflexive form. Whatever applies to sensation must apply likewise to physiology, wrote Müller, and whatever applies to physiology must apply likewise to sensation. The original Principle of Nomination permits us only to predict the mental from the physical, its singleness of direction thereby smacking of a materialism. By way of contrast, the principle's reflexive form permits us to predict in both directions, with an evenhandedness that gives greater ontological weight to mental activity. Not only must sensation be constant whenever neural behavior is constant, but some neural behavior must be constant whenever sensation is constant.

The trouble with the Principle of Nomination (as I will call the original, one-directional form) is that, while it is virtually indubitable, at the same time it does not take us very far. (And at least one philosopher of acumen has suggested that it is dubitable [Wittgenstein, 1967].) From it, we can say that when Stimuli A and B produce the same neural response, they will yield the same perceptual experience; but we cannot say that because A and B produce the same perceptual experience, they necessarily produce the same neural response. To deduce the latter requires the principle's reflected version.

This problem crops up in the scheme formulated by Brindley (1960). In order to go about correlating visual physiology with visual perception, he relied on a notion similar to the Principle of Nomination. In his formulation, Brindley distinguished what he called Class A and Class B psychophysical operations. Class A comprises all of those manipulations of stimuli that yield invariant sensations. When different stimuli produce sensations that are absolutely identical, it is possible to look for a neural response that is also absolutely identical. Only from such invariances, Brindley argued, is it possible to establish links between perception and physiology. This *reductio ad nominatum*, however, is insufficient. As Boynton and Onley (1962) pointed out, even when the empirical evidence relies on Class A operations, inferences about physiological correlates to perception require the use of a reflexive Principle of Nomination.

Where does the reflexive principle stand? Boring (1941), for one, questioned its general validity. As he indicated, some differences among neural states may not be available to consciousness or to behavior.

More fundamental is the following question: Can wholly different physiological states underlie the same perceptual experience? Boring noted that some very small difference between neural states might have no conscious counterpart; he considered circumstances where the neural states are, for the most part, the same—and that small differences might have no mental analogues. But what about neural states that are vastly different? Could such states underlie identical perceptions?

To answer these questions, it is crucial to be explicit about the stage of neural processing being considered. If two stimuli produce exactly the same effect at the sensory receptors, then they must also produce the same effect at every neural stage thereafter. This yields the sort of invariance that most concerned Brindley. But the converse is not necessary; two stimuli that affect receptors differently might still arouse identical sensations. The question is how they do this. One possibility is that different peripheral signals might end up producing identical neural responses somewhere further along in the nervous system.

What we want to know is not just whether physiological processes differ at the periphery, but also whether they differ wherever in the central nervous system perception takes place. Phenomenal identity need not rely on wholly identical mechanisms. Kolers (1972) demonstrated that real movement and apparent movement may be phenomenally indistinguishable yet rely on different sequences of processing. Even so, when real and apparent movement do appear identical in perception, they may do so because they arouse identical central neural processes. Indeed, the reflexive Principle of Nomination says that they do: When all is said and done, the identity of two sensations entails the identity of some physiological process. Unless we invoke the principle's reflexive form, the task of correlating perceptual experience with physiology is probably hopeless. At the very least, we need a reduced form of the reflexive principle, a form that applies to specific perceptual properties like brightness, pitch, size, duration. This mini-principle says: Whenever some perceptual property is constant, some property of the physiological state must also be constant.

The search for neural correlates readily embraces multisensory events, and, in doing so, leads directly to a second main principle, the *Principle of Convergence*. Whenever perception combines inputs from different sense modalities, as when one sees the object felt in hand, or whenever thought compares such inputs, as when one hears and sees the strident colors of a peacock, the nervous system must be combining or comparing information derived from two or more sensory channels. Somewhere in the nervous system, eye, ear, tongue, and skin talk to each other. And part of the sensory physiologist's job is to decipher the senses' secret language.

There is a third principle. According to the *Principle of Correspondence*, psychological events mimic physiological processes. Not only do mental events and brain processes match up, one for one, but they may even share fundamental characteristics. Underlying the gallery of analogies and common principles operating in different senses, there may exist, each for each, analogous and common neural mechanisms. Crucial here is the qualifier "may," for the third principle serves more as guide to the perplexed scientist than as a priori to the inquiring metaphysician. A good example—one that will be considered in detail later in the chapter—is the representation of sensation magnitudes by neural firing rate, which is an intensity-like property of nerve activity.

A Principle of Correspondence cannot legislate analogy. It is possible that correspondence is a principal rule of nature, that some fundamental properties of the natural world do forge, even demand, structural similarities between physical and mental states. But whether these fundamental properties exist and what they are if they do, we are ignorant. If structural analogies exist between mental and neural states, these must be gleaned through careful experimentation; their existence cannot be laid down by fiat.[2] What the principle provides is a heuristic.

Yet, one may inquire, why elevate mere heuristic to the status of fundamental axiom? The reason is, I suspect, more psychological than logical. As far as I know, analogy is not demanded. At the same time, it is often assumed, presumably because analogy satisfies the scientific impulse for simplicity and similarity: Whatever the relation is between mind and brain, it should "make sense"; Nature or God would not assign mental states to physical states capriciously. To search for a

---

[2]Some may disagree. G. E. Müller's (1896) psychophysical axioms, especially his second, explicitly charge mental and physical events to be analogous:

To an equality, similarity, dissimilarity in the constitution of sensations . . . corresponds an equality, similarity, dissimilarity in the constitution of the psychophysical processes, and vice versa. And, indeed, to a greater or smaller difference in sensations corresponds also a greater or smaller similarity in the psychophysical processes, and vice versa [pp. 1–2].

neural process that resembles a perceptual process is to carry the banner of the metaphorical imperative—the same imperative, I suspect, that has led to such diverse opinions as the Swedenborgian doctrine of correspondence between the physical and spiritual worlds and the Platonic doctrine that the ideal expresses the physical and mental in mathematically-statable, structural relations.

The Principle of Correspondence manifests the metaphorical imperative, the urge to discover or create similarities. But it is not a natural law, which is to say that scientists are not bound to build only analogue models. An example that is relevant here is G. T. Fechner's (1860) theory of inner psychophysics. When Fechner proposed his famous logarithmic "law," he hoped to say something deeply philosophical as well as psychological; in the process, he distinguished between two domains of psychophysics: outer and inner. Outer psychophysics was the subject of Chapter 4; it refers to the relation between external stimulus and sensation. Outer psychophysics comprises two parts. The first is a transformation that takes place when sensory receptors react to external stimuli. This Fechner believed to consist of linear, not logarithmic functions. The second part of outer psychophysics is inner psychophysics, and it refers to the transformation that takes place between the brain and the mind: It is this relation that Fechner believed to be logarithmic. In other words, Fechner tried to account for the overall nonlinear behavior of sensory systems not in terms of peripheral neural processes, not even in terms of central neural processes, but in terms of a lack of complete isomorphism between the physical and mental aspects of the universe.

I resurrect Fechner's theory because it so nakedly rejects obeisance to the Principle of Correspondence. By and large, this part of his thesis fell on deaf ears. Many present-day scientists, like Fechner's contemporaries, tend to assume linear relationships in inner psychophysics, while seeking nonlinearities in physiological processes. I suspect that most hold this view not because they specifically reject Fechner's proposal, but rather because the metaphorical imperative exerts a strong, if unseen, hand. If we are to reject Fechner's solution, the rejection should be conscious and explicit.

Through the Principle of Correspondence, analogy is compounded on top of analogy. Our new set of analogies—neural analogies—work at two levels: first, parallel to their psychological counterparts, and second, analogous to them. To find that different sensory nervous systems use similar mechanisms for discriminating intensity would be to uncover an analogy wholly at the neural level; to find a neural equivalent to Weber's law in different senses would be to uncover an analogy between psychophysics and neurophysiology. Analogies themselves beget analogies.

As often happens with proposals that wander beyond the gates of logical demands, this third principle is rich in potential, thus attractive both as doctrine and as theory. Bear in mind, though, that the two aspects of the unity of the senses—one psychological, the other neurological—are not the same. Similar properties in behavior do not demand similar neural mechanisms, nor do analogous attributes demand analogous neural codes. Despite the generality of the psychophysical power law relating the strength of sensation to the intensity of stimulation, all modalities need not use a single process of neural transduction; despite the generality of brightness as an attribute of sensation, all modalities need not code brightness in the same way.

NEURAL CHARTS OF THE COMMON SENSE

How do neural mechanisms tie in to their corresponding psychological processes? The linkup can take different forms, depending on the type of intersensory relation. For convenience, I shall divide the psychological phenomena into three broad classes. First, different senses provide common information about features of environmental stimuli: When eye and hand tell us about an object's size, neural inputs from the different sensory systems *must* converge. Second, different senses display analogous perceptual attributes: When sounds are loud and lights are bright the neural codes *may* be similar; if, moreover, the analogy itself is appreciated, then the sensory information *must* also converge somewhere in the system. Finally, different senses display common psychophysical properties: When all of the senses obey Stevens's law, the neural mechanisms *may* be analogous. The point is that what we need to look for on the physiological side will naturally be influenced by what we find on the psychological side.

What philosophers call primary qualities—more precisely the perceptual representations of primary qualities—may well have neural counterparts different from those of secondary qualities. The presence of primary qualities—features of the environment, like shape and size, that can be perceived through several senses—leads us to seek one sort of map in the brain, namely a set of heteromodal representations of objects. That is, we look for places in the brain or systems of neurons where inputs from different modalities converge; we look for individual nerve cells or functional groupings of cells that pick up information gleaned through several senses. One goal of perceptual physiology is to discover where and how the nervous system meshes the way a pen looks with the way it feels, where and how it welds a ventriloquist's voice to the dummy's mouth.

Sensory experience presents us with universal dimensions, such as brightness, and these universals lead us to seek a second sort of map. In this case, the Principle of Correspondence induces us to look for neural processes that seem similar in different sensory systems. Might the brightness of colors, tones, and touches be coded the same way? Perhaps the common neural code is even isomorphic—structurally similar—to the attribute itself. Could brightness be, in part, the perceptual face of what is in the neurosensory system a rise in nerve activity that is sudden, rapid, and, so to speak, correspondingly bright?

It is one thing to find similar neural codes in different senses, quite another to find unitary mechanisms receiving inputs from several senses. But first appearances can deceive. The very fact that we are capable of appreciating phenomenal similarity in visual and auditory experience means, if we follow the guidelines set by the Principle of Convergence, that somewhere the nervous system must receive and compare converging inputs. How else could we appreciate "music bright as the soul of light"?

Because people can perceive that music as well as light can be bright, the common sense must include a mechanism that receives multisensory information about brightness, regardless of whether different modalities code brightness differently. Imagine now that brightness does not have a single code, but is represented one way in vision, another way in hearing, still another way in touch. This means that some higher-level neural device, a physiological comparator of some sort, oversees visual, auditory, and tactual brightness. No matter how far removed from the senses the comparator is, nevertheless it has to receive inputs that ultimately derive from the eye, the ear, and the skin.

DIFFICULTIES AND LIMITATIONS

So much for principles and organization, now for some caveats. Voyages that fascinate are often fraught with difficulty; and a tinge of the dangerous, I suppose, enhances their seductive power. This chapter's discourse on the neural foundations of the unity of the senses holds together only as well as the proverbial weakest link. Do we know enough about neurosensory functioning to draw solid conclusions about the foundations of perception? And if not, why not? Two reasons for a negative answer recommend themselves: First, it is difficult to fathom how the nervous system works, especially, what properties of nerve cells correlate with perception. The Principle of Nomination does not take us very far. Second, much of what is surmised about the physiological underpinnings of human sensation comes by extrapolating from studies on lower animals. Sometimes, this is a questionable procedure.

The major impediment is not, I suspect, merely a shortage of data. Some modalities, to be sure, suffer from a paucity of knowledge—the receptors themselves that are responsible for initiating temperature sensations remain partly shrouded in mystery. But other systems—the visual, for instance—fare well. A good deal is known about structure and process in vision at all levels, from the retinal tapestry to the cerebral cortex. Despite such a steadily increasing and imposing body of neurosensory data, the journey from physiology to sensation remains long and treacherous; it does so not just because the path is hard to follow, but also because so many enticing avenues lie before us. Perhaps the main difficulty comes from the fact that each body of data—one neurophysiological, one psychophysical—is so greatly self-contained; each body talks to itself, but the two hardly talk to each other. Often it is easier to ask whether neural processes are similar across the senses, or whether neural processes operate on information from more than one sense, than to ask what it is in perception that correlates with the neural processes.

One need not look very far into the neurophysiology of sensory systems in order to find *potential* correlations. The central nervous system teems with cells that are activated by stimulation of two or more senses. Nonspecific (multisensory) neurons can be found all through the brain—in the so-called association areas of the cerebral cortex, which are thought to be responsible for complex behavioral and cognitive functions; in the primary sensory projection areas of the cortex, which are the first cortical regions to get input from the sense organs; and in subcortical regions too. Let me give a few examples. Murata, Cramer, and Bach-y-Rita (1965) discovered neurons in the visual cortex of cats that responded not only to light, but also to sound and to pinprick of the skin. Horn (1965) described neurons of the cat's visual cortex responsive to electrical shock of the skin as well as to light. Neurons that react to light, sound, and touch have been located in subcortical sites including the caudate and red nuclei (Fessard, 1961), the cuneate nucleus (Atweh, Banna, Jabbur, & To'mey, 1974) and the trigeminal nucleus (Dubner, 1967). Figure 5.1 points out these sites of multimodal neurons.

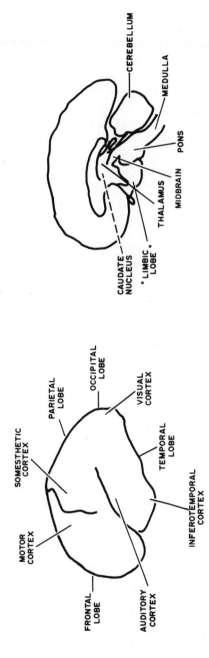

Figure 5.1. Schematic diagrams of the brain, showing, on the left, a surface view of the major lobes, and on the right, a cross-section of the major internal structures.

Finding nerve cells that react to stimulation of several senses is one thing. Assessing what sorts of perceptual information, if any, these nerve cells convey is quite another. Can we hope to understand the articulate dialogue among thousands, sometimes millions of nerve cells?

Let me start at an elementary level: Which characteristics of nervous activity are crucial? Attention typically centers on neural impulses—the nervous system hums with electrical impulses that weave intricate patterns in space and in time. By patterns in space, I mean patterns across different neurons; by patterns in time, I mean the number and spacing of impulses in a given interval. These patterns define, somehow, perception and other mental activities. But alternate possibilities should not be neglected. Recently, considerable interest has emerged in graded electrical potentials; electrical currents need not be quantized or fixed in size but can very continuously in an individual nerve cell and, moreover, can sum their effects with those of nearby nerve cells (Schmitt, Dev, & Smith, 1976).

To make inferences about neural functioning demands extrapolation and interpolation from the available data. The prime matter of concern here is sensation in humans. Unfortunately, most empirical analyses of physiological processes, especially analyses that require invasion of the body, are necessarily directed at lower animals. A guiding principle, to which many sensory scientists subscribe, asserts that some basic sensory processes operate throughout the phylogenetic scale—which is to say that analogous processes operate in various species. Nevertheless, certain processes are specific to individual species. Let me give a concrete example: Electrical potentials recorded in cats from the frontal portion of the cerebral cortex show convergence of inputs from vision, hearing, and touch (Thompson, Johnson, & Hoopes, 1963). Nerve-cell responses recorded from homologous regions in squirrel monkeys behave similarly (Bignall & Imbert, 1969). But responses measured in rhesus monkeys show less convergence (Bignall & Imbert, 1969) or none at all (Albe-Fessard & Besson, 1973). A difference like this is hard to interpret. Does it mean that the common sensory mechanism in rhesus monkeys differs qualitatively from that in squirrel monkeys and cats? Or do the mechanisms differ only quantitatively? Which species, if any, provides the best model for man? Given the evidence that lower animals show less in the way of cross-modal perceptual behavior than humans do, does any infrahuman species provide a good model?

Coding Perceptual Information

SPACE AND TIME

The brain is complex and complicated, enormously so. At times its interconnections seem hopelessly entangled, its operations unfathomable, even mysterious. Still, the brain is a physical device, an organ whose parts extend in space, whose actions extend through time. In theory, if far from present practice, it should be possible to specify all of the brain's activities in terms of physical and chemical processes that take place in four dimensions—like viewing a nickelodeon, each of whose snapshots captures events in three dimensions of space at a moment in time. Space and time are basic dimensions of physics, of perception, and of physiology. Size, shape, duration, motion—these "primary qualities" are molded out of space and time. According to a primitive psychology, the way people perceive space and time bears at least a rough isomorphism to physical space and physical time: The passage of time "in one's head" resembles real time; the spread of the visual world captures the spread of objects in space. Should not the physiological intermediate, the neural bridge between the external world and our perception of it, also maintain some of this structural similarity?

Köhler's (1947) theory of isomorphism is an outstanding example of an affirmative answer. He suggested that spatial relationships in perception are basically similar to relationships in the brain: "Experienced order in space is always structurally identical with a functional order in the distribution of underlying brain processes [Köhler, 1947, p. 61]." The visual cortex of the brain is laid out to map external space, so that certain spatial relations in the visual field have corresponding spatial relations in the brain. The relations need not be identical. The central portion of the visual field, the portion that stimulates the fovea of the retina, has a disproportionately large representation in the cortex, far exceeding its fair share as calculated in terms of its fraction of the whole visual field. A reasonable psychophysiological hypothesis is that the abundance of cortical cells representing the fovea allows the fine acuity that central vision is noted for. But the expansion of foveal vision in the cortex does not make a pencil look any bigger when it is viewed straight on than when it is viewed from the corner of the eye.

What about other senses? Somewhere, the brain may contain a spatial representation of auditory space (Jeffress, 1948). So too for haptic space. Given that spatial information from sight, hearing, and haptic touch are integrated perceptually, the heteromodal inputs may converge on a single spatial representation. Perhaps all inputs are referred to visual space.

The view that perceptual space maps neurosensory space is, I think, persuasive; even more persuasive is the view that perceptual time maps neurosensory duration. Duration is a characteristic of external stimuli, of neural responses, and of percepts. The common sense presumably looks at how long events last, regardless of the modality through which they are perceived—that is, the common sense assesses activity in the visual, auditory, somesthetic, and other sensory systems, perhaps along with some repetitive internal activity, and integrates all of the information in its "time center." The common sense, therefore, probably must shoulder the blame for illusions that occur in several senses—for example, intervals filled with sensory events appear longer than empty intervals. On the other hand, the common sense probably is not responsible for disagreements between the senses—for example, sounds appear to last longer than lights of the same physical duration. This disagreement is presumably due not to an error made in the common sense, but to an intrinsic difference between certain temporal response properties of the visual and auditory systems.

TWO PARADIGMS

To form a coherent theory of the neural mechanisms underlying multimodal perception is not possible without at the same time specifying what sorts of mechanisms underlie unimodal perception. I will take this opportunity to sketch two paradigms.

One paradigm views perception in terms of the activation of highly specific nerve cells, where each cell represents some important attribute of sensation or feature of the environment (some secondary or primary quality, respectively, to adopt crudely John Locke's terminology). This paradigm applies most readily to visual perception, which has seen a good deal of success in discovering "feature detectors." Empirical evidence comes in large measure from the signal work of Hubel and Wiesel (e.g., 1962, 1968), who described the functional properties of cells in the visual cerebral cortex of cats and monkeys that respond to lines and edges in specific orientations, to corners, and so forth. The inferotemporal cortex of monkeys contains cells responsive to complex visual stimuli (including at least one, now well-known, cell that reacted vigorously to a pattern shaped like a monkey's hand) (Gross, Bender, & Rocha-Miranda, 1969). A model of perception might be built on sets of feature detectors—actual or hypothetical neurons that convey appropriate information—without the need for placing a large burden on integrating systems. Barlow (1972) has tried to characterize such a model. If something along this line is correct, then some of the feature detectors would be multimodal.

Can perception be specified in terms of activating a set of feature detectors? One difficulty this approach faces is that the sensory world continuously undergoes transformation, yet certain objects and events remain stable. Consider what happens when you see and hear someone cross the room: The visual image moves across the retina, and as it does it changes its shape, its orientation, its size. The accoustical image shifts in quality, maybe decreases in overall intensity, shifts from the left to the right ear. Yet what is seen and heard is but the same person in different places.

To account for invariant perception in the face of varying stimulus input, what seem to be needed are not just detectors of relatively simple features like edges and corners of objects, or formants of vowels, but at the least some higher-order integrators that can put together information over time and over space (cf. Rock, 1975). Possibly this is accomplished by a relatively small number of nerve cells, but more likely the perceptual invariances depend on complicated circuitry that reflects the use of "heuristic" rules, which at the same time build up percepts from elementary information and evaluate them according to what "makes sense."

Hence the second paradigm tends to view perception as a *process* consisting of patterned activity in a large number of interconnected nerve cells. No one perceptual feature or quality can be attributed necessarily to a small set of specialized neurons. Instead, complexity of interaction is the hallmark, as neurons chatter and debate. This is not to deny the existence of neurons that act like feature detectors, nor to deny that nerve cells selectively responsive to spatial and temporal characteristics of stimulation provide indispensible ingredients to perception. What the second paradigm does deny is that feature detection at an elementary level is enough.

What is the evidence?

Some nerve cells are so precisely tuned to properties of the external world that they can respond to invariant features of the environment despite apparent flux in sensory input. Horn, Stechler, and Hill (1972) studied the behavior of cells, in the visual cortex of cats, that responded selectively to lines with specific orientations. Most of these cells answered simply to the orientation of the line relative to the eye: If the orientation of a line was held constant in space, and the animal was tilted (so the spatial representation of the line on the cat's retina shifted), these cells' responses changed, and they changed just as if the animal had been held stationary and the orientation of the line shifted. But a few cells—14 of 224 to be exact—behaved in a very different manner: When the animal was tilted, these cells' responses to orientation themselves changed, and they changed in just such a way as to compensate for the tilt. Presumably, visual information and vestibular information converge at the level of individual neurons so as to provide a constant response to a high-level invariance in the external environment.

MECHANISMS OF EQUIVALENT INFORMATION

Let us see what happens if we take to its logical conclusion the notion that certain nerve cells are equipped to respond selectively to particular features of external stimuli. The next step is to suggest that certain nerve cells serve as specific mediators of common sensory properties. What results is the following (hypothetical) picture: Each of Aristotle's common sensible attributes—shape, size, motion, rest, unity, number—has its neural analogue. That is, the *sensus communis* or common sense, wherever it may be in the nervous system, comprises a body of neurons that respond to stimulation of all or several sense modalities. By joining Aristotle's doctrine of common sensibles with the paradigm of neural specificity, it follows that specific neurons in the common sense should respond to rest, others to motion, others to unitariness, others to constant number, others to constant size, others to constant shape, regardless of the sense modality that is stimulated.

This is a rather heady theory, to say the least. Is there any evidence for it? Some possible support appears in a study conducted by Thompson, Mayers, Robertson, and Patterson (1970) of cells in the association cortex of cats. The association areas of the cerebral cortex are regions that neither receive primary sensory information nor control motor activity directly. Instead, these areas are believed to play a major role in organizing behavior. In the cat's cortex, Thompson *et al.* located a few multisensory cells that appear to respond to number—that is to say, these cells "count." A "counting cell" will discharge only if the animal is stimulated by a fixed, constant number of external events that occur consecutively. Of 500 brain cells examined, only a small proportion (1%, or 5 cells in all) responded to number: One cell responded to "2," another to "5," two to "6," and one to "7." It mattered not whether the stimulus was delivered to the ear, to the eye, or to the skin. As long as the right number of stimuli was presented, the appropriate cell discharged. Thus when stimuli were presented (at a rate of 1/sec) to a "number 6" cell, the maximal discharge occurred at the appearance of the sixth item in the stimulus sequence.

Do "counting cells" count? Do they mediate the perception of numerousness? As Thompson *et al.* (1970) cautioned, "It remains to be demonstrated that these 'counting' cells function to code number of stimulus events in the organism under conditions of normal behavior [p. 273]." Their caution was well founded, for these results should be interpreted in the light of Blank and Bridger's (1964) finding that young children have great difficulty transferring from one modality to another discriminations of number (number of flashes of light versus number of pulses of sound). Indeed, children 3 to 6 years of age have considerable difficulty discriminating among different numbers of items presented to a single sense modality: For young children, success at discriminating number seems to require the use of language.

In the association cortex, as well as in many other parts of the brain, reside various other multisensory cells besides ones that "count." Neurons that are triggered by stimulation of several senses form only a small fraction of all sensory cells, but nonetheless they are pervasive and readily discovered. The association cortex of the frontal lobe in cats contains precisely demarcated areas that respond to light, sound, and touch. Multisensory activity shows up both in relatively gross electrical potentials (Thompson *et al.*, 1963) and in responses of single nerve cells (Dubner & Rutledge, 1964). There is, however, some question as to whether the neurons respond equally well to all these modalities. According to Thompson *et al.* (1963), the spatial distribution and waveforms of electrical responses evoked in frontal cortex are identical, regardless of the sense organ stimulated; according to Dubner and Rutledge (1964), individual cells in this region do not respond equally well to all, but instead respond primarily to visual stimulation.

What might be the functional significance of multisensory cells in the frontal cortex? As I mentioned earlier in the chapter, squirrel monkeys as well as cats show converging sensory inputs on neurons in the frontal lobes, whereas rhesus monkeys show little such convergence (Albe-Fessard & Besson, 1973; Bignall & Imbert, 1969). Nevertheless, the frontal cortex seems to play an important functional role in cross-modal perception: When the frontal cortex is removed, rhesus monkeys lose their ability to match objects from touch to vision (Petrides & Iversen, 1976).

Can we extrapolate a finding like this to perceptual processing in man? Cortical association areas—of the frontal lobe and elsewhere—have long been implicated in the mediation of complex behavior, particularly, in recent years, in the mediation of cross-modal relations.

Man's capacity to interrelate information gleaned through different sensory channels appears to depend, at least in part, on language. Language helps transfer information from modality to modality and perhaps is largely responsible for the vast superiority that humans display in performing cross-modal tasks.

Geschwind (1965) has argued that cross-modal perception depends significantly on language, and in this function he has implicated the inferior parietal lobe of the dominant cerebral hemisphere (usually the left hemisphere in right-handed people, often the right hemisphere in left-handed people). The inferior parietal gathers visual, auditory, and somatosensory information. Its importance to cross-modal perception was demonstrated by Butters and Brody (1968), who looked at language functioning and cross-modal matching ability in people who had suffered neurological damage, mainly from strokes. Patients with damage to the posterior parietal lobe showed a notable loss in their ability to match tactual to visual stimuli. The degree of deficit exceeded the loss in their ability to make purely visual or purely tactual matches. When the damage to the parietal was severe, these patients found cross-modal matching more difficult than intramodal matching; by contrast, patients with brain damage elsewhere found intramodal tactual matching most difficult of all. Along with their excessive loss in cross-modal matching ability, patients with parietal damage also displayed the most marked aphasia (loss of language).

As the functions of various brain regions become better established, the role of multisensory cells can sometimes be inferred. Consider the superior colliculus and visual cortex. A small proportion of collicular and cortical cells respond to auditory and even tactile, as well as visual, stimulation. What may we surmise about their functional significance?

The superior colliculus is an important subcortical station in the visual railroad. Functionally, it appears to play a role in the control of movements of the head and of the eye. The superficial layers of cells in the colliculus receive visual information. Much of this information is direct, that is, it comes straight from the eyes via the optic nerves. But the deeper collicular layers receive auditory and tactile as well as visual information. Probably most of this information is indirect; it does not come straight from the auditory nerves, for example. Instead, these deeper layers receive auditory inputs by way of the inferior colliculus and the temporal cortex, tactile inputs by way of the spinal cord and the trigeminal nuclei. B. Gordon (1972; Wickelgren, 1971) found cells in the superior colliculus of cats that respond to both auditory and visual stimulation—to pure tones, tonal sweeps, and noises; to light and dark shapes. About 80% of the cells in deep layers that reacted to light also reacted to sound or touch. Furthermore, most of these cells were sensitive to movement in particular directions and had restricted receptive fields; that is, each cell discharged only when the stimulus came from a limited portion of space. Perhaps of greatest significance was the fact that the cells that responded to both sound and light did so when the visual and auditory stimuli came from the same location in space. That is, the bimodal cells had receptive fields that were highly correlated spatially—in a given neuron, the borders of the visual and auditory fields tended to coincide.

B. Gordon (1972) noted that some cells in the cat's colliculus also responded to touching the skin. A similar finding was previously reported by Jassik-Gerschenfeld (1966), who suggested that the superior colliculus may, consequently, play a role in the control of visually guided behavior—in integrating sight, touch, and movement. More recently, Stein, Magalhães-Castro, and Kruger (1975) demonstrated a correspondence between the spatial organization of neighboring visual and tactile cells in the colliculus. Visual cells that responded to stimulation of the retinal center were located above tactile cells that responded to stimulation of the midline of the face. Visual cells that responded to visual stimulation more and more eccentric were located above tactile cells that responded to tactile stimulation correspondingly more eccentric from the midline. This result suggested that "the colliculus may serve as a means of extracting the most salient sensory cues that indicate stimulus location, regardless of the specific modality [Stein *et al.*, 1975, p. 225]."

Cells that respond to sound as well as to light appear in the visual cortex; here too, as with multimodal cells in the superior colliculus, the spatial location of the stimuli is critical. Morrell (1972) and Fishman and Michael (1973) found cells in the striate and parastriate (visual) cortex that could be excited by both light and sound: The receptive fields of these cells were closely aligned visually and acoustically in the horizontal dimension.

These examples provide a few clues to the neural basis of multimodal spatial localization. Neurons in other parts of the brain, in pathways of senses besides the visual, may play a similar role. The inferior colliculus of the midbrain and the medial geniculate nucleus of the thalamus are important centers of the auditory system. Syka and Straschill (1970) made the interesting observation that electrical stimulation of the inferior colliculus of cats (an important station in the auditory system) caused movements both of the eyes and of the pinnae (external ears). The medial geniculate in cats contains cells that react not only to sounds, but also to tactile, thermal, and vestibular stimulation (Love & Scott, 1969; Wepsic, 1966). These cells may serve to "integrate somatic, auditory, and vestibular information pertaining to the localization of sounds of significance to the animal [Aitkin, 1973, p. 282]."

How much can we say—in summary—about the neural substrate underlying the interrelation of information from different senses? We should not be surprised to learn that at present the answer is, not very much. Hints there are, but not nearly enough to build substantive models. Especially worrisome is the need often to extrapolate from results obtained on a variety of nonhuman species, for cross-modal perception is far from equivalent in all animals.

The evidence at hand does imply that the integration of multisensory information begins within the sensory systems themselves. But a good deal of the perceptual elaboration undoubtedly takes place higher up in the stream of processing. Not nearly enough is known to decide whether individual neurons, or even small clusters of neurons, mediate each of Aristotle's common sensible attributes. Indeed, the common sense might consist of a rather diffuse set of neural pathways and connections extending over large portions of the cerebral cortex—and probably over subcortex too. Perhaps, as some (e.g., W. A. Wilson, Jr., 1965) have suggested, subcortical areas legislate the more primitive intersensory functions, whereas higher, which is to say cortical, areas legislate more complex and abstract functions. If so, then the frontal and parietal cortex of the brain might well play a significant role in conceptually integrating the information that comes from different modalities (Butters & Brody, 1968; Geschwind, 1965; Walter, 1964).

Coding Sensory Attributes

Not all sensory attributes convey information about spatial–temporal features of the environment. Though sensory experience arises out of interactions between stimulus events and sensory receptors, the qualities of sensation are themselves determined by the makeup of the organism, not by the qualities of the stimulus. Or at least so states Johannes Müller's (1838) famous "doctrine of specific energies of nerve." Müller's doctrine serves as a physiological counterpart to Locke's doctrine of secondary qualities. Secondary qualities, argued Müller, are determined by properties of the sensorium not by properties of the external stimuli. Sweet and bitter, red and green, high pitch and low pitch are properties of sensation, hence properties of nervous action, not properties of objects.

Sensory qualities of one modality can resemble those of another. From dim whisper to glaring shout, the visual dimension of brightness lines up alongside the auditory dimension of loudness. Such resemblances—similarities in phenomenal appearance—need not reflect any common object in the environment. Brightly illuminated objects can ring out sounds soft or loud, bright or dull. Even pungency to the nose gives no clue whether a liquor will be sharp to the tongue.

What is of concern in the present section is, purely and simply, phenomenological similarity, and specifically, the neural basis of resemblance across the senses. By and large, this boils down to assessing the physiological underpinnings of sensory intensity. The qualities themselves—pitch, hue, touch, taste, and odor quality—resemble each other far too little to justify inquiring, in this work, as to the neural basis to whatever similarity exists. And of brightness's physiological basis in different modalities we know virtually nothing. By way of contrast, studies on the intensity of sensation have held a preeminent place throughout the history of sensory physiology.

Given that every perceptual dimension has a counterpart in a physiological mechanism of some sort, we may ask two questions. First, What is the physiological mechanism that corresponds to or codes a sensory dimension such as intensity? And second, Do all modalities use the same code? Is the brightness of lights, neurophysiologically speaking, like the loudness of sounds?

SENSORY INTENSITY:
THE METAPHORICAL IMPERATIVE

Immanuel Kant (1781) said that quantity or "how much" is an a priori concept of human understanding, a basic factor in the way we "size up" the world. Both phenomenological and experimental evidence suggests that of all sensory dimensions, it is intensity that displays the strongest cross-modal similarity. Many sensory scientists almost take it for granted that the neurophysiological correlate of sensory intensity is frequency of neural discharge. Why this tacit acceptance of the Doctrine of Correspondence? The answer lies, I presume, in scientists' own human penchant for analogy. It seems reasonable to expect of whatever it is in the brain that parallels or underlies sensory experience, that its properties in some ways mimic those of sensation—that processes in the brain do more than just represent sensations and perceptions in a nominal way, do more than just identify them in a form so arbitrary as to demand a detailed codebook to decipher the psychophysiological relations. Properties of brain processes may actually resemble the sensory events: When the perceived strength of a sensation is low, then the level of the neural process will accordingly be weak; when the strength of sensation is great, the level of the neural process will perforce be high.

As I indicated earlier in the chapter, this eminently reasonable thesis is by no means necessary and, conceivably, could be untrue—though I strongly suspect that it is correct. If it is correct, it is a powerful and important principle of psychophysiology. But it is not a necessary principle. The only principle that elementary assumptions demand is the much weaker Principle of Nomination, namely that for every unique psychological state there is a corresponding, unique physiological state or set of states. This unremarkable postulate merely affirms that when percepts differ, neural processes must differ. Nothing in it requires that a systematic change in perception have as its neural counterpart a similar change or even a systematic change.

Despite this disclaimer, it is hard to avoid the stronger Principle of Correspondence—that psychological processes mimic physiological ones. The second of G. E. Müller's (1896) psychophysical axioms, for instance, says that systematic changes in physical states give rise to analogously systematic changes in sensations. Historically, this sort of principle has held sway, both in guiding research and in suggesting interpretations. The strength of its grip attests to the potency that analogy has in thinking, particularly in scientific thinking.

CODING SENSORY INTENSITY

Let me focus on the main point, which is the notion that the strength of sensory experience has some neural counterpart that resembles it. This notion itself has had a long history, tracing back to preexperimental speculation. It appears, for example, in the work of David Hartley (1749), the eighteenth-century physician and psychologist who is best known as an exponent of associationism, the doctrine that attempts to explain mental activity in terms of sequences of associated ideas. Hartley's opinion influenced not only psychologists of his own day and later, but also the poets Coleridge and Wordsworth. Hartley proposed that sensations arise out of physical motions in the environment that are transmitted to nerves. From his statement that the neural vibrations vary in vigor with the strength of the stimulus, we may infer the premise that the amplitude of "neural vibration" is the counterpart to the strength of sensation. As a matter of fact, these sensory vibrations, once aroused, leave lingering remnants, which he termed "vibratiuncles"; and the remnants, according to Hartley, constitute ideas or images.

Only in the mid-nineteenth century did physiology establish the electrical nature of nerve action. For several decades thereafter, a prevailing pair of opinions held by sensory scientists were (a) that the electrical discharge in a sensory nerve can vary in magnitude, and (b) that accordingly, the magnitude of a sensory experience relates directly to the magnitude of the neural discharge. These opinions dissolved, or at least transmuted, when it was demonstrated that individual sensory nerve cells fire in all all-or-none fashion: The discharge of a nerve cell is not graded; when a neuron does fire, the size of its electrical impulse is always the same (Adrian, 1914). So the all-or-none law says that the discharge must be constant in size. But it need not be constant in rate. Forbes and Gregg (1915) proposed, and Adrian (1926) later confirmed, the frequency theory: As stimulus intensity increases, so too increases the number of neural impulses generated in a given interval of time. An intense stimulus may not be able to produce bigger neural impulses, but it can produce more of them.

The general notion that sensation intensity somehow resembles the level of neural activity gained credence in the nineteenth century when physiologists noted that neural activity tends to increase in a nonlinear fashion with increasing intensity of the stimulus. The relation between magnitude of neural electric responses and magnitude of stimulation appeared to be roughly logarithmic (e.g., Waller, 1895), in that a given multiplicative increase in the stimulus produces, roughly, a constant arithmetic increase in neural response. This is (perhaps) as it should be if Fechner's (1860) hypothesis concerning stimulus and sensation were correct. Many examples of sensory activity, recorded from peripheral nerves and from nerve cells in the central nervous system, seem at least roughly in accord with a logarithmic formulation. At the same time it is doubtless true, as Rosner and Goff (1967) noted, that scientists reported logarithmic functions at least partly because scientists sought them. In recent years, evidence has mounted to accord with the view that some neural responses are at least equally consistent with a power function (S. S. Stevens, 1970), (again perhaps) as they should be if S. S. Stevens's (1957) generalization is correct: With a power function, a given ratio increase in the stimulus leads to a ratio increase in the neural response. Sometimes, the very same neural measurements find themselves supporting one claim or another. A well-known example comes from Adrian and Matthews's (1927) study of optic nerve fibers in the eel: Adrian and Matthews concluded that the frequency of neural impulses grew as the logarithm of light intensity, whereas S. S. Stevens (1970) concluded, from the same data, that the impulse rate grew as a power function of intensity.

As I indicated, these two alternative neurophysical laws have counterparts in two psychophysical proposals—in Fechner's hypothesis that equal stimulus ratios produce equal sensation increments and in S. S. Stevens's hypothesis that equal stimulus ratios produce equal sensation ratios. But in either case, to jump directly from a psychophysical law to a mathematically similar neurophysical law is to assume that mental magnitude and neural magnitude are related to each other simply and proportionately. Interestingly, Fechner (1860) did not think so: He believed that the logarithmic transformation takes place not in the way the physical stimulus converts to nerve response, but instead in the way the neural converts to the psychological. Fechner rejected the notion that there is a perfect isomorphism between mind and body (see Woodward, 1972). Contemporary scientists tend to eschew Fechner's approach, and often expend a good deal of energy trying to find the "right neurons," that is, the neurons whose neurophysical function corresponds mathematically to the analogous psychophysical function.

Neurophysical functions do not always agree with psychophysical functions. This troubles some people. How, then, do sensations get to match up with neural responses? MacKay (1963) suggested a possible way to reconcile Stevens's power law of sensation with a logarithmic law for sensory receptors. According to MacKay's theory, perception involves the activity of an internal mechanism, which generates a response that is matched to incoming sensory information. If the stimulus is a light, for instance, the mechanism generates a train of neural impulses whose rate matches the rate of impulses coming from the visual system. Brightness as a sensory magnitude corresponds to the "effort" that the internal mechanism expends in producing the matching signal. This effort is related to the frequency of neural impulses generated, but is not necessarily proportional to it. If the rate of impulses varies logarithmically with the effort, then MacKay's model will accommodate both a neurophysical logarithmic function and a psychophysical power function. In the final analysis, MacKay's theory proposes the matching operation and its mathematical properties purely in order to make sensation fall directly porportional to some physicochemical activity of the nervous system.

But is this necessary? One alternative is to escape the Principle of Correspondence's iron fist and reject complete isomorphism. Another is to seek neurophysical and psychophysical functions that do agree.

If the goal is to correlate perception with processes in those neurons that "give" perception, then the most immediate concern should not be activity in peripheral nerves, but, presumably, activity somewhere in the brain. A possible somewhere is the primary sensory cortex. With the advent of devices capable of recording small electrical potentials on the scalp, research has extended so as to make it possible to try to correlate the intensity of a stimulus presented to the sense receptor with the size of the electrical potential transmitted through the skull from the cerebral cortex. Again, however, the relation between stimulus intensity and neural response is ambiguous, to say the least. Some data suggest a logarithmic formulation, some a power formulation. Rosner and Goff (1967) surveyed much of the literature, and they and H. Davis (1974), among others, have cautioned against concluding too readily that an evoked potential reflects in any simple and direct manner the subjective intensity of sensation. Although evoked potentials, like sensations, often appear to follow a rule of constant ratios, quantitative agreement between physiological and psychological measures has not generally been good. Take as an example the typical psychophysical function that relates the loudness of a pure tone to its acoustical intensity. Under many conditions, when sound energy increases about tenfold, loudness doubles. What happens to the size of the electrical potential measured at the scalp? When sound energy increases tenfold, the auditory evoked potential may not quite double, but instead may increase by only an additional one-half or one-fourth. That is, evoked potentials often follow a power law, but not the same power law that governs sensation (H. Davis, Bowers, & Hirsh, 1967). Other times, evoked potentials appear to obey not a power law, but a logarithmic law.

The senses transmit information along several paths. Most or all senses send information both through modality-specific systems to primary receiving areas of the cortex and also through a diffuse system to widely distributed areas in the cortex. H. Davis, Osterhammel, Wier, and Gjerdingen (1972) discovered cross-modal interactions in electrical potentials (recorded at the scalp) evoked by light, sound, touch, and shock. Mechanical and electrical stimulation of the skin excite the same primary projection area. Thus the particular combination of touch and shock might be expected to yield greater interactions than, say, touch and light or shock and sound. It did not: All cross-modal combinations of stimuli produced interactions of about the same size. This outcome suggested that the evoked potentials may be mediated not by specific projections, but instead by a diffuse, nonspecific system. H. Davis (1974) concluded that at least some evoked potentials arise from a pathway in the sensory system that differs from the pathway where sensory magnitude is determined. To a good extent, evoked potentials seem to reflect processes of selective attention and discrimination (see, for example, Ford, Roth, Dirks, & Kopell, 1973; Galambos, 1974).

STAGES IN PROCESSING INTENSITY

In this section, I will assume that the processes mediating the intensity of sensory experience are themselves intensity-like. Do the same sorts of processes appear in different modalities?

A general scheme for coding sensory intensity appears in Figure 5.2. First, there must be some process at the sensory receptor by which stimulus energy is transduced into an electrical potential. The term *transduction* identifies a process whereby energy is converted from one form to another—as a microphone transduces sound into electricity. The relation between the intensity of the stimulus (stimulus energy) and the amplitude of receptor potential is usually curvilinear, as shown by the prototype in Figure 5.3. Lipetz (1971) has pointed out how quantitatively similar this relation appears to be from one sense to another, and he has presented a model that may be capable of describing the primary receptor process that underlies the relation in many sense departments.

After the receptor transduces stimulus to electrical potential, the continuously varying electrical potentials are converted to discrete, all-or-none neural impulses. The available evidence suggests that this second process is linear, in that the frequency of neural impulses is proportional to the amplitude of the receptor potential. As Lipetz (1971) and Fuortes (1971) have noted, if this conversion process is linear, then the mathematical form of the function relating stimulus intensity to neural firing rate must be the same as the form of the function relating stimulus intensity to magnitude of the receptor potential.

Finally, if all of the subsequent links in the neural chain behave linearly—that is, if the transmission across synapses, from neuron to

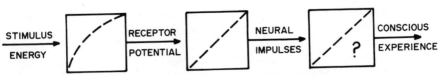

Figure 5.2. A scheme for the coding of sensory intensity. Transduction processes at the receptors convert stimulus energy to graded electrical activity, according to a nonlinear function. The receptor potentials translate linearly into frequency of neural impulses, and this frequency is transmitted, sometimes linearly, sometimes nonlinearly, to more central sites in the nervous system.

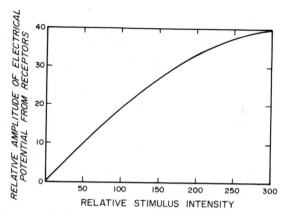

Figure 5.3. The relation between stimulus intensity φ and the magnitude of the electrical potential recorded from receptors. The curve is drawn according to the formula $R = a\varphi/(b + \varphi)$, where R is receptor potential and φ is stimulus intensity.

neuron, does not change the *relative* frequency of neural discharges—then the mathematical function that describes receptor potential and firing rate will continue to operate throughout the sensory system. Add to this the Principle of Correspondence and it follows that the same equation will also describe the psychophysical function relating sensation to stimulus. G. Werner and Mountcastle (1965) and Harrington and Merzenich (1970) argued this to be the case for the somesthetic (touch) system; they reported that the neurophysical power function obtained from first-order, tactile neurons in cats and monkeys is the same as the psychophysical power function obtained from magnitude estimates of touch intensity in humans. And S. S. Stevens (1970) suggested that linear transmission may apply to several modalities.

If a three-stage system like the one just sketched adequately described the way all senses operate, it would help to tie together a large number of facts. First, it would provide a sensible basis for the phenomenal, cross-modal equivalence of sensory intensity. Qualitatively different sensations can be alike with regard to their apparent intensity "because" psychological intensity depends on a single, common physiological principle. Second, the scheme would "explain" why numerous psychophysical principles are common to many senses: (*a*) The primary receptor process often would parallel the psychophysical function—that is, the neurophysical function that relates receptor activity to stimulus intensity would be analogous to the psychophysical function that relates sensory magnitude to stimulus intensity. The elemental power transformations would take place, as indicated, at the sense receptors;

and (*b*) Because intensity relies on a similar code in different modalities, the discrimination of intensity often would follow similar rules. For instance, G. Werner and Mountcastle (1965) claimed that one can treat a constant *increment* in neural firing as the analogue to a just-noticeable-difference (JND) in sense perception: The neurophysiological discriminability function they derived from data on single mechanorecep-tive fibers was very much like the discriminability function derived from human psychophysical data. The same assumption—that percep-tual discriminability is constant whenever there is a constant increment in the magnitude of some underlying physiological quantity—also ap-pears in several models of sensory function (for example, in a model for discrimination of visual stimuli proposed by Matin, 1968).

It is noteworthy, however, that at least one general theory of inten-sity discrimination asserts that a JND consists of a constant *proportional* change in sensation magnitude (R. Teghtsoonian, 1971). This rule fol-lows from combining Weber's law with Stevens's law. If, moreover, neural activity is proportional to sensation magnitude, then, according to this theory, the physiological underpinning of a JND must be a constant *percentage* change in neural activity, not a constant increment.

Cross-modal correlations between neurophysiology and sensation might also apply to other psychophysical events and processes, such as adaptation and inhibition. Several models postulate recurrent feedback as a mechanism of visual light adaptation (Matin, 1968; Rushton, 1965; Sperling & Sondhi, 1968). Appropriate physiological circuits can be found in the visual system (Dowling, 1967), and, interestingly, similar circuits are found in other senses, such as olfaction (Reese & Brightman, 1970). Figure 5.4 depicts schematically how a feedback circuit can ac-count for a decrease in sensory magnitude over time, that is, for sensory

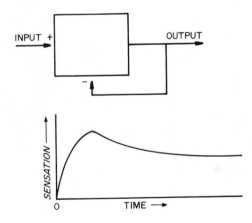

Figure 5.4. A model of feedback that can help explain sensory adap-tation. Part of the output from some stage in sensory processing feeds back on itself to exert an inhibitory effect on that stage. When the ex-citatory and inhibitory effects stabilize, the sensation is at a steady state.

adaptation. Stimulation first produces a positive, excitatory effect on the sense organ—but as time goes on the excitation begins to feed back on itself in a negative, inhibitory fashion, thereby reducing the size of the excitatory effect. After sufficient time elapses, excitation and inhibition come to balance each other, and the sensation attains a steady level.

If this model is correct, adaptation exemplifies what may be called self-inhibition. Inhibitory processes similar to the one just described do seem involved in certain other perceptual interactions, for instance, in brightness contrast. Békésy (1967b) suggested that lateral inhibitory mechanisms might underlie the phenomenological observations of sensory inhibition in many sense departments.

The prototype of sensory inhibition is spatial brightness contrast, where stimulation of one part of the visual field depresses brightness in another part. Lateral inhibitory interactions are now relatively well understood, thanks to the intensive research that goes back to the classical studies by Hartline (1949; Ratliff & Hartline, 1959) of neural impulses in optic nerve fibers of the horseshoe crab, *Limulus*. Excitation of any one fiber leads to depression in the responses from nearby fibers. "Cross-talk" among neural elements likely provides one component to brightness contrast. Whether or to what extent functionally similar neural processes take place in other senses remains to be clarified. There is some evidence for spatial inhibitory mechanisms, similar to those of vision, in the somesthetic system (Carreras & Andersson, 1963; G. Gordon & Manson, 1967).

Unfortunately, the scheme just outlined will most surely fail to be universally satisfactory in detail. For one thing, despite encouraging results like those of Borg, Diamant, Ström, and Zotterman (1967)—which showed that numerical estimates of taste magnitude were linearly related to neural activity recorded in the human chorda-tympani nerve—there has been only limited evidence that receptor processes account for all of the nonlinear transformations between stimulus and sensation. Additional nonlinearities, based on processes that come into play more centrally in the nervous system, may well occur, as Lipetz (1971), for one, has considered.

Let us take the example of neural coding of visual brightness. Visual information is kneaded through a sequence of transformations in the retina, from the receptors through bipolar cells to ganglion cells, apparently with the assistance of "cross-talk" and feedback via horizontal cells and amacrine cells. The power transformation from stimulus energy to sensation intensity can be modeled by a series of stages whose input–output characteristics become nonlinear through feedback (Marks, 1972). Mansfield (1974) proposed that fundamental information about brightness is coded at the level of ganglion cells (the final stage of processing in the retina), and that optic nerve fibers relay this information linearly to more central stations in the brain. Nevertheless, it is worth noting that a lot of processing has taken place by the time information reaches the ganglion cells; it takes several neural stages in the retina to establish the final form of the neurophysical function.

Sometimes it is possible to deduce properties of neural coding from psychophysical experiments. For example, it is well known that the afferent neural messages for touch, temperature, and pain in the skin of the face are carried by the two trigeminal (fifth cranial) nerves. Each nerve carries signals from one side of the face only. So, if like-sized patches of skin on the two sides of the face are, for instance, heated equally, the stimuli will trigger two equivalent sets of nerve impulses, one set carried by each cranial nerve. Psychophysical evidence on the perception of warmth demonstrates that these two sets of signals interact in a nonlinear way, much as they do when the heat stimuli trigger both sets in a single nerve (Marks & Stevens, 1973). Because the two cranial nerves merge only when they reach the brain, some of the warmth sense's nonlinear transformation presumably takes place in the central nervous system.

Special mention should be made of the way sensory magnitude is coded in the auditory system. When an auditory stimulus increases in intensity, perhaps as important as the concomitant increase in the frequency of neural discharge is the increase in the number of neurons activated (Galambos & Davis, 1943). S. S. Stevens and Davis (1936) and H. Davis (1961) argued that what counts in determining loudness is the number of active nerve fibers, not the average rate in all of the active fibers. A similar conclusion was reached by Whitfield (1967). Recently, Goldstein (1974) sought to demonstrate that loudness parallels the activity in fibers of the auditory nerve. To do this, he had to postulate an increase in the number of active fibers as stimulus intensity increases.

Is it possible to salvage the hypothesis that loudness is coded simply by rate of discharge within individual neurons? Perhaps only a certain number, a relatively small number, of fibers code loudness; if so, then different fibers may code different portions of the subjective range. A few fibers could code soft sounds, others medium sounds, still others loud sounds. Brugge and Merzenich (1973) examined the properties of neurons in the auditory cortex of macaque monkeys. One of their most intriguing findings was that different neurons responded maximally to different ranges of sound intensity; some responded best to low, others to moderate, others to high intensities. We might want to entertain the hypothesis that a small subset of auditory neurons code loudness. A similar hypothesis—stating that some fibers are specialized to signal sensory intensity—also appears reasonable in the somesthetic system (Harrington & Merzenich, 1970).

The same hypothesis may help to explain the frequent finding, already mentioned, that gross measures of neural activity (such as electrical potentials recorded at the scalp) often fail to follow along with sensation intensity; for if only a portion of the activated neurons are actually coding intensity, then the overall level of neural activity will tap not only intensity, but the pool of neural responses to a variety of sensory characteristics. This interpretation is attractive. Much processing of auditory information takes place in the peripheral part of the system. The auditory system—like the visual system—mediates many perceptual functions (think of pitch and timbre patterns in music, of phonetic structure and voice quality in speech); and, because it does, loudness, the perceived intensity of sounds, makes up only a small part of auditory information. Auditory neurons do not just take sound energies at various frequencies and turn them into loudnesses at various pitches, just as visual neurons do not just take light energies at various points in space and turn them into an array of brightnesses. Unlike some sense departments, such as temperature and taste, the so-called higher senses—hearing and vision—select and organize spatial and temporal information.

The senses order themselves in a distinct hierarchy—at the bottom huddle the thermal senses, sending a few bits of information about intensity, a couple about temporal characteristics, even fewer about spatial ones; at the top perch hearing and vision, providing virtually all of the ingredients that go into higher cognitive processes. Is it not likely that most neurons in the temperature senses serve up information about intensity, whereas only a relatively few neurons in the higher senses do? Concomitantly, perhaps the code for intensity itself changes—from an analogue system using frequency of nerve impulses in the lower senses to a more efficient digital system using range-sensitive neurons in the higher senses. This possibility leads to an even more basic question: How, neurophysiologically speaking, is it that sensory intensity is appreciated as an attribute common to all modes of sensation? If all modalities use the same code, a simple solution recommends itself: The common sense looks at the frequency of neural impulses, regardless of modality. If, however, some modalities employ highly selective neurons that are specialized to interpret intensity, the solution could be more complicated: The common sense might first have to translate the babel of different senses into a universal language.

Perhaps some common neural centers assist in the appreciation of sensory magnitudes in all modalities, even while other, specific centers rule individual sense departments. Rosner and Goff (1967) concluded that both specific and nonspecific neural pathways mediate the perceived intensity of somesthetic sensations: "If nonspecific responses play such a crucial role in perception of intensity in all modalities, the neurophysiological basis for cross-modality intensity matching becomes a bit clearer. Different modalities feed information into the diffuse systems, which then can organize and compare data arriving over different channels [p. 214]."

WHERE MIND AND BRAIN MEET

What matters most to the search for neural correlates? As I mentioned earlier, it is not the initial, peripheral processes, nor any of the succeeding stages through the penultimate. What matters most is that final, still largely hypothetical, stage where mind faces brain.

Fechner, I think it significant to point out, held a monistic view of the universe. To Fechner, the mental and the physical were two aspects of one reality. Thus to say that Fechner believed there is a nonlinear process of conversion at the interface between mind and brain is to say no more than that he believed a nonlinear function intervenes between two aspects of the same process (see Woodward, 1972). One need not even consider the transformation to be a conversion from one kind of "stuff" to another. What matters first and foremost is the idea of a functional relationship between two quantifiables.

At the heart of the issue of correspondence between brain and sensation is the question of how to measure perceptual quantities themselves. In order to ask whether changes in the brain parallel, in a quantitative way, changes in sensation, one must be able to measure both the neurophysiological and the perceptual changes. In order to ask whether a sensation doubles its strength every time some neural process doubles its strength, one must be able to say when sensation doubles. Rules for measuring physical quantities are well established, while rules for measuring mental quantities have eluded general acceptance. Thus the more basic question is, Can sensory magnitudes be measured unequivocally?

In the last chapter, I argued that procedures whereby people try to tag numbers onto the magnitudes of their sensory experiences often come very close to yielding valid measures of sensation. The argument rests partly on finding instances where the magnitude of a sensory experience that is compounded of two or more parts can be described as the linear sum of the magnitudes of the components (Marks, 1978).

When pure tones are introduced to the two ears, the overall loudness (as assessed by the method of magnitude estimation) equals the loudness of the component in the left ear plus the loudness of the component in the right ear. Underlying this outcome, I would hypothesize, is the following process: Stimulation of each ear produces a loudness that relates nonlinearly to the level of stimulus energy that impinges on that ear—and farther downstream, in the brain, the signals from the two ears combine in simple proportion. If one were to seek a physiological correlate to binaural loudness summation, one would look for nerve cells whose inputs come from both ears and whose overall response to binaural inputs equals the linear sum of the responses to left- and right-ear inputs. A schematic follows.

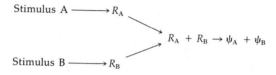

$$\text{Stimulus A} \longrightarrow R_A$$
$$R_A + R_B \rightarrow \psi_A + \psi_B$$
$$\text{Stimulus B} \longrightarrow R_B$$

At the left, Stimulus A and Stimulus B are the physical stimuli impressed on the two ears. Each stimulus undergoes some transformation in the nervous system, yielding physiological responses R_A and R_B. Ultimately, these responses converge to produce a unified sensory event. The property of linear addition of sensations means that if Stimulus A is presented alone (B = 0), the sensation has a magnitude ψ_A; if Stimulus B is presented alone (A = 0), the sensation has a magnitude ψ_B. If both are presented together, the total sensation has a magnitude $\psi_A + \psi_B$. Because the psychological addition is linear, it should be possible to find the neural correlate to sensation magnitude —some physiological response to Stimulus A + B that equals the simple sum of the responses to A and to B alone.

Does this mean that Fechner must have been wrong, that no nonlinear transformation can possibly intervene between brain and mind, that the Principle of Correspondence must apply with full, unshackled vigor to the mental and physiological aspects of at least this one dimension of sensation? Perhaps, but to see whether it must, it helps to try to construct a scenario where the Principle of Correspondence fails. What I show next is one way that the neural state underlying sensation need not follow the analogous psychological rule: If Stimulus A yields state R_A, and Stimulus B yields R_B, Stimulus A + Stimulus B need not yield $R_A + R_B$. Following this, I will show how to retrieve the Principle of Correspondence.

I shall work within the model of summation just described. And though the model described is one of summation between the two ears, keep in mind that the same reasoning can apply to a variety of other paradigms where sensory channels combine their effects linearly (and, by extrapolation, to paradigms that do not even use additivity as a criterion).

First, let Stimulus A produce a particular sensation with a magnitude defined as unity ($\psi_A = 1$). Next, let Stimulus B produce a sensation equal to that of A, hence also unity ($\psi_B = 1 = \psi_A$). Simultaneous stimulation of both ears (A + B) gives a sensation with a magnitude equal to $\psi_A + \psi_B = 2$. Now, it is a straightforward matter to find a new stimulus to the left ear alone, A*, whose sensation has a loudness that matches the loudness of the binaural A + B. Stimulus A*, then, gives a sensation with loudness of 2. For most sound frequencies, the physical intensity of A* turns out to be about 8 to 10 times the physical intensity of A or B, as it should if an eightfold to tenfold increase in physical intensity gives a doubling of loudness.

What happens in the corresponding physiological state? Stimulus A yields response R_A, whose magnitude presumably equals that of R_B produced by Stimulus B. Define each of these neural magnitudes as unity ($R_A = R_B = 1$). The central question is, What is the neural response to the compound Stimulus A + B? Does $R_{A+B} = R_A + R_B = 2$? If it does, then neural and perceptual responses are fully proportional to one another, contra Fechner.

R_{A+B} need not equal 2. It could equal some other value perfectly well. What it must equal, though, is the value that is produced by Stimulus A*. This may be deduced from the reflexive form of the Principle of Nomination: Sensory events that are equal psychologically are equal physiologically. R_{A+B} and $R_A{}^*$ need not equal 2; they could equal 1.5, or 3, or 100. Invariant psychological states demand invariant physical states. So $R_A{}^*$ must equal R_{A+B} if $\psi_A{}^*$ equals ψ_{A+B}. But the magnitude of the physiological response $R_A{}^*$ or R_{A+B} need not take on a value exactly twice that of R_A or R_B.

What we seem to have at this point, then, is the possibility that Fechner's claim is correct. Nonlinearity may intervene between body and mind. A myriad of functional relationships could possibly bridge the gap between the physiological and psychological sides of sensation. Within each domain, the crucial invariances hold fast, but the mapping from one to the other—so it would seem—need not progress in a direct, proportional manner. Psychological magnitudes could equal the square or square root, the cube or the cube root, of physiological magnitudes, indeed could equal any of an infinite number of continuous, single-valued mathematical functions.

Or can they? Perhaps I should say, Or need they? The final turn of the river takes us full circle in its run, back to the issue of quantifying the psychological side of sensation, of measuring sensory experience. What does it mean to say that a nonlinear formula translates brain process to sensory experience? Does this very fact not imply that the gap between physiological and mental is bridged through a simple mathematical conversion, a transformation from one scale of numbers to another? And what is this bridge, except a renaming of the values in an appropriate fashion, so that the invariances are retained but the two scales line up anew, in a manner that makes the physical and mental scales proportional? [3]

I can put this another way. It is not necessary to say that a nonlinear relationship between brain and sensation describes a change from physical to mental "stuff," or even that it describes a change of "viewpoint." Why not, instead, incorporate the function into the realm of one of the states, namely the psychological? What this boils down to is redefining the numbers on the sensory scale so that all of the equalities remain, but the quantitative properties now fall in line with the numbers derived from the physiological responses. Unless some absolute criterion can be established so that once mental magnitudes are defined nonlinear transformations are forbidden, it will always be possible, within the constraint set by invariances, to submit to the imperative set by the Principle of Correspondence and bring the mental and physiological magnitudes into simple register.

[3] I owe much of this argument to discussions with Barry G. Green.

6

The Unity of the Senses

"It appears," wrote Suzanne Langer, "that light, smoothness and especially movement are the natural symbols of life, freedom and joy, as darkness and immobility, roughness and hardness are the symbols of death and frustration [1967, p. 193]." Sensations from different modalities, she concluded, at once are charged with resemblance when they arouse a common feeling, and, through resemblance, symbolize the feeling. By means of the language of resemblance, sensory qualities speak to one another and, as it were, talk over their common feeling; and by the same language of resemblance, their voices carry beyond the sensory realm, invading qualities that are not primarily sensorial, again to share, in metaphor, a common feeling. To give one of Langer's examples, the word "light" extends from the "light of the sun" to the "light of reason." Such metaphors, like some translations across sensory modalities, rely on common feeling–tones, and thus share parentage with intersensory analogies. And, as I have argued through the last four chapters, intersensory analogies come in large part through an intrinsic unity of the senses.

Evolution and Development

The unity of the senses reveals itself in a variety of ways: in sensory processes, where the psychophysical behavior of different senses shows marked similarities; in perceptual processes, where different senses provide common information about the world and where characteristics of sensory experience resemble one another; and in cognitive processes, where verbal metaphors describe or suggest similarities among sensory phenomena. In these many forms, the unity of the senses reflects fundamental facts of phylogenetic and ontogenetic development. All of the senses, it is commonly believed, trace their evolutionary history back to a single primitive sense, a simple undifferentiated responsiveness to external stimulation. It is not difficult to imagine some early form of life, a relatively simple agglutination of cells that wriggled or withdrew when bombarded with virtually any sharp stimulus, whether mechanical, radiant, or chemical. Indeed, even today most cells seem to be responsive to light energy, which acts to regulate or modulate biological processes such as cellular metabolism. The evolution of a visual system out of an undifferentiated sensitivity took one of its most important early steps with the development of special light-sensitive pigments.

Over the ages, the primitive, unitary sense differentiated into the various modalities—into photosensitive organs of vision, mechanosensitive organs of touch and hearing, chemosensitive organs of taste and smell. To some extent, ontogeny captures this differentiation, as the sensory systems of embryos elaborate themselves from ectodermal tissue. It perhaps should not be too surprising to find that different sensory systems, when fully developed, use similar mechanisms, for the senses are, after all, constructed of similar neural tissue. Receptors differ, to be sure, because peripheral organs are specialized for transducing different types of stimulus energies into neural activity; but farther downstream—in the central nervous system—there is little in the microstructure of neural tissue to distinguish one sensory pathway from another. A neuron is a neuron.

The senses of hearing and of vision, it has been hypothesized, both evolved from an earlier touch sense. That there is presently a close kinship between hearing and the modern touch sense is clear. Both modalities are excited by mechanical energy, that is, by changes in patterns of pressure at the receptors, and both show phenomenological as well as psychophysical similarities. One theory of the auditory system's evolution projects its ancestry back through lateral-line organs of fish. On either side of a fish's body, starting near each eye, runs a longitudinal groove—the lateral line—in which are embedded sensory cells that respond to mechanical stimulation, especially low-frequency vibration. Lateral-line organs may provide a link between the most primitive system of touch and the advanced system of hearing. In primitive touch, sensitivity to mechanical stimulation, it may be presumed, used to provide primeval fish with information about movements of objects and fluid at the site of stimulation, that is, at the skin surface; in the advanced system of hearing, sensitivity to mechanical stimulation provides modern vertebrates with information about movements of objects some distance away from the sense organs (but see van Bergeijk, 1967).

It is not difficult to picture an auditory system evolving out of primitive tactile or lateral-line organs. Less obvious is the possibility that vision too may have evolved directly from touch. Yet just such a phylogenetic history was suggested by Gregory (1967), who proposed that the earliest visual system—the first eyes—emerged out of a tactile system, then developed independently as a means to process information about objects at a distance. Gregory's scheme rests firmly on his acceptance of the Berkelian hypothesis—the hypothesis that each of us develops visual perception early in life through feedback from touch and movement, that is, by dint of correlations between visual experience and touch stimulation:

> What is true for development of perception in the individual should also be essentially true for the development of vision in evolution, for touch must have preceded vision if touch information is required to make retinal images effective signals of the non-optical world of objects [Gregory, 1967, p. 372].

The big "if" is, of course, "if touch teaches vision," a questionable "if" to say the least (see Chapter 2, pp. 30–31).

The senses' common phylogenetic heritage pervades the world of sensory quality. Heinz Werner (1934) attributed both mutual interactions among sensory processes and the synesthetic unity of sensory attributes to mechanisms that linger on as remnants of the senses' common heritage. The way children, especially, perceive the world recaptures part of the way that the single, primordial sense functioned in the distant past. As evidence to support the notion that sensory unity has a primitive basis, H. Werner (1940) pointed out three conditions where synesthesia often appears—in childhood, in the language and thought of so-called "primitive" peoples, and in the behavior of individuals who have suffered brain damage. Analogies among attributes in sensation, and in particular the blossoming of these analogies in synesthesia, express the organism's primary, undifferentiated responsiveness to sensory stimuli, a response of the *whole* organism to activation of receptor systems:

> The senses' intimate bond—the existence of intersensory qualities like brightness, intensity, roughness, etc.—all of this is based on the fact that the psycho-physical organism reacts as a whole [H. Werner, 1934, p. 202].

The crux of Werner's theory is that the primordial unity of the senses involves the entire organism. Synesthesia, according to this view, is not just a sensory phenomenon, but an organismic one. An outgrowth of this viewpoint, and—as seen in retrospect—a natural outgrowth at that, was the empirical research that Werner and his colleagues conducted under the formulation of their sensori-tonic theory of perception (H. Werner & Wapner, 1949). This theory states that sensory stimulation—stimulation of any and all sense modalities—produces undifferentiated, tonic muscular responses, whose effects, in turn, can be readily measured in the way a person perceives the orientation of his body relative to objects and the position of objects relative to his body. For example, a person sits in a dark room, views a luminescent rod, and at the same time listens to a loud tone played through earphones. When the loudness at one ear is greater than that at the other, the person perceives the rod's orientation to shift (Chandler, 1961). Asymmetrical electrical stimulation of muscles in the sides of the neck produces a similar shift in perceived orientation (Wapner, Werner, & Chandler, 1951). There is, then, a *functional equivalence* to shock, visual tilt, and sound, at least with respect to certain perceptual events. This interrelation among the senses involves the whole body, not just the sensory systems alone.

Out of the primordial unity of the senses come a few of the ingredients that go into the expression of dynamic properties—of physiognomic properties, to use H. Werner's (1940) term. A thundercloud appears threatening, a skylark's song sounds joyful, a drawing of pointed lines looks hard, silvery, and cold. William Butler Yeats (1924) apprehended this evocative nature in sensory equivalence:

> All sounds, all colours, all forms, either because of their preordained energies or because of long association, evoke indefinable and yet precise emotions, or, as I prefer to think, call down among us certain disembodied powers, whose footsteps over our hearts we call emotions; and when sound, and colour, and form are in a musical relation, a beautiful relation to one another, they become as it were one sound, one colour, one form, and evoke an emotion that is made out of their distinct evocations and yet is one emotion [pp. 192–193].

Emotions can involve the entire organism, including essential patterns of muscular activity. When people are asked to express an emotion, such as love, grief, or anger, by pressing one finger on a key, they exert regular, reliable patterns of pressure that characterize the particular emotion beckoned (Clynes, 1973).

Holistic and synesthetic properties may characterize the first wave of a sense's response, but only the first. Specific, modal properties follow on their heels. The various senses are, after all, different and differentiated; each end organ is specialized both in molar and molecular structure to receive and transduce its own form of energy, whether chemical, electromagnetic, or mechanical. The senses should be viewed as biological systems, as adaptations to the requirements for survival and productivity in the world, and once they are viewed in this way, it becomes apparent how their diversity itself enhances the organism's ability to cope, how it provides the potential to signal and inform the organism about a wide scope of environmental activities. Though they probably descended from a single, primitive organ, the several senses diverged enough to stake out their individual claims. The purview of every sense is limited, in that each demands a particular kind of energy (light for vision, sound for hearing, chemicals for smell and taste) and each focuses on a particular kind of information (vision on arrays of objects in space, and changes in these arrays over time; hearing on sequences of events in time). The domain of each sense is limited, but not wholly distinct: Sensory domains overlap, for the world about which the senses inform us is, in itself, a unitary one, and so usually is our conception of it.

At the level of perception, the five or seven or however many external senses serve admirably to hold together our knowledge of the world. We do not apprehend the world as a grab-bag of different entities—we do not see one world of sight, hear another of sounds, taste or smell another or yet another. Instead, we know one world, a world of sunsets and trees and baseball games, of ice cream cones and thunderstorms and brushing teeth, all of which make themselves known to us through the instruments of sight and sound and touch and taste and smell. Imperfect instruments, to be sure, not always trustworthy or completely informative, and, indeed, not always in perfect harmony with each other, yet, nevertheless, what an admirable job they do!

Perceptual processes provide the bricks and mortar from which we construct our conceptual representations of the world. Sense perception gives meanings, meanings that are organized, recorded, remembered. As Arnheim (1969) has eloquently argued, perception captures the essence of cognitive acts. And inextricably tied to human perception we typically find language. The unity of the senses operates here too, and we should not be surprised to find it. Thin indeed are the partitions between sense and thought.

On Similarity

To say that the senses are unified because of their functional equivalence—whether this is an equivalence of information about objects and events, an equivalence of sensory attributes, or an equivalence of organismic, sensori-tonic states—is first and foremost to aver that the effects of sensory stimulation have something in common, that sensory and perceptual responses in different modalities share some elements or features, some characteristics or relationships. This elementary property of sharing, where activities that are not identical overlap in some way and to some degree, is *similarity*. Similarities arise at many psychological levels: from relatively simple perceptual processes involved in recognizing a sensory likeness, like that between middle and high C on a piano or between turquoise and aqua colors; to much more complex cognitive processes involved in constructing a scientific model, like that between the brain and a computer; or a literary metaphor, like that between aging, with its intimations of approaching death, and winter's "boughs which shake against the cold, / Bare ruined choirs."[1]

The concept of similarity has had a long and eminent history in psychology, for the principle that ideas link one to another by their similarity has been a staunch bulwark of theories of associative processes ever since Aristotle postulated that memory operates, in part, though association of similar ideas. Many, though by no means all, of the subsequent proponents of associationism set the principle of similarity high on their list of fundamental processes. David Hume, John Stuart Mill, and Alexander Bain did, though David Hartley and James Mill did not. To simplify grossly the general doctrine of associationism, I will sum up as follows: Complex thought and behavior are the products of two components—the current perceptual input plus the *mélange* of remembered associations, which are traces of items previously connected to identical or similar input. Put another way, our present perceptions and thoughts bring to mind past perceptions and thoughts that previously were associated either with the same perceptions and thoughts or with *similar* ones. When psychology became behavioristic and less introspective, the principle of similarity found itself wrapped in a new terminological cloak. The appropriate descriptive expression became *stimulus generalization*, a term that refers to the quasitautological notion that responses conditioned under one set of stimulus conditions may also be evoked or emitted under the appearance of other, similar conditions.

---

[1] William Shakespeare, Sonnet 73.

When we say that two items—a pair of objects or events—are similar, we imply that they share some common properties or characteristics.[2] What it is that may be shared is almost limitless, bounded only by the farthest reaches of the human mind. What can make things similar? Identical elements can—parent and child may have "the same nose." So can proximity along an intrinsic dimension—both elephants and whales are large in size. So can common relationships, which may be internal—both Beethoven's "Eroica" and Dvorák's "From the New World" are symphonies—or external—both ice cream and steak may be eaten. Some examples, which by no means exhaust the range of possibilities, appear in Figure 6.1. The trio of sketched faces illustrates similarity through identical elements; the trio of single circles illustrates similarity through proximity along a single dimension; the trio of double circles illustrates similarity through common structure.

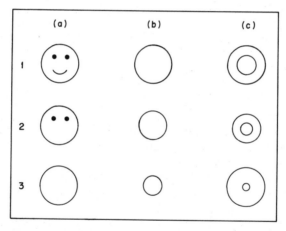

Figure 6.1. Some examples of similarity: (a) similarity through common elements; (b) similarity through proximity along a single dimension; (c) similarity through identical relationships.

To say what it is that is shared is not always an easy task. Take as an elementary example two notes played on the piano. Their similarity depends on their pitch, their loudness, their harmonic structure. When percepts are compared within a given sensory modality, how similar they are depends on their values along the several attributes. Two piano notes that differ in pitch, but not in loudness, sound more alike than

---

[2] When several items are said to be similar, it sometimes can be difficult to find a single characteristic or set of characteristics common to all. Instead, the items may display a "family resemblance" (Wittgenstein, 1953), linking up one to another through a variety of characteristics, each of which is common to a different group of items. Still, one may wonder whether the very process of categorizing items as similar itself imposes a common characteristic: Are similarities discovered or constructed?

two notes that differ as much in pitch and also differ in loudness. Within a single sense modality, sensations can vary continuously, or at least in very small steps; that is, two different sensations may, at least in principle, be brought closer and closer together until they become identical. It is possible to vary the proportion of sugar and salt in a solution so that the taste of their mixture falls anywhere from wholly sweet to wholly salty, or to bring the frequency spectra and intensities of two sounds closer and closer to each other until they are indistinguishable. This operation reveals the very essence of what it is that, according to Helmholtz (1879), delineates a *modality,* namely the capacity to make transitions from one quality to another.

Similarities across the senses, however, are another story. No unitary sensory experience spans the chasm between sight and sound, or between warmth and smell. Despite the many concurrences among modalities, analogies among the senses cannot completely overcome their ontological isolation. Even in unity, the senses show diversity.

A sound, a light, an odor may all be phenomenally bright—perhaps it can be meaningful to say equally bright—but they remain nevertheless a sound, a light, and an odor. The pen that I see is the same as the pen that I hold, but even though the pen is unitary the sight and the touch are not the same. Similarity across the senses must necessarily be one step removed from similarity within a sense, for there is, by definition, no continuity between modalities. If the senses were truly continuous there would be only one sense. But there is no way that we can gradually modulate a chord played on a piano until it becomes indistinguishable from the fragrance of a rose, just as there is no way the sight of the pen can become the feel of it.

So similarity betwixt stands a quantum step removed from similarity within. But, I would like to argue that this quantal step plays a singularly important role: For similarities among the senses not only establish the senses' own consanguinity, a sharing of essential properties that comes through a common phylogenetic heritage and an innate biological substructure, but go even further in that they transform, perhaps even transmogrify, similarity itself, turning it from potential identity into analogy. To pass from similarity within one sense to similarity between two senses is to undergo a metamorphosis, to establish a new process, which provides an elementary basis for metaphoric resemblance.

I find it valuable to distinguish between two classes of similarity: One class refers to the experiencing individual, the other to the scientific description. Similarity is part and parcel of both, at once a psychological phenomenon and a scientific style, a subject matter and a language. The Doctrines of the Unity of the Senses—all of the doctrines elucidated in the preceding chapters—comprise *descriptions* of similarities, models of behavior that are extracted from empirical investigations. Both verbal descriptions and mathematical descriptions are scientific models; both are representations founded on distilled observations of phenomena in nature; both are creations of the scientific mind. When we establish the generality of certain relationships in sensory psychology like Weber's law and Stevens's law, we ought to realize that these exist as formulations put together by an experimenter–theoretician. It is the scientist who sees the similarity in different senses. To the perceiver, the laws themselves usually are wholly unknown.

Certain expressions of sensory unity, however, do impress themselves on the perceiver's phenomenal experience: Examples, familiar by now, are the similarity between loud, high pitched sounds and bright colors; between soft, slowly played melodies and rounded, pale figures; in sum, the synesthetic and synesthetic-like resemblances among sensory qualities. These directly perceived, phenomenologically given analogies straddle the two sides of the scientific and ontological fence, because they are at once conscious content to the percipient organism and data to the perceptive scientist.

Analogy is a quintessential property of mental activity, and is a fundamental property of scientific inquiry. An analogy is a model, a representation of one system by another, a working metaphor in which the attributes and relationships in one domain are seen or made to parallel those in another, thereby providing the continual hope that more attributes or relationships discovered in one will predict observations made on the other. The expansion of knowledge is in large measure the proliferation of metaphors.[3] One of the most powerful scientific metaphors involves applying mathematics to the results of empirical operations. To construct a mathematical science is to represent observations by numbers, to construct an analogy between a formal system and the results of empirical operations. Mathematical science is a theory, and every time one performs a new computation, whose outcome is confirmed, the theory is fulfilled. The development of models, analogies, representations, is one of the themata (to use Holton's [1975] term) of scientific history.

[3] An interesting case of intersensory representation is the familiar translation of music into written notation. For one, musical notation gives a nice example of translating temporal sequences of sound into spatial sequences of sight. For another, musical notation gives a curious blend of analogue and digital codes. Pitch gets a spatial code—with "high" notes appearing higher on the staff; duration, however, both of notes and of rests, gets what might be called primarily a "nonrepresentational" code. Pitch is represented by a visual *analogue*, whereas duration is not.

To repeat, the path from similarity to analogy to metaphor has its origin in phenomena of the senses—in sensory processes, in sensory experiences, in perceptions of objects and events. Metaphorical language is replete with the use of words that are primarily sensory; words that denote qualities of individual senses and words that denote qualities of several. Some adjectives in English that first referred to sensations in one sense department came later to refer to sensations in others. According to the *Oxford English Dictionary*, "sharp" applied first to touch, then subsequently to taste (*ca*. 1000), visual shape (1340), and hearing (1390). "Bright" originally applied to luminous objects, but already by the year 1000 came also to describe sounds. When words that describe sensory qualities slip from one modality to another, they seem to do so in specific and limited ways, as Williams (1976) has catalogued. In particular, the linguistic history of synesthetic transfer tends to display a hierarchical progression, from most primitive to most advanced. A modified version of Williams's scheme may be diagrammed as follows:

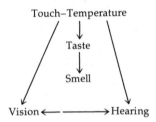

Touch—which Williams uses in an Aristotelian way to encompass all of the skin's senses—he calls the most primitive of sensory systems, and words that originally described qualities of touch expanded, over time, to describe gustatory, visual, and auditory experiences as well. Examples are *dull sounds, soft colors, sharp tastes.* But rarely does the reverse occur; we do not talk, for instance, of *loud* or *fragrant touches.* When counterexamples do occur, Williams notes, they tend to fall out of use quickly. This conclusion fits well with my discovery that the expression *loud stench* passed briefly in and out of the English language in the last century. Williams's evidence is suggestive, to say the least, and does support his generalization that "sensory words in English have systematically transferred from the physiologically least differentiating, most evolutionary primitive sensory modalities to the most differentiating, most advanced, but not vice versa [Williams, 1976, pp. 464–465]."

Words that originally described sensory qualities frequently spread through the sensory order, then spill their meanings out beyond the sensory realm itself. We speak not only synesthetically of warm and cool colors, but also metaphorically of warm and cold personalities, of bright ideas, of bitter failure. Emotions have their hues, when we become green with envy, purple with passion, or just plain blue. Asch (1955) noted how we often describe people by means of sensory words, calling them shallow or hard or dull or sweet or slippery. Multiple use of sensory words, including their metaphorical extension to describe people, Asch found, occurs in languages as diverse as Biblical Hebrew, Homeric Greek, Chinese, and Hansa (the language of the Sudan), as well as English.

A psychological chain links intramodal similarity to synesthesia, synesthesia to metaphor. Similarities among the qualities of a single sense progress to similarities among qualities of different senses, which in turn progress to similarities and resemblances that transcend simple sensory properties and partake of the myriad relationships that the mind can construct. A prime characteristic of this progression is the way the correspondences become increasingly abstract. A gulf grows between the events, objects, or thoughts that are conjoined. Steeped with a strong synesthetic flavor is a placid and quiet dusk, where, in Robert Browning's words, "the quiet-coloured end of evening smiles."[4] A similar mood, albeit one where the reader feels the metaphorical sinew stretching, is captured by William Wordsworth's

> *beauteous evening, calm and free*
> *The holy time is quiet as a nun*
> *Breathless with adoration*[5]

and, an even more soporific one, by T. S. Eliot:

> *When the evening is spread out against the sky*
> *Like a patient etherized upon a table.*[6]

According to the classical view, for instance, Aristotle's, metaphor is simply a bridge constructed of resemblance. But it is more, as Max Black (1962) argued. Not only does metaphor connect, but sometimes, as with Eliot's evening and etherized patient, it may even transform the conjoined images to create new meanings. It is, presumably, metaphor's capacity to organize a new reality that led Wallace Stevens (1957) to remark, with seeming whimsey, that, "In the long run the

---

[4]"Love among the Ruins."

[5]"It is a Beauteous Evening, Calm and Free."

[6]From "The Love-Song of J. Alfred Prufrock" by T. S. Eliot. In *Collected poems, 1909–1935*, Harcourt Brace Jovanovich, Publishers.

truth does not matter [p. 180]." To the poet, at least, what does matter is the reality created by metaphoric imagination.

The final two chapters will deal with the expressive and the metaphorical in literary language. The first of them deals with the way that the unity of the senses reveals itself through physiognomic properties in speech sounds of poetry, the second with the way that the unity of the senses reveals itself through synesthetic metaphor in poetry.

7

Sound Symbolism in Poetry

If the unity of the senses is, as I have tried to show, pervasive and profound, then we should not be surprised—indeed, we might well expect—to discover its threads running through the very fabric of human thought, revealing themselves in the articulate web of images, ideas, and concepts that go into cognitive activity. And most important, perhaps, to cognitive activity is language. Language does more, after all, than just help us reach out to others; it also helps give coherence and structure to mental life. This being so, verbal behavior should show clear evidence of sensory correspondences. And it does, Into the stream of language run synesthetic analogies whose murmur echos resemblances among sense modalities. The final two chapters will explore some of the ways that intersensory phenomena, mainly synesthetic relations, express themselves through language.

One of these ways is through sound symbolism: The sounds of speech can intimate meanings, in part because all types of sounds can suggest, synesthetically, other sensory qualities. The present chapter explores a few of the intersensory relations that are revealed by sound symbolism in poetry.

Analogue and Formal Representation

Ernst Cassirer (1953) proposed that the development of language proceeded through three stages, which he termed the mimetic, the analogical, and the symbolic. As we pass from stage to stage, we find a shift in the basic relationship between speech sound and meaning, a shift from an intrinsic and nonarbitrary relationship to an increasingly extrinsic and capricious one. The mimetic stage corresponds to the onomatopoeic use of speech—the representation through speech of some acoustical event in nature by means of direct imitation. The relationship between sound and meaning is essentially intrinsic. Imitations of animal sounds, like "cockadoodle doo," "moo," and "quack" are familiar examples; only slightly more sophisticated are onomatopoeic words like "crack," "thud," and "ping." In mimesis, language acts as a relatively simple analogue system.

At the opposite end of Cassirer's scale lies the third or symbolic stage. Here, the relationship between the meaningful units of speech and the objects and events they represent is fundamentally arbitrary: Language functions abstractly, as a formal system of semantic representation. At the symbolic level, representation is a matter of definition, a mutually accepted convention—naming an object by one word is as good as naming it by another, a fact perfectly clear to Humpty Dumpty if not to Alice. It makes no real difference, from this point of view, whether a winged, warm blooded animal is called "bird," "oiseau," "flügel," "avis," or "blix." With Shakespeare we must at least partly concur that

> that which we call a rose
> By any other name would smell as sweet.[1]

Between the mimetic and the symbolic falls the analogical. Here, as in the mimetic stage, speech mediates meaning in a fashion that is not wholly arbitrary—but with a crucial difference: In the mimetic, speech sounds represent other sounds by mimicking them; in the analogical, speech sounds suggest objects or qualities that are not themselves sounds. Both mimicry and sound symbolism (as I prefer to call sound analogy) are analogue systems, but in sound symbolism the referents stand an additional step removed from the speech sounds. An example is the use of low and high pitched vowel sounds to suggest large and

[1] *Romeo and Juliet*, II, ii.

small objects. The reader may note that the present distinction between mimetic and analogical representation embodies the distinction made in the last chapter between within-modality and cross-modality similarity. Both distinctions rest on the dichotomy between the kind of similarity that can approach identity and the kind that cannot. Onomatopoeia expresses similarity within a sense; sound symbolism, similarity across the senses.

Actually, language provides two very different ways of expressing interrelationships among the senses. One of these is analogical, the other symbolic, to go back to Cassierer's terminology. First of all, language comprises a set of behaviors that themselves are stimulus events, by which I mean, behaviors that have sensory components. Language production—the act of speaking and the act of writing—involves movements of muscles and joints, and these acts have concomitant sensory effects mediated through the kinesthetic system. Language reception—the act of listening and the act of reading—involves auditory and visual experience. Kinesthetic, visual, and auditory sensations alike are able to kindle synesthesia-like experiences. Perhaps most significant is the fact that speech serves as an auditory stimulus, rousing sensations of sound whose suprasensory attributes become the medium for suggesting qualities and attributes for other modalities. In general, suprasensory attributes form a basis for synesthetic translation; and in particular, suprasensory attributes of sound form one basis for analogical sound symbolism.

There is a second way that language can mediate concordances among the senses. Not only does speech, as sound, embody suprasensory qualities, but language, as formal representation, makes it possible to communicate cross-modal equivalence. Simply said, we can talk or write about sensory correspondences. In this, the penultimate chapter, I shall restrict attention to sound symbolism, and defer considering synesthetic metaphor to the last chapter.

Sound and Meaning

The notion that the words of a language may bear some intrinsic, that is, some nonarbitrary, relation to their meanings, is certainly not new; it appeared at least as early as Plato's *Cratylus*. To repeat, by sound symbolism I do not mean onomatopoeic expression. Onomatopoeic words like "buzz," "hiss," and "moo" clearly bear an intrinsic relation to their referents: A couple of well-known examples from poetry are

Tennyson's "murmuring of innumerable bees"[2] and Joyce's "Wind whines and whines the shingle / The crazy pierstakes groan."[3] But onomatopoeia is not my major concern. What is, is a more analogical, though nonetheless often intrinsic relation between sound and meaning—a relation where the sound and the referent are not identical, or even nearly so. Sound symbolism is attained when meaning expressed by sound reflects some nonacoustical property of nature.

It is only fair to point out that sound symbolism—or physiognomic sound, to use Heinz Werner's (1940) terminology—is not always salient in speech. Mostly, we listen for abstract meanings, which is to say nonanalogical meanings. In listening to ordinary conversation, for instance, we tune in largely on the formal meanings, the symbolic meanings that are expressed through the lexical, semantic, and syntactic structures. (To be sure, these meanings are modulated through patterns of intonation, but the inflections of voice that characterize declarative, plaintive, and interrogative tones work on the formal content of speech, and so they are specific to the linguistic properties of speech.) What about the meanings conveyed by sound symbolism? Speech sounds have the potential to suggest meanings; they have, not because they are speech, but because they are sounds. Because speech carries "abstract" information, the suggestiveness of speech as sound may go unnoticed, surfacing only on special occasions. When an acoustical waveform—a pattern of sound—is perceived as speech, it is processed in a special way: The perceptual apparatus chops up the acoustical waveform and segments it into discrete phonological units. So dominant are the phonological characteristics of speech that, unless attention is directed toward sound quality, the speech characteristics usually overwhelm the physiognomic. Sometimes, in order to tune in on the suggestiveness of sound, one almost has to tune out the linguistic character.

Because sound symbolism is, in prosaic speech, evanescent and shadowy, it needs a showcase to display its goods. Such a showcase is often found in poetry, for the poet's stock of acoustical devices—stresses, rhythms, sheer repetitions of units as small as single sounds or as large as whole phrases—can call attention not just to the lexical meanings of words, but to their phonetic and acoustic character, and thus set the stage for analogical meanings. Poetry is speech heard in a special way, where sound itself takes on a central role.

Students of poetry as well as poets themselves have testified to the intimate ties between sounds and nuances of meaning. The poetry of

---

[2] "The Princess."

[3] From "On the Beach at Fontana" by James Joyce. In *Collected poems*, copyright 1936 by The Viking Press. Reprinted by permission.

Edith Sitwell welds rich sound textures to synesthetic images; one of her best-known verses reads "Jane, Jane / Tall as a crane, / The morning light creaks down again."[4] In the introduction to her collected poems, Sitwell (1954) went on at considerable length to describe and explain her attempts at shading meaning through repetitions and contrasts of sound. When carried out to its limit, this sort of verbal play can lead to a poetry of pure sound, a montage of utterances that are formally meaningless but endlessly suggestive, as, for instance, in some of the late poems of Antonin Artaud.

Is pure sound enough to give poetry meaning? William Empson (1947) described, and rejected, what he called the Cult of Sound, the view that poetry conveys its impressions through sound alone. In its place, he recommended Alexander Pope's more moderate opinion that "the sound should seem an echo to the sense."

Not all agree even with this conservative posture. To Pope's dictum, Samuel Johnson (1778) replied that just the reverse is true: Sound, according to Johnson, does not engender words with meaning; instead, the sounds absorb the meanings that surround them. Meanings may pass from a word to the word's constituent sounds. Consider the opening lines of Sitwell's poem "The Drum":

> *In his tall senatorial*
> *Black and manorial*
> *House where decoy-duck*
> *Dust doth clack—*
> *Clatter and quack*
> *To a shadow black . . . .*[5]

Wrote the poet, " 'Black,' 'duck,' 'clatter,' and 'quack,' with their hard consonants and dead vowels, are dry as dust, and the deadness of dust is conveyed thus, and, as well by the dulled dissonance of the 'a's, of the 'u' in 'duck' followed by its crumbling assonance 'dust' [Sitwell, 1954, p. xxiii]." To which Johnson might have responded that the repeated "d" and "ck" sop up the meanings of "dust" and "black."

It is not easy to say when sounds take on meanings from the immediate semantic context, as opposed to when they impart meanings by dint of inherent evocative powers. When I recite aloud

smooth, smooth, smooth

---

[4]From "Aubade" by Edith Sitwell. In *The collected poems of Edith Sitwell*, copyright 1954 by Vanguard Press. Reprinted by permission.

[5]From "The Drum" by Edith Sitwell. In *The collected poems of Edith Sitwell*, copyright 1954 by Vanguard Press. Reprinted by permission.

the words flow one into another like freshets after an April rain, while

bumpy, bumpy, bumpy

springs along like a child on a pogo stick. Where does this difference in rhythm come from? Do the sounds themselves impose it? Perhaps. The very sound of Paul Verlaine's "Chanson d'Automne" seems to me to impart a slow, limpid melancholy that may be perceptible even to one ignorant of the language:

> *Les sanglots longs*
> *Des violons*
> > *De l'automne*
> *Blessent mon coeur*
> *D'une langueur*
> > *Monotone.*

As I said earlier, the poet's repertoire contains several devices that serve to highlight particular sounds; these devices include alliteration, assonance, rhyme, and stress. From time to time, certain poets will methodically repeat sounds in order to emphasize a mood or image, a perception or thought. Sitwell's often rococo repetitions, taken together with the poet's self-analysis, imply a clear motivation to use acoustical devices. Nevertheless, it is worth pointing out that, although a given verse may exhibit acoustical effects, we cannot always infer that the poet was motivated, either consciously or unconsciously, to use them. Even a poet's claim of intent may be post hoc. Still, imputing intention to Sitwell seems appropriate, largely because sound repetitions occur so often in her poetry.

This point is significant—to argue that a poet selects certain combinations of sound implies that those combinations show up more often than would be expected by chance. After all, even randomly chosen sequences will occasionally alliterate or rhyme. Shakespeare's sonnets, for instance, reveal some repeated consonants, but Skinner (1942) calculated that the number of alliterations is about what would be expected by chance. On the other hand, Skinner showed that Swinburne's "Atalanta in Calydon" contains many occurrences of contiguous consonants (alliteration), many more than in Shakespeare's sonnets and well beyond what could be accounted for by chance. Even so, some instances of alliteration in Swinburne's poem are presumably "accidental." To the reader, though, it may not be possible to tell the fortuitous from the intended.

Dimensions of Sound Symbolism

Speech sounds and meanings are, at times, closely associated. How do they get that way? Sometimes, as Dr. Johnson suggested, the semantic context does it; but this cannot be the whole story, for even nonsense words can conjure up reliable impressions. What are the other possibilities? Individual sounds, may, of course, bring to mind meanings that the sounds had picked up previously, meanings of other words that contain those sounds; this is what Masson (1953) called a *lexical* process of evocation. Alternatively, the relation may be an intrinsic one, with meanings coming either from sensations aroused in moving the mouth and tongue when the sounds are spoken, by a *kinesthetic* process; or from the sounds themselves, by an *acoustical* process. I want to concentrate on this last process—on the sounds themselves: Sounds can suggest meaning through those of its perceptual attributes that are suprasensory.

That sounds can generate meanings wholly apart from what they pick up in the immediate semantic context is supported by a number of experimental findings that used nonsense material. Some of these were recounted in Chapter 3; others will be described now. One way that sounds symbolize meaning is by means of affect. Hevner (1937) systematically varied the vowel and consonant structure of pseudoverse (stanzas constructed out of nonsense words) and had readers report on the "meanings" of the stanzas. Pseudoverse containing "light, open, thin vowels"—/i/, /ai/, and /ei/, as in he*a*t, he*igh*t, and h*a*te—was consistently judged more serene, playful, delicate, and happy than pseudoverse containing "dark, full, rounded vowels"—/u/, /a/, and /o/, as in wh*o*m, h*o*t, and h*o*me. The dark vowels, however, produced pseudoverse that was judged more dignified, exciting, and vigorous. Interestingly, differences among consonants, and among combinations of consonants, yielded only small variations in affective responses.

To illustrate the difference between the delicate and playful vowel sounds on the one hand and the fuller and more dignified vowel sounds on the other, I will contrast two poems on the theme of love—Leigh Hunt's "Jenny Kissed Me" and Robert Burns's "John Anderson My Jo." The two are similar not only in that both poems center on love, but also in that both focus on the encroachment of age. Yet these similarities strike the reader as superficial; for the tones of the poems are vastly different, in large measure because of the striking differences in their patterns of sounds, especially their vowels (cf. Macdermott, 1940). Hunt's poem bounces with the gaiety and playful lightness of repeated high vowels, especially /i/ and /ɪ/. For its sound alone, few other names compare to "Jenny":

> *Jenny kissed me when we met,*
> > *Jumping from the chair she sat in;*
> *Time, you thief, who love to get*
> > *Sweets into your list, put that in!*
> *Say I'm weary, say I'm sad,*
> > *Say that health and wealth have missed me,*
> *Say I'm growing old, but add,*
> > *Jenny kissed me.*

Burns's poem, though less consistent in its pattern of vowels, nevertheless contrasts well with Hunt's. "John Anderson My Jo" exhibits a greater use of the more serene /ɔ/, the flat /a/, /ɑ/, and /æ/, and the dignified, even solemn /o/:

> *John Anderson my jo, John,*
> > *When we were first acquent,*
> *Your locks were like the raven,*
> > *Your bonnie brow was brent;*
> *But now your brow is beld, John,*
> > *Your locks are like the snow*
> *But blessings on your frosty pow,*
> > *John Anderson my jo!*

> *John Anderson my jo, John,*
> > *We clamb the hill thegither,*
> *And monie a cantie day, John,*
> > *We've had wi' ane anither;*
> *Now we maun totter down, John,*
> > *And hand in hand we'll go,*
> *And sleep thegither at the foot,*
> > *John Anderson my jo!*

Certain speech sounds even appear more pleasant or unpleasant than others. Among vowels, reported Roblee and Washburn (1912), /a/, /ɛ/, and /o/ (as in got, get, and goat) are judged more pleasant than /ʌ/, /ɔ/, and /u/ (as in sup, saw, and soup). Experiments have shown that glottal consonants—those, such as /k/ and /g/, produced near the back of the mouth—are judged less pleasant than apical or labial consonants— those, such as /f/ and /p/, produced near the front of the mouth (Folkins & Lenrow, 1966; Roblee & Washburn, 1912). Garver, Gleason, and Washburn (1915) found that they could account for many of the differences in pleasantness among consonants in terms of, first, the associations between the consonants and the pleasantness and unpleasantness of words that contain them, and second, the degree of difficulty in articulating them. But though such an account was possible for consonants, it was not possible for vowels. Vowels, it seems, have a natural pleasantness and unpleasantness. Perhaps we should not be surprised to find that vowels can be intrinsically pleasant or unpleasant. There is reason to believe that musical notes can be. Might the inherent pleasantness of vowels and musical notes come from a single source, as evidenced, perhaps, by the fact that certain sounds may be perceived both as vowels and as notes played by musical instruments? Slawson (1968) showed that complex sounds—specifically, computer-generated sounds that were constructed to mimic vowels—could readily be heard either as vowels or as musical notes.

Vowel Symbolism in Poetry

Studies of poetry frequently allude to the ways that changes in meaning are associated with changes in sound pattern. Barber (1960) commented as follows on Shakespeare's use of vowels in the sonnets: "When we shift from quatrain to quatrain . . . part of the newness is often the sound of a fresh set of dominant vowels; or again, we sometimes recognize a set of sounds carried all the way through a sonnet to give it its distinctive tune [p. 17]." In this regard, I would like to juxtapose and contrast two of William Shakespeare's sonnets, 73 and 97. Though both contain strong images of wintery cold, how different they are! In Sonnet 73, the cold is deep and vast, resonating with intimations of growing old,

> That time of year thou mayst in me behold,
> When yellow leaves, or none, or few, do hang
> Upon those boughs which shake against the cold,
> Bare ruined choirs

a cold whose profundity is in some measure reinforced by the emphasis of the /o/, repeated in "behold" and "cold," and /au/, repeated in "thou" and "boughs."[6]

How much sharper and more penetrating (in a piercing way, though not in the profound way of Sonnet 73) is

---

[6]This assumes the phonology applies to Elizabethan pronunciation. A note of caution: The questions, "When does sound symbolism work?" and "What are its rules?" need to be answered through experimentation. Is the / o / of cold itself "cold?" Sitwell thought not: She claimed that / o /—and / au /—are warm!

How like a winter hath my absence been
From thee, the pleasure of the fleeting year!
What freezings have I felt, what dark days seen,
What old December's bareness everywhere!

Here we find the acuteness of the /i/, repeated five times in these four lines: in "thee," "fleeting," "freezings," "seen," and "everywhere."

Hilda Doolittle's (H. D.'s) "Sea Gods" uses vowels in a somewhat similar way:

We bring hyacinth-violet
sweet, bare, chill to the touch—
and violets whiter than the in-rush
of your own white surf.[7]

Of these lines, Babette Deutsch (1935) remarked that " . . . the repeated 'i' in 'hyacinth-violet,' 'violets,' 'whiter,' 'white,' give the lightness of the flowers themselves, while the 'in-rush of . . . surf' carries the sibilance of foamy waters [p. 68]."

Among the most potent physiogonomic expressions of speech are the undercurrents of brightness and darkness, of sharpness and dullness, of smallness and voluminousness, in sum, the expressions of suprasensory attributes. Part of the effectiveness of "Sea Gods," and this is what Deutsch alluded to, comes from the intimation of brightness through the repeated use of high pitched "i" (though it is also possible that the high pitched "i" picks up some of its brightness through the word "white"). With some trepidation at the idea of belaboring the point, let me also quote from James Joyce's *Ulysses* (1934) a passage where Joyce veritably flaunts this device with self-conscious abandon:

Bob Cowley's twinkling fingers in the treble played again. The landlord has the prior. A little time. Long John. Big Ben. Lightly he played a light bright tinkling measure for tripping ladies, arch and smiling, and for their gallants, gentlemen friends. One: one, one, one: two, one, three, four.

Sea, wind, leaves, thunder, waters, cows lowing, the cattle market, cocks, hens don't crow, snakes hissss. There's music everywhere. Ruttledge's door: ee creaking [p. 277].

Speech sounds can represent gradations in brightness, and variations in size. This has been demonstrated in numerous experiments, beginning with Sapir's (1929) classic study and continuing through subsequent investigations by Bentley and Varon (1933), Newman (1933), Tsuru and Fries (1933), and Czurda (1953); much of the evidence

[7] From "Sea Gods" by Hilda Doolittle (H. D.). In *Collected poems;* copyright 1925, 1953 by Norman Holmes Pearson. Reprinted by permission of New Directions Publishing Corp.

was reviewed earlier (Chapter 3, pp. 75–83). To summarize it, high pitched vowels like /ɪ/ and /i/, /ɛ/ and /e/ tend to suggest bright, small referents, whereas low pitched vowels like /o/ and /u/ tend to suggest dark and large ones. This mirrors the psychoacoustic properties of the vowels themselves—the way they partake of the suprasensory attributes of brightness and size. High pitched sounds are phenomenally bright and small, while low pitched sounds appear darker and larger.

Sound symbolism may, therefore, in part be treated as a branch of psychoacoustics. This approach is predicated on the fact that the dimensions of brightness and size that sounds can "symbolize" or designate are actually properties of the sounds themselves. Indeed, this seems to be precisely what H. Werner (1940) meant when he said that language has a physiognomic property, namely that there are meanings carried directly and inherently by sounds themselves.

Sounds are able to "symbolize" features like size and brightness because certain characteristics of sensory experience are shared by several modalities. That is, there exist common, intersensory dimensions through which sounds can invoke, for example, visual and tactile impressions. There are equivalences among the attributes high pitched, bright, and sharp, among the attributes high pitched, small, and delicate. It is useful to distinguish two types of equivalence: One is intrinsic, a property of sensory systems that probably reflects invariant aspects of the primary physiological responses to stimulation in different modalities; the other is extrinsic, a property that depends on mediational processes that are to a large extent derived and to some extent cultural. Though both types of equivalence undoubtedly can play a role in sound symbolism, it is the former that is of concern here.

SIZE AND BRIGHTNESS

According to Coleridge (1847), the poet must be able to put into practice "the *vestigia communia* of the senses . . . the excitement of vision by sound and the exponents of sound [p. 142]." The psychoacoustic relationships between size and brightness on the one hand and sound frequency on the other exhibit themselves in numerous examples of poetic sound symbolism. Sometimes, onomatopoeia and physiognomic sound symbolism run together, as in William Collins's description of the way

> *the weak-eyed bat*
> *With a short shrill shriek flits by on a leathern wing.*[8]

[8]"Ode to Evening."

The repetition of high frequency consonants, like /sh/, and vowels, like /i/ and /ɪ/, serves to highlight smallness, brightness, compactness. e. e. cummings's lines

> *what if a keen of a lean wind flays*
> *screaming hills with sleet and snow*[9]

exhibit many of the same repetitions of sound, emphasizing again smallness, sharpness, brightness.

It is interesting to contrast these lines of cummings with other lines in the same poem:

> *what if a dawn of a doom of a dream*
> *bites this universe in two.*[10]

The repetition of /d/ places emphasis on the vowels /ɔ/ of "dawn" and /u/ of "doom," and the /u/ is carried forward to the next line, where it is twice repeated, in "universe" and "two." Both /ɔ/ and /u/ are low frequency vowels that convey darkness, profundity, massive bulk.

Symbolism of size and brightness by sound appears in the poetry of Edith Sitwell. To take one instance, let us go back to the opening verses of "The Drum," where the vowels of the "tall senatorial, / black and manorial / House where decoy-duck / Dust doth clack—clatter and quack / To a shadow black" echo bulk and darkness. Actually, as important to the poem's overall effect as its vowel symbolism is its rhythm— the strong pulsation that mimics the subject matter of the verse. A rhythm of this sort is also found in what will be this chapter's final example of sound symbolizing size and brightness.[11]

Perhaps the finest single example of the merger of physiognomic sound symbolism and onomatopoeia is Edgar Allan Poe's "The Bells." The poem is a model of the genre, as Buranelli (1961) noted: "World literature can scarcely show a more triumphant handling of onomatopoeia—suggestiveness and meaning conveyed through the medium of sounds [p. 108]." Each part of Poe's poem not only conjures up auditory images of the particular sounds (onomatopoeia), but also invokes visual images (sound symbolism) of the bells that produce the sounds.

"The Bells" divides into four stanzas, one each allotted to sleigh bells, wedding bells, alarm (martial) bells, and funeral bells, a sequence

[9]From "what if a much of a which of a wind" by e. e. cummings. In *Complete poems, 1913–1962*, Harcourt Brace Jovanovich, Publishers. Reprinted by permission.
[10]*Ibid.*
[11]For further examples of size symbolism in poetry, see Moynihan (1958).

that clearly represents a chronology from childhood through adulthood to death. A striking feature of the poem is the variation from stanza to stanza in the patterning of speech sounds. Some of the differences in patterns may even be ascertained through a statistical tabulation: Table 7.1 lists the relative frequencies of the major vowel sounds. (Distributional differences also appear in the way consonants are used; for example, /t/ and /k/ appear often in the early stanzas, /b/ and /d/ often in the later ones.) A table like this by no means does justice to the detail of the sound patterns, since it glosses over the effects that arise from local stresses and repetitions, to say nothing of the powerful, hypnotic rhythms. (Note, though, that the pattern of vowels is similar for stressed and unstressed syllables.) Nevertheless, an idea of the vowel distributions that Poe employed may be gleaned from the table.

The first stanza of the poem begins by beckoning the reader–listener to

> Hear the sledges with the bells–
> Silver bells!

At once the image is conjured up of lightness, of dancing movement, to

Table 7.1

Relative frequencies of vowel sounds in Edgar Allen Poe's "The Bells."
Each entry is the vowel's probability[a]

Vowel			Stanza		
		I	II	III	IV
/a/	(m*o*p)				
/ɑ/	(m*a*r)	.07	.13	.14	.13
/æ/	(m*a*p)				
/ɛ/	(m*e*t)	.16	.15	.14	.14
/e/	(m*a*te)	.04	.03	.08	.03
/ei/	(m*ay*)				
/ɪ/	(m*i*tt)	.12	.06	.07	.06
/i/	(m*ee*t)	.23	.18	.12	.14
/o/	(m*oa*t)	.03	.06	.02	.09
/ɔ/	(m*o*re)	.03	.01	.02	.03
/u/	(m*oo*t)	.02	.08	.03	.05
/au/	(m*ou*se)	.01	.04	.05	.01
/ai/	(m*i*te)	.07	.03	.05	.06
/iu/	(m*u*se)	.02	.01	.01	.01
/ə/	(th*e*)	.20	.21	.28	.25

[a] Frequency in the stanza divided by total number of vowels in the stanza.

the ear as well as to the eye. The image is reinforced by the repetition of sound, especially repetition of whole words

> *What a world of merriment their melody foretells!*
> *How they tinkle, tinkle, tinkle,*
> *In the icy air of night!*
> *While the stars that oversprinkle*
> *All the heavens, seem to twinkle*
> *With a crystalline delight;*
> *Keeping time, time, time,*
> *In a sort of Runic rhyme*
> *To the tintinnabulation that so musically wells*
> *From the bells, bells, bells, bells,*
> *Bells, bells, bells—*
> *From the jingling and the tinkling of the bells.*

It is only these silver bells—their jingling and tinkling—that give tintinnabulation; tintinnabulation is, of course, a word Poe coined specifically to carry the tune of the sleigh bells.[12] The first stanza displays the most frequent use of the high pitched vowels /i/ and /ɪ/ and the least frequent use of the low pitched /u/. The abundance of high pitched sounds, and in particular the repetition of them, as "they tinkle, tinkle, tinkle," serves the dual purpose of imitating the high pitched ringing and symbolizing the physical smallness of the sleigh bells.

The last three stanzas find none of the extraordinary use of high pitched vowels; instead, the second and fourth stanzas especially show an increasing frequency in the "a" vowels /a/, /ɑ/, and /æ/, as well as in /o/ and /u/. These are deeper, that is, low register vowels, which convey both the lower pitches and greater physical size of the wedding bells, the alarm bells, and the funeral bells.

The second stanza opens with the call to

> *Hear the mellow wedding bells*
> *Golden bells*

and the reader–listener is soon immersed in mellow sounds of /o/ and /u/

> *From the molten-golden notes,*
> *And all in tune,*
> *What a liquid ditty floats,*
> *To the turtle dove that listens, while she gloats*
> *On the moon!*

---

[12] Coincidental, perhaps, is the suggestiveness through repeated sound in another poem—"The Windhover" by Gerard Manley Hopkins: "I caught this morning morning's minion, kingdom of daylight's dauphin, dappledawn-drawn Falcon, in his riding / Of the rolling level underneath him steady air, and striding / High there, how he rung upon the rein of a wimpling wing / In his ecstasy!" The windhover is a small falcon, technically known as *Falco tinnunculus.*

Stanza three digresses a bit. The alarm bells are larger and louder, but, onomatopoeically either somewhat higher in pitch

> In the startled ear of night
> How they scream out their affright!
> Too much horrified to speak,
> They can only shriek, shriek,
>   Out of tune,

or else discordant, "twanging," "clanging," "jangling," and "wrangling." Verbs, nouns, and adjectives speak in the voice of the bells.

The last stanza returns to the vowel pattern of the second, and is perhaps the most notable in its acoustic effect. For in the large, iron bells—the funeral bells—every "tone" is a "groan":

> For every sound that floats
> From the rust within their throats
>   Is a groan.
> And the people—ah, the people—
> They that dwell up in the steeple,
>   All alone,
> And who, tolling, tolling, tolling,
>   In that muffled monotone
> Feel a glory in so rolling
>   On the human heart a stone—
> They are neither man nor woman—
> They are neither brute nor human—
>   They are Ghouls:—
> And their kind is who tolls:—
> And he rolls, rolls, rolls,
>   Rolls
>   A paean from the bells!

The repetitions of "tolls," "rolls," "tolling," and "rolling" lead inexorably to the somber climax in "the moaning and the groaning of the bells." What could contrast more, in physiognomic meaning, to "tintinnabulation"?

EXPRESSION OF MULTIPLE MEANINGS

In this chapter, I have placed special attention on the way particular vowel sounds can suggest differences in size and brightness. But sound symbolism goes much further. Even if we stick to the vowels, and even if we look solely at the contrast between high pitched and low pitched, we can discover a whole gamut of meanings that appear to be associated with each type of vowel. Poe's lost Ulalume is not only dark, but also sad and mysterious, and her name could hardly substitute for that of Chaucer's delicate Madame Eglentyne, the

> *Prioresse,*
> *That of hir smyling was ful simple and coy.*[13]

Macdermott (1940) investigated the subject matter of several dozen poems and, on a line by line basis, correlated meanings with the use of low and high pitched vowels. A sample of her results appears in Table 7.2. Even though each set of attributes shows a wide range—from relatively simple sensory qualities like warm versus cool and black versus white, to complex affective responses, like deep, mature love versus light-hearted, youthful love, the two sets are cohesive. Each set of attributes seems to form a cluster because all of the members share some properties or characteristics. In the sensory realm, this means sharing supramodal attributes: Angular objects are like sharp cold, heavy objects are like heavy odors, warmth is like warm colors. But there is more. The shared characteristics transcend sensations. Not only white colors, but also upward movement, gaiety, and even light-hearted love speak the language of brightness.

Subsets of the attributes listed in each column of Table 7.2 also form

Table 7.2
Connotations of low pitched and high pitched vowels, as
determined from passages of poetry

Low pitched vowels	High pitched vowels
Low in space	High in space
Downward movement	Upward movement
Heavy and rounded objects	Light and angular objects
Strength	Weakness
Heavy odors	Delicate odors
Warmth	Coolness
Dull cold	Sharp cold
Warm colors	Cool colors
Black	White
Roughness	Smoothness
Slow movement	Quick movement
Greatness	Smallness
Solemnity	Gaiety
Deep, mature love	Light-hearted, youthful love

Source: Modified and abridged from Macdermott (1940).

[13]*The Canterbury tales.* "Prologue."

clusters in data that Osgood and his colleagues collected by the method of semantic differentiation. Recall that Osgood, Suci, and Tannenbaum (1957) asked people to evaluate the connotative meanings of words on a large number of bipolar scales. They found, to take examples relevant in the present context, that treble (versus bass), high (versus low), white (versus black), light (versus heavy), and smooth (versus rough) tended to group together in that all showed high loading on a factor of *evaluation*—good as opposed to bad. Large (versus small), sharp (versus dull), hot (versus cold), angular (versus rounded), and fast (versus slow) grouped together in that they were high on a factor of *activity*—active as opposed to passive. This suggests an explanation as to why high and low vowels evoke so many different attributes: Many different attributes share, with high or low pitch, similar affective connotations. Osgood, May, and Miron (1974) point to the pervasive role of three semantic factors—evaluation, activity, and potency—in sound symbolism and in verbal metaphor.

To some degree this surely is so, though verbal metaphor, including synesthetic metaphor is, I think, much more complex than simply shared affect. Still, to the extent that sound symbolism and metaphor do spring from shared connotative meanings, one major source is the well of intermodal attributes of sensation, the attributes that are common to several or all sensory modalities.

8

Synesthetic Metaphor in Poetry

Language teems with synesthetic metaphor. Everyday expressions like "loud colors," "dark sounds," "sweet smells" are basically synesthetic, in that they transfer meanings from one sensory mode to another. Yet so commonplace are these expressions and others like them that their cross-modal characteristics may escape notice, the synesthetic undercurrents to their meanings having fallen victim to their very prevalence: For even though verbal images start out fresh and new, potent and vigorous, often they end up stale and old, tired and sapped of meaning. Because they capture some essential cross-modal relationship, they become popular heroes in the language game; and because they are popular, their meaning fades. Once exhausted, they become dead metaphors, leaving us hardly aware that these phrases we continue to speak, hear, or read actually connect different senses, drawing analogies between different modalities.

One of my favorite examples is the expression "bitter cold." It is an expression that most of us toss off carefreely, usually when we want to signify a cold that is extreme. Yet in a literal sense the conjunction of bitter with cold is synesthetic, for it transports a meaning to the thermal realm from the gustatory. Even so, it is probably a good bet that most people say "bitter cold" without ever recognizing that the phrase crosses two senses. Frequent repetition has bled the metaphor of meaning. Doubtless there was a time when "bitter cold" was strikingly fresh and rich—in the Elizabethan age, when William Shakespeare wrote, "Freeze, freeze, thou bitter sky,"[1] perhaps even three centuries later, when Robert Burns wrote of

> bleak December's winds ensuin'
> Baith snell [= bitter] an' keen![2]

More on this later.

Unity of the Senses and Synesthetic Metaphor

The Doctrine of the Unity of the Senses provides a good starting point for interpreting synesthetic metaphor. In a nutshell, the doctrine says first, that there are meaningful similarities across different sense modalities, and second, that some of these similarities are appreciated by virtually everyone. From these two principles, we can produce a general scheme for classifying and interpreting examples of "synesthesia" in language. To do this, a couple of distinctions should be made. For one, a synesthetic metaphor may—but need not—rely on universally understood similarities. For another, a metaphor may be full, partial, or nondescriptive, by which I mean that it can identify the qualities on all, some, or none of the senses involved.

What are the main categories of synesthetic metaphor? First and foremost, there is a class of *appropriate* metaphors, metaphors in which the two or more sensory elements are tied together by a natural bond. The arrival of spring reminded Joseph Auslander of "the silver needle-note of a fife."[3] Whether or not this metaphor aptly describes spring, the metaphor's own internal structure hits its target. The bright note of a fife does have the sharpness of a needle, the shininess of silver. In a similar vein is Conrad Aiken's "shrill bells of silver."[4] Here, the analogy is perhaps based on a different intersensory relation, namely an equivalence between the absence of rich timbre from certain sounds and the paleness of silvery colors. Regardless of the exact basis for the analogy,

---

[1] *As you like it*, II, vii.

[2] "To a Mouse."

[3] "Steel." Compare Swinburne's "loud as marriage bells that peal, / Or flutelike soft, or keen like steel, / Sprang the sheer music": "A Ballad of Appeal."

[4] "The House of Dust."

the significant point is that there are relatively few colors that may be deemed proper to go with shrill sounds. Silver stands out. Consider, by way of comparison, shrill blue, shrill black, or, worse yet, shrill purple.

Most synesthetic metaphors that are perceived immediately as appropriate (and maybe even some that are not) derive largely from the same primordial unity of the senses that expresses itself in sensory synesthesia. Such metaphors typically convey intrinsic correspondences through dimensions like brightness or affect that are common to many or all sense modalities. Auslander's "silver needle-note of a fife" shows how brightness can unify the three senses of hearing, touch, and sight, with an emphasis on the sharp, tactile quality. Nafe (1927), on the basis of introspective evidence, not only suggested that brightness is a common property of different modalities, but in addition implied that its nature is quintessentially tactile. Williams (1976) has presented linguistic evidence that suggests a parallel in the evolution of language—adjectives whose meanings originally applied to tactile sensations (e.g., "sharp," "dull") came later to apply to other senses. Many of these adjectives have a notable brightness component.

Full synesthetic metaphors in this first category specify relatively unambiguously, if not always with great precision, the sorts of sensory qualities that are said to correspond. When the qualities agree, the metaphor is appropriate—it expresses an intrinsic correspondence, to continue the terminology introduced earlier: Silver colors are in some way like the brisk notes of a fife.

Sometimes, though, a synesthetic metaphor runs wholly or partly against the grain of an intrinsic cross-modal relationship. Metaphors of this sort form a second category. Given that loud sounds are deemed bright, soft ones dark or dull, it may be difficult to comprehend how

> silence undisturbed might watch alone,
> So cold, so bright.[5]

Silence epitomizes softness in sound, and as such should not be associated with brightness. It is possible that the mediation between modalities is indirect, that silence resembles cold, and cold can be bright. Regardless of whether one can uncover a satisfactory interpretation of this particular metaphor, the point is that synesthetic metaphors need not be wholly appropriate.

All of the metaphors that I have talked about so far are *full* metaphors; they tell the reader–listener which sensory qualities are

---

[5] Percy Shelley, "Queen Mab."

supposed to correspond to which others—for instance, that cold is silent is bright. In another class, the metaphors are not fully stated. *Partial* synesthetic metaphors like "loud colors" and "bright smells" identify the sensory qualities of only a single modality. Because the metaphor is specified incompletely, the analogy is, in consequence, defined or created in part by the metaphor itself. As long as an intrinsic correspondence underlies the metaphor, its meaning will probably transfer effectively. Indeed, we may infer that the use of partial, intrinsic metaphors finds its justification in the existence of natural intermodal correspondences. It is presumably because people can comprehend what bright or silvery sounds are—that they are high pitched, relatively loud (in the case of bright sounds), perhaps staccato—that these phrases have communicative value. Shelley could not have meant just any music when he wrote of "undernotes / Clear, silver, icy, keen, awakening tones."[6] To speak of "music bright as the soul of light,"[7] as Swinburne did, is really to describe certain features of auditory experience as well through the visual mode as through the auditory mode itself, hence to rely on a tacit understanding of a fundamental unity of the senses.

Not all synesthetic metaphors carry their meanings so deftly. While one can readily appreciate what is meant by "bright cold" or "large rumble," it is much less apparent what is meant by "white flavors" or "loud stenches." Williams (1976) noted that expressions like these do crop up in the language from time to time, but tend to drop out of use. That they originate at all is interesting; perhaps their existence comes from the same creative spring of idiosyncrasy and individualism that often characterizes sensory synesthesia. In the present terminology, it is not that short-lived synesthetic transfers of meaning are uninterpretable; it is that they define rather than exemplify. The "loud perfumes"[8] that John Donne wrote of three centuries ago has not lasted as a description, whereas the (admittedly more recent) "loud colors" has. When metaphors do not endure, it may be because they have no very clear or strong synesthetic partnership. It is not obvious, for instance, whether there are such things as white flavors—Would people agree on the colors of tastes? Or maybe partnerships do exist, but are just not very salient. When Arthur Rimbaud alluded to "black perfumes,"[9] he was saying, in effect, "There exist certain odors that partake of qualities akin to blackness." In fact, when I consider what is meant by black perfumes, the

[6] "Prometheus Unbound."

[7] "Astrophel."

[8] *Elegy*, III, "The Perfume."

[9] "Le Bateau Ivre."

other adjectives that come to mind tend also to be borrowed from foreign modalities: thick, heavy, dull, etc.

Finally, there is a class of synesthetic metaphors so bereft of any explicitly stated quality that they consist primarily of a checklist, naming modalities but indicating hardly or not at all how they interrelate. Conjunctions of this sort may be called nondescriptive, in contrast to either the full and intrinsic or the partial and defined metaphors. Loud purple, bright cold, white flavor are all descriptive, in that they consist of adjectives taken from one modality and applied to another. (Note that the explicit use of adjectives per se is not necessary in order for a metaphor to be descriptive. The descriptors can be implicit, as in Kipling's analogy between dawn and thunder.) In nondescriptive metaphor, however, there is not even an implicit quality or characteristic that can readily be pointed to. Metaphors of this sort seem to fall more in the domain of poetry than of everyday speech—as exemplified by Shelley's

> *every motion, odour, beam, and tone*
> *With that deep music is in unison.*[10]

What rules characterize the synesthetic transfer of meaning? One way to analyze synesthetic transfer is in terms of suprasenory attributes like brightness, intensity, and affect. Osgood has suggested that both sensory synesthesia and verbal metaphor come about through shared connotative or affective meanings, where these meanings comprise a triumvirate of bipolar dimensions: evaluation, potency, and activity (Osgood, 1960; Osgood, Suci, & Tannenbaum, 1957). Osgood, May, and Miron (1974) suggested that both synesthesia and metaphor are likely to occur when shared affective features override contradictory denotative features. This view is correct, but, I believe, incomplete. To be sure, metaphor presupposes that something is shared, and often what is shared is a mutual connotation of good or bad, strong or weak, active or passive. But many metaphors—even some relatively simple sensory metaphors—transcend description in terms of bipolar scales.

Take the achromatic colors white and black. The difference between their assessed meanings shows up almost entirely in terms of evaluation—white as positive, black as negative (Osgood, 1964; Osgood *et al.*, 1957). But achromatic colors also bear a psychological attribute of intensity; this attribute, however, may not be picked up when only the scale's end points—white and black—are considered. The reason is that

---

[10] "Epipsychidion."

people assess both white and black as relatively intense or potent colors, gray as a nonintense or weak color (see Osgood, 1960). Hence the achromatic series black–gray–white passes from intense through weak back to intense. And so it is that in a cross-modality matching task, people may equate both black and white colors with loud sounds, but equate gray colors with soft sounds (Marks, 1974a). A simple bipolar representation is insufficient to capture this down-and-up pattern.

Both ends of the lightness domain project to a single point on an underlying ruler of intensity. This, I believe, has implication for the creative aspects of metaphor. Since a loud sound may be represented as either white or as black, the choice of representation must be determined by other considerations, such as relatively minor nuances of connotation or even denotation. Through multiple determination comes originality and creation.

Affect in Synesthetic Metaphor

If synesthetic metaphor springs from the same source as sensory synesthesia, then many of the same intersensory relationships should operate in both domains. And it is the case that suprasensory dimensions like intensity and brightness frequently do turn up in synesthetic metaphor. But in examining verbal expressions, one is struck foremost by the great many intersensory connections that are made through a common affective dimension. On the pleasant side, we find perhaps the largest single example of synesthetic transfer of meaning in the multiplied usage of the word "sweet." From the "Goodnight, sweet prince" directed at Hamlet to the pipes on Keats's Grecian urn whose "heard melodies are sweet," poetry is as chock full of sweets as the nearly extinct neighborhood candy store. As a matter of fact, it is hardly possible—for me, at least—to read much of Keats, Shelley, or especially Swinburne, without feeling inundated by sweets. Sounds and sights can be as sweet as the taste of rich chocolate, and hardly an eyebrow lifts. The usage is so common, so clearly an attempt to supply a pleasing flavor, that it may hardly be proper to speak of the metaphors as synesthetic. Only when the metaphor is drawn out, and thereby makes itself obvious *as* metaphor, does the synesthesia even become apparent, as in Swinburne's

> *Fine honey of song-notes, goldener than gold,*
> *More sweet than bees make.*[11]

[11] "Thalassius."

An entire verbal edifice may be constructed from multisensory elements held together with affective glue. Thomas Campion provides an example in his poem to rose-cheeked "Laura," a paean to visual beauty played in sound. In the first stanza appears Laura, commanded to sing

> *smoothly with thy beauty's*
> *Silent music, either other*
> *Sweetly gracing.*

The beauty (visual) sings a music (auditory) in a manner that is smooth (tactual). The poem continues by describing forms flowing in music and notes of concord and discord—assuredly a structure of sensations steeped in affect.

The pleasant taste–quality sweet has unpleasant counterparts in sour and bitter. Let me return to that timeworn expression "bitter cold." An obvious way to interpret the conjoining of these two sensory qualities is in terms of affect. According to this interpretation, the analogy between extreme cold and bitter taste resides in their common unpleasantness. Hence "bitter cold" implies unpleasantly cold. Several other usages of bitter support this contention—"with a great and exceeding bitter cry,"[12] "a bitter pill to swallow," and so forth.

Is this all? Perhaps not. If bitter is used metaphorically solely because of its unpleasant connotation, we may inquire, why is sour not used similarly? People never, or hardly ever, say "sour cold," yet sour does not seem very different, hedonically, from bitter. On the purely verbal level—and that, of course, is where we are at present—sour and bitter seem to be about equally unpleasant, at least according to the semantic judgments obtained by Osgood *et al.* (1957). It seems clear that location on the dimension of pleasantness and unpleasantness is not enough to predict why we say "bitter cold" but not "sour cold." We must search deeper into the nuances of these gustatory adjectives. For instance, when we modify the word "note" with "sour," not only do we suggest something unpleasant, but in addition we suggest something askew or awry, a quality of "just-missed" that is absent from the expression "bitter note."

What does bitter suggest that transcends mere unpalatability? What additional attribute does it share in common with cold? Burns called the cold winds of December both "snell" and "keen." Perhaps he used "keen" specifically to reinforce a second quality that applies to both bitter and cold sensations—besides unpleasantness—namely their

[12]Genesis [27:34].

sharp, biting character. According to this interpretation, bitter and cold are united, or unitable, through their common tactile quality.

Only after writing this last paragraph did I discover the curious linguistic history of "bitter" (see the *Oxford English Dictionary*). In line with the interpretation of "bitter cold" given above, the word "bitter" appears to come from the root "bîtan," which meant "to bite"; hence the root originally referred to the quality "sharp." But the word "bitter" itself came to apply solely to taste and, moreover, wholly lost its reference to a tactile property, not to regain this until Shakespeare's days when it began to modify "cold."

Of course, my interpretation of "bitter cold" may not be correct. But even if it is not right, nevertheless the main point here surely is: The nuances of the phrase "bitter cold" go beyond simply the element of common hedonics. Another example that seems to follow this notion is Keats's

> To one so friendless the clear freshet yields
> A bitter coolness.[13]

Despite the limitations just noted, there is little doubt that the gustatory adjectives sweet and bitter often are used in a cross-modal fashion at least partly because they connote pleasantness and unpleasantness. Indeed, language, especially poetic language, frequently employs the adjectives "sweet" and "bitter," much more frequently than sensory synesthesia involves the sense of taste. The transfer of taste qualities to other modalities is more often conceptual than perceptual.

Warm and Cool Colors

There is another type of cross-sensory translation that appears often in verbal metaphors, only occasionally in a true sensory form. Thermal qualities are often attributed to colors, leading to the well-known dichotomy between warm colors (yellow and red) on the one hand and cool colors (green and blue) on the other.

In the case of warm and cool colors, as in the case of sweet and bitter sounds, sensory correspondences are being expressed, but in neither case must one invoke the existence of sensory synesthesia. To speak of a sweet sound or a warm color does not demand that one taste

[13] "Endymion."

the sweetness of a violin note or feel the warmth of a yellow daisy. This is not to deny the existence in sense perception of synesthetic relations between temperature and color. Such relations do occur, as evidenced by Ginsberg's (1923) and Collins's (1929) reports of synesthetic subjects who perceived cold as white and heat as red. Some investigators have even found evidence for sensory interactions between thermal and visual stimuli. Mogenson and English (1926), for instance, reported that the color of an object held in the hand influences its apparent temperature, and Kearney (1966) noted that ambient temperature influences preferences for hue. Nevertheless, the fact that yellow and red colors are called warm, green and blue ones cool, does not seem to have its main basis in sensory synesthesia. Children are not as reliable as adults in the way they assign warmth and coolness to colors, and for this reason it has been suggested that relations between color and temperature are learned (Morgan, Goodson, & Jones, 1975). Blue–green is, after all, the usual color of lakes and oceans, red and yellow the colors of fires and heated objects. Warm and cool colors are unlike many sensory synesthesias, for the latter, I have argued, typically begin in childhood and express intrinsic cross-modal equivalences. If warmth and coolness in color do express intrinsic relations, the expressions are nevertheless as much conceptual as sensory.

Metaphors of temperature and color pervade poetry. Allusions to the "cold moon" often exemplify cool colors. For one, there is the contrast between the colors of moonlight and of sunlight, between the paler, whiter light from the moon and the yellower light from the sun. Perhaps even more basic is the regular connection between moonlight in the cool of night and sunlight in the warmth of day. Edgar Allan Poe's moonlight—the "brighter [than the stars], cold moon,"[14] the moon with "her cold smile"[15]—may represent little more than coldness of the night when the moon happens to be present.

This interpretation readily extends to metaphors of temperature and moonlight that appear in works of other poets. I discovered 11 such synesthetic metaphors in Shelley's poetry, 9 of which display a connection between moonlight and coldness: "the cold white light of morning,"[16] "the pale moonbeam . . . / Sheds a flood of silver sheen . . . / As the cold ray strays / O'er thy face,"[17] "icy moons most cold

---

[14] "Evening Star."
[15] *Ibid.*
[16] "Alastor."
[17] "To the Queen of My Heart."

and bright,"[18] "the pale, the cold, and the moony smile,"[19] "cold light of the moon,"[20] "the cold chaste Moon,"[21] "the frozen and inconstant moon,"[22] and "the cold moon sharpens her silver horn."[23] Two of Shelley's metaphors, however, suggest warmth instead—one apparently by dint of the moon's peculiar color at the time

> *yellow light, warm as the beams of day—*
> *So warm*[24]

the other apparently because of the warmth of the evening itself

> *warm light is flowing*
> *From the young moon into sunset's chasm—*
> *O, Summer eve!*[25]

This variation in metaphor is reminiscent of the way people can associate loud sounds with both black and white colors and is consistent with the idea that some correspondences between color and temperature are metaphors not based on rigid associations.

Synesthetic Metaphor in Poetry

Aside from the commonplace, prosaic, dead synesthetic metaphors of everyday speech, poetry probably is the most fruitful source of verbal synesthesia. To the extent that verbal expressions of cross-modal correspondence reflect important sensory equivalences—equivalences that are part and parcel of the nature of sensory qualities—we might expect poets to be especially well attuned to them. Poets do use synesthetic metaphors for a variety of reasons—to emphasize, to modulate, to set the tenor of a poem, or even to suggest that fundamental unifying principles operate in the universe, which may be the universe of material things, of thoughts, or of discourse. In some instances, poets generate sensory correspondences that do not reflect basic or commonly held analogies, but instead correspondences that create new meanings or illuminate previously unfamiliar relationships.

[18] "Ode to Heaven."
[19] "On Death."
[20] "The Triumph of Life."
[21] "Epipsychidion." "Moon" is probably capitalized here to symbolize Mary Godwin Shelley.
[22] "Prometheus Unbound."
[23] "The Revolt of Islam."
[24] *Ibid.*
[25] "Prince Athanase."

Synesthetic metaphor in poetry, or literary synesthesia as some call it, has come under occasional but erratic scrutiny in the past. Most investigations have focused on literary and esthetic issues (e.g., Fischer, 1907; Margis, 1910; O'Malley, 1957; Silz, 1942), although a few have been undertaken from a semantic (Ullmann, 1947, 1957) or psychological vantage point (Downey, 1912). Perhaps the most significant, and certainly one of the most detailed and comprehensive literary analyses, was performed by Siebold (1919; Erhardt-Siebold, 1932), whose major concern was the use of synesthetic imagery in the English Romantic poetry of the nineteenth century. Ullmann's (1947, 1957) work is of interest because of its general conclusion that literary synesthesia displays one main direction of semantic transfer: Words or phrases that primarily describe touch come to describe other, higher senses, especially hearing. This observation is of special relevance because it parallels Williams's (1976) conclusions about the linguistic history of synesthetic adjectives.

June Downey's (1912) study is noteworthy because of its clear psychological bent. Besides analyzing cross-sensory metaphors of several poets, Downey applied experimental method in an attempt to characterize the way readers respond to synesthetic passages. She presented synesthetic and nonsynesthetic fragments from several poets (Blake, Keats, Poe, Shelley, and Swinburne) to subjects, who were asked to judge each fragment's pleasantness. Synesthetic passages were, on the whole, judged slightly the more pleasant, but the average difference was not great. The failure to discover a sizable difference in pleasantness complements Downey's (1911) finding in a study conducted on a sensory synesthesia—colored taste. In the earlier study, Downey had concluded that affect did not provide the primary basis for the synesthetic connections between colors and taste qualities.

Yet it must be reiterated that affect sometimes *does* play a role both in sensory synesthesia and in synesthetic metaphor. A synesthetic passage might not arouse strong affective responses in readers, but affect could nonetheless form part of the passage's content. Verbal expressions of synesthesia may be so strongly steeped in affect that the emotional component serves as the link among different senses. This is true of the way that taste adjectives like sweet and bitter apply to modalities other than taste, and partly helps explain those transfers.

The linking of modalities through affect need not rely only on taste. In the following lines from Swinburne's "Birthday Ode"

> *Sounds lovelier than the light*
> *And light more sweet than song from night's own bird*

sight and sound congeal primarily on their own. As with expressions like "bitter cold," these verses hardly even deserve to be labeled as synesthetic, at least not to the extent that sight and sound are considered. For the two modalities connect not directly, but indirectly—through their common actualization of a pleasure that is potential, but not necessary. Swinburne's poetry is replete with synesthetic images, especially associations between sight and sound.

Synesthetic allusions are paradoxical. Even though synesthesia—especially what I have termed intrinsic synesthesia—reflects basic analogies and correspondences between different senses, even though it conveys some meaningful intersensory similarities, and hence entails a universal undercurrent, at the same time synesthesia is fundamentally illogical, improper, a violation of common sense (to give that term its popular meaning, not Aristotle's definition). Perhaps the character of synesthesia is a microcosm of metaphor itself, going as it does beyond ordinary meaning to new meaning. Synesthesia is a model for metaphor, as metaphor is a model for poetry.

Inherent in the use of synesthetic allusions is the danger of taking them too far, of surpassing paradox and embracing absurdity. So it is when the novelist J.-K. Huysmans (1884) has the character Jean des Esseintes orchestrate the flavors of liqueurs. So it even can be with sensory synesthesia proper; to the untutored, its patent abnormality may be not only striking but overwhelming and sometimes, it is easy enough to imagine, even amusing—as it is, for instance, when Luria's (1968) mnemonist S. describes the taste aroused by a loud, 2000-Hz tone as that of a briny pickle.

Synesthesia implies a "derangement of the senses," which in turn furnishes the potential for humor, a potential that poet or novelist may capitalize upon and use as a source of mockery. Saying this serves as a prelude to mentioning William Shakespeare's (1564–1616) funny and clever use of synesthesia in *A midsummer night's dream*—in the first scene of the fifth act, where Bottom and company undertake their play-within-a-play, the production of "The most lamentable comedy, and most cruel death of Pyramus and Thisby." As the characters carry out the play, in the finest tradition of slapstick comedy, Pyramus blunders through a mixed auditory–gustatory–visual synesthesia, focused through an alliterative lens:

> *I see a voice; now will I to the chink,*
> *To spy an I can hear my Thisby's face . . .*
> *Sweet moon, I thank thee for thy sunny beams;*
> *I thank thee, moon, for shining now so bright;*
> *For, by gracious, golden, glittering streams,*
> *I trust to taste of truest Thisby's sight.*

In the hands of Pyramus, synesthesia is humorous and ridiculous, but it is largely because Pyramus himself is ridiculous. That is, synesthesia in Pyramus sounds ridiculous, though synesthesia per se need not be. To the extent that we laugh at Shakespeare's "I trust to taste of truest Thisby's sight," but not at Keats's "The same bright face I tasted in my sleep,"[26] it is because both poets have succeeded in the poetic use of a particular cross-sensory equivalence, but they have succeeded at different tasks. Viewed in this way, there is a sense in which Shakespeare and Keats did not deal inherently with the same phenomenon. For is not Pyramus, at least in part, a predecessor of Mrs. Malaprop, a practitioner of erroneous diction, therefore not even "really" synesthetic? Is not, then, the synesthetic imagery spun by Pyramus's words a convenient device for characterizing Pyramus, rather than characterizing synesthesia?

Still, one might ask, why this device?

Relevant here is the fact that Shakespeare also used a more straightforward, which is to say nonhumorous, type of synesthetic imagery in his poetry. In Sonnet 18, for example, we discover the lines

> *Yet nor the lays of birds, nor the sweet smell*
> *Of different flowers in odour and in hue.*

And, in a similar vein, the opening scene of *Twelfth night* discloses

> *That strain again;—it had a dying fall;*
> *O, it came o'er my ear like the sweet south,*
> *That breathes upon a bank of violets,*
> *Stealing and giving odour.*

In both examples odor and music appear as central—in the former, odors are the focus, while music lies in close contiguity; in the latter, odor and music share the center stage. No trace of humor here: Instead, the second example gives a wholly serious attempt to convey the feeling of a strain of music in terms of its olfactory equivalent. A fine example this of defined synesthesia; the passage leaves little doubt about the character and style of the music—slowly executed, softly played, a distinctly Elizabethan air. Three centuries later finds its descendant in Sidney Lanier's "The Symphony," where

> *From the warm conclave of that fluted note*
> *Somewhat, half song, half odor, forth did float,*
> *As if a rose might somehow be a throat.*

Again, music is embodied in odor.

---

[26] "Endymion."

It is exceedingly rare to find olfactory experience forming a component of synesthesia in sensation. Yet odors often play a role in poetry's synesthetic metaphor. For one poet, at least—Charles Baudelaire—odors played a primary role.

Synesthesia as Doctrine—Charles Baudelaire

If there is any poet for whom the unity of the senses was a matter of doctrine, it is Charles Baudelaire (1821–1867). The intimate analogies among different senses were, to Baudelaire, a main theme. His poem "Correspondances" occupies an early location in *Les fleurs du mal*— number three in the first edition, number four in the second—and it played an important role subsequently in the history of the Symbolist movement. Central to the poem are analogies among sight, sound, and smell; I use the word "central" in two ways—both literally, in reference to the physical location of the crucial lines in the poem, and interpretively, in reference to the philosophical position that the lines express:

> *Comme de longs echos qui de loin se confondent*
> *Dans une ténébreuse et profonde unité*
> *Vaste comme la nuit et comme la clarté*
> *Les parfums, les couleurs et les sons se répondent.*

> *Il est des parfums frais comme des chairs d'enfants,*
> *Doux comme les hautbois, verts comme les prairies.*

Qualities of sense correspond because, presumably, they reflect or manifest the same underlying reality. Scents may be as fresh as children's skin, as sweet as the music of oboes, as green as fields. Odors are named first, and by dint of this primacy they become the vortices about which the analogies rotate. Perhaps the very impalpability of odors, their evanescence, made them seem to Baudelaire to be the closest that phenomenal appearance ever gets to noumenal reality. Some commentators, like Chaix (1919), have suggested that Baudelaire may actually have had an inherently superior sense of smell, or possibly that he had cultivated its use. My own suspicion is that Baudelaire was acutely aware of the peculiar, intangible character of odors. In any case, Baudelaire's doctrine is philosophical as well as psychological: Not only do sensory qualities correspond to each other, they also correspond to that ultimate reality that underlies them. Each sense serves up its own symbols of reality, but, discovers the poet, all symbols reflect a singular reality.

Similar cross-sensory analogies appear elsewhere in Baudelaire's poetry. In "Harmonie du Soir"

Les sons et les couleurs tournent dans l'air du soir.

And "Tout Entière" concludes

O métamorphose mystique
De tous mes sens fondus en un!
Son haleine fait la musique
Comme sa voix fait le parfum!

No doubt, Baudelaire's doctrine of sensory correspondences was influenced by the work of E. T. A. Hoffmann (author of the well-known *Tales*). In his own *Salon de 1846*, Baudelaire quoted, with clear approval, from Hoffmann's *Kreisleriana*:

Not only while dreaming, and in the faint delirium that precedes sleep, but also while awake, when I hear music I find an analogy and an intimate connection among colors, sounds, and odors. It seems to me that every thing has been ignited by the same ray of light, and that all reunite in marvelous concert. The odor of red and brown marigolds, above all, produces a magical effect on me. It causes me to fall into a profound reverie, whereupon I hear as from afar the dark and deep sounds of the oboe [Baudelaire, 1889, p. 93].

Here are the colors, the sounds, and the ever present, ever prominent odors.

Lest it be thought that odors always form the focus of Baudelaire's synesthetic metaphors, let me note a more "traditional" example: in the same *Salon de 1846*, an analogy between color and sound, where hues take on the characteristics of music

But immediately great blue shadows rhythmically pursue in front of them the throng of orange and fragile rose tones, which are like the distant, enfeebled echo of light. That great symphony of yesterday, that succession of melodies, where infinity generates variety, that complex hymn goes by the name of color.

In color there is harmony, melody, counterpoint [p. 89].

Still, odors often are implicated in Baudelaire's synesthetic analogies. In this respect, the Hoffmannian triplet of color, sound, and odor is typical of Baudelaire's own literary imagery, and may have been a source. One might even opine that the intersensory analogies of Baudelaire were totally derived. I suspect, however, that this is not so, but instead that Baudelaire found mirrored in Hoffmann's work a striking reflection of his own sensibility.

My suspicion is based largely on Baudelaire's account of synesthesia induced by hashish. Baudelaire appears to have been a participant, if not an actual member, of the *Club des Hachichins*, which met at the Hôtel Pimodan, on Ile Saint-Louis by the Seine in Paris, during the years shortly before the middle of the nineteenth century. The Hashish Club's illustrious members included the literary figures Théophile Gautier, Victor Hugo, Honoré de Balzac, Alexandre Dumas *père*, and Gérard de Nerval, in addition to Baudelaire. (For a lucid account, see Grinspoon, 1971.) In the strange and exotic atmosphere of the Pimodan, they ate hashish and, it would seem, some of them some of the time experienced synesthesia. That psychoactive drugs, especially mescaline and hashish, can induce synesthesia has been noted time and again (Beringer, cited by H. Werner, 1940; Delay, Gérard, & Racamier, 1951; Simpson & McKellar, 1955). Assuming that Baudelaire did, as he reported, take hashish, it is quite likely that he underwent the synesthetic experiences that he described so vividly.

Baudelaire's description of the synesthesia he experienced under hashish strongly resembles the analogies he expressed in his poetry. Of his perception under hashish, he wrote in *Les paradis artificiels*, 1860, "Odor, sight, hearing, touch participate equally . . . . Sounds cloak themselves in colors, and colors contain music [Baudelaire, 1923, p. 218]."

Should we conclude that when Baudelaire described sensory correspondences in his poetry, he did nothing more than relate real synesthetic experiences, perhaps hallucinations (a term that Baudelaire himself used), that he had while in a drugged state? Perhaps. But the source of the poetic analogies was probably deeper and less serendipitous than this. Baudelaire, much more analytical and insightful than Gautier about his synesthetic adventures, recognized clearly that nothing can be created from nothing, not even in a drugged state. What hashish does is to make more vivid those analogies that exist, albeit dormant, in normal perception:

> Sounds cloak themselves in colors, and colors contain music. This, one will say, is only natural, and every poet's brain, in its normal and healthy state, comprehends these analogies with ease [p. 218].

Baudelaire's interpretation is sympathetic with the view expressed here, namely that fundamental similarities exist across different senses, that these similarities form a basic unity of the senses, and that from them derive true synesthetic experiences as well as the perception and comprehension of elemental analogies among sensory qualities.

To Baudelaire, synesthesia did more than just illuminate the unity of the senses; in addition, it symbolized the unity of reality—as expressed, for instance, in "Correspondances." The correspondences of odors, colors, and sounds had a quasi-religious significance, or so we might conclude from Baudelaire's approbatory references to the writings of Emanuel Swedenborg, who also believed that "everything corresponds"

> There is a spiritual world, and . . . there is a natural world . . . . Natural things represent spiritual things and . . . they correspond . . . . What is natural cannot at all exist except from a cause prior to itself; its cause is from the spiritual . . . . All natural things represent things pertaining to the spiritual, to which they correspond [Swedenborg, 1751/1840, p. 56].

Swedenborg's philosophy seems to have struck an especially responsive chord in Baudelaire. In *L'art romantique* of 1846, he wrote

> [Swedenborg showed that] all form, movement, number, color, odor, in the *spiritual* as in the natural, is signifying, reciprocal, converse, *corresponding* [Baudelaire, 1923, p. 126].

The secrets of the natural world lurk in a "forest of symbols." For Swedenborg, understanding the spiritual world comes with revelation of its correspondences to the natural world. To this, Baudelaire added synesthesia—correspondences among the senses, that is, correspondences within the natural world, and hence also within the spiritual world: To decode correspondences in the natural world is simultaneously to decode correspondences in the spiritual world.

Is it surprising that descriptions of synesthesia appear prominently in the writings of several members of the Hashish Club? Like Baudelaire, Théophile Gautier (1846) wrote of his encounter with the drug. He rendered his experience of the synesthesia of musical colors in effervescent and flowery language, evidencing none of Baudelaire's critical acumen, but instead an exuberant glory in what Baudelaire called the "unaccustomed vivacity" of multimodal perception:

> The notes quivered with such power, that they entered my breast like luminous arrows; then the air being played seemed to come out from my self; my fingers moved over a nonexistent keyboard; the sounds gushed out blue and red, in electric sparks; Weber's soul had been reincarnated in me [Gautier, 1846, p. 530].

As I mentioned, Honoré de Balzac and Gérard de Nerval were members of the Club, and they too aired principles of intersensory equivalence; theirs, however, contained no direct references to hashish intoxication (nor, in fact, even any very specific cross-modal corre-spondences). What their writings do show is the quasi-religious notion of a fundamental unity between the physical and metaphysical worlds. Like Baudelaire, Balzac acknowledged Swedenborg. In the mystical novel *Séraphita*, 1835, Balzac wrote, with reference to Swedenborg,

> The Spirits exist in the secret of the harmony of creations; they resonate with the spirit of sounds, with the spirit of colors [1961, p. 96].

Similar expressions appear in Gérard de Nerval's *Aurélia*—first published just after its author's death in 1855—expressions that MacIn-tyre (1958) and Leakey (1969) noted as resembling Baudelaire's "Corre-spondances":

> From arrangements of pebbles, from angled forms, from cracks or holes, from cut-out leaves, from colors, from odors and sounds, I saw harmonies emerge that were previously unknown.
> —How, I said to myself, have I been able to live so long outside of nature, without identifying with it? Everything lives, everything acts, everything corre-sponds [Nerval, 1897, p. 93].

Surely this is not all coincidental. Something was in the air. Was it that potent green paste served in the Hôtel Pimodan? Or was it some-thing more pervasive, something in the *Zeitgeist* of the first half of the nineteenth century? Though two decades remained to pass before one saw the surge in the number of clinical reports on synesthesia, still, a few case studies had already appeared. Moreover, Swedenborg's phi-losophy had disseminated and Castel's color organ was already a cen-tury old.

In any event, to Baudelaire, as to Nerval and to Balzac, a central theme was that everything corresponds. On the phenomenal level, sounds, colors, odors correspond to one another, and, at the underlying noumenal level, there is a corresponding unity of reality, just as in Swedenborg's terms the spiritual and natural worlds correspond. Thus one might wish to interpret Baudelaire's literary doctrine of sensory correspondences not simply as the poetic expression of a Doctrine of Analogous Sensory Attributes, but as a more far-reaching and encom-passing Doctrine of Equivalent Information. The κοινα αἰσθήτα, or common sensibles, were for Baudelaire almost coextensive with sensory perception itself.

Baudelaire, if we can take him at his word, exemplifies a writer whose use of synesthetic imagery was based at least in part on primary perceptual experiences, perceptual experiences powerful and lasting enough not only to impress themselves indelibly on Baudelaire the man's consciousness but also to find their way into Baudelaire the philosopher's view of the universe. In a letter to Alphonse Toussenel dated January 21, 1856, he declared,

> Long ago, I said that the poet is *supremely* intelligent, that he is intelligence itself— and that *imagination* is the most scientific of faculties, because it alone understands *universal analogy*, or what mystical religion calls *correspondence* [1947, p. 368].

This from one who, as man and as poet, was condemned in his day as satanic, immoral, and obscene.

The unity of nature as it is apprehended through the unity of the senses was to Baudelaire more than mere metaphor; it was fundamental truth. In this respect Baudelaire stands unique among the writers whom I shall consider here. I take leave of him now, to examine the use of synesthetic language by other poets, ones who, by and large, employed multimodal imagery as metaphor.

Auditory Companions of Light and Dark—Edgar Allan Poe

The writings of Edgar Allan Poe (1809–1849) strongly influenced Baudelaire. This being so, perhaps it is not surprising to discover that synesthetic images appear prominently in Poe's poetry and prose. Though it may remain a matter of debate whether Poe's synesthetic allusions and images were actual precursors of Baudelaire's, we certainly are perfectly well able to examine Poe's multisensory imagery in its own right.

Many of Poe's synesthetic metaphors are concentrated in a single work, his early poem "Al Aaraaf." Especially notable in that work are strong associations between sound and light. For the most part, Poe's synesthetic metaphors—in "Al Aaraaf" and elsewhere—coincide with the most commonly found forms of perceptual synesthesia, reviewed in Chapter 3. A good example, from the fantastical "Al Aaraaf," is

> *All nature speaks, and ev'n ideal things*
> *Flap shadowy sounds from visionary wings*

with its allusion to sight engendering sounds. Though J. Crépet (cited by MacIntyre, 1958) mentions Poe's verses as a possible source for "Correspondances," neither in style nor in content do they resemble the synesthetic expressions of Baudelaire. The content of Poe's metaphor differs vastly from Baudelaire's. Poe's lines describe the sounds as "shadowy," as dark sounds, a far cry from the sweet sounds of oboes in Baudelaire's poem.

Sounds of darkness, sounds *as* darkness, seem to have been prominent in Poe's thought, at least as his thought is revealed in "Al Aaraaf." Later in the same poem, Poe further developed the metaphorical theme of sounds as darkness

> *Sound loves to revel in a summer night;*
> *Witness the murmur of the gray twilight*
> *That stole upon the ear in Eyraco,*
> *Of many a wild star gazer long ago—*
> *That stealeth ever on the ear of him*
> *Who, musing, gazing on the distant dim,*
> *And sees the darkness coming as a cloud—*
> *Is not its form—its voice—most palpable and loud?*

The gray twilight begins subtly, as a murmur—a dark murmur that takes shape and grows increasingly loud. The metaphor of sound giving birth to light expresses, basically, a correspondence between the increasing intensity connoted by blackness in sight and by loudness in hearing. Perceptually speaking, black is as much a sensation as is white. Blackness can be potent and intense, can "shout out" just as loudly as sound can.

Other passages in Poe's writings suggest that he was acutely sensitive to the analogies between sound and light, and in particular to the auditory accoutrements of the metamorphosis of day into night. In a footnote to Part II of "Al Aaraaf," he confided that "I have often thought I could distinctly hear the sound of darkness as it stole over the horizon." The thought resounds in "Tamerlane":

> *and will list*
> *To the sound of the coming darkness.*

Similarly, in "The Sleeper," the dim, "opiate vapor" of the "mystic moon"

> *Softly dripping, drop by drop,*
> *Upon the quiet mountain top,*
> *Steals drowsily and musically.*

Should we conclude from these statements that Poe, like (presumably) Baudelaire, perceived the world, at least on occasion, synesthetically? Maybe. But if the images of "Al Aaraaf" are representative, then Poe's synesthesia was of an extremely specific and limited sort, consisting exclusively of the association of sound with darkness. Downey (1912) considered Poe's auditory–visual metaphors to be idiosyncrasy. In this regard, one of the most interesting and, for present purposes one of the most valuable, synesthetic images to appear in Poe's writings is found in his prose dialogue "The Colloquy of Monos and Una," 1845, where, again, he acknowledges correspondences between sound and light:

> The senses were unusually active, although eccentrically so—assuming often each other's functions at random . . . . [The effect of rays of light that fell on the retina] was so far anomalous that I appreciated it only as *sound*—sound sweet or discordant as the matters presenting themselves at my side were light or dark in shade—curved or angular in outline [1938, pp. 447–448].

What is most striking here is the similarity between the nature of these intersensory bonds and the nature of intersensory bonds found in sensory synesthesia. In essence, what Poe is saying in the passage just quoted is that a *dimension* in the perception of sounds corresponds to several *dimensions* in the perception of lights. The way in which one sensation engenders another is consistent with that stated in "Al Aaraaf," in that visual stimuli provide the primary sensory qualities, whereas the auditory qualities are derivative and secondary. This order, which defines auditory vision, so to speak, is opposite to the visual hearing most often encountered in sensory synesthesia. Even though in Poe it is the visual that arouses the auditory, nevertheless the cross-modal relations themselves consist of dimensions, aligned with one another in the manner typical of synesthesia. The association between sweet and discordant sounds on the one hand, lightness and darkness on the other, suggests a common affective basis, equivalence along an evaluative dimension (cf. Osgood *et al.*, 1957). To this extent, Poe expressed not only his personal conception of cross-modal similarity (whether truly synesthetic in his sense perception or not), but also, and more importantly, an intrinsic cross-modal correspondence that strikes the reader as appropriate for the mutual reinforcement of meaning.

Insofar as Poe's synesthetic imagery conjures up these sorts of universally appreciated analogies, their effect, and the interpretation of them, differs notably from that of Baudelaire. When, for instance, Baudelaire wrote of "Odors as fresh as children's skin / Sweet as oboes, green as prairies," he did not express a multisensory correspondence that can be *directly* and *immediately* appreciated as appropriate. For the analogy with the sounds of oboes, the green grass of prairies, serves as much if not more to define what is meant by the freshness of odors—an otherwise vague description—as the quality of freshness in odors serves to arouse the appropriately analogous auditory and visual qualities. Poe's metaphors of light and sound are more fully descriptive, to use the terminology introduced earlier in this chapter.

To dichotomize in this manner presents a danger of being simplistic. There are gradations in the effectiveness with which meanings are conveyed, and there are gradations in the style of synesthetic metaphor—from fully delineated, wholly appropriate representations of intrinsic relations between sensory qualities to vague statements about the existence of correlations between different sensory modalities or sensory events. In the vast in-between sits a fertile plain of latent meanings, where various perceptual dimensions may engage one another in various ways. This is the property that H. Werner and Kaplan (1963) called "plurisignificance." From the multiplicity of pathways connecting the senses springs the possibility of creativity, of generating meaning through descriptive metaphors that select one actual from several potential cross-modal relations.

Much synesthetic language in poetry is of this sort: A sensory experience—a quality of touch or taste, of hearing or sight—is sent forth to tap some experience proper to another sensory modality, so that the one appropriates features or properties of the other, or both appropriate characteristics of each other. Neither, however, automatically or mechanically elicits the other. The transfer of meaning is defined, at least in part, by the poet's command of words, by the particular or peculiar attributes of experience that are described or suggested. Dusk adopts not any sound: Edwin Arlington Robinson beckons us to see and hear the

> Dark hills at evening in the west,
> Where sunset hovers like a sound
> Of golden horns.[27]

Falling rain comes in many varieties, but Conrad Aiken meant only one when he wrote that he "heard one night the rain / Weaving in silver an intricate pattern of pain."[28] Cross-modal meanings are selected or imposed as well as expressed, may be defined or proposed, culled out

[27] From "The Dark Hills" by Edwin Arlington Robinson. In *Collected poems*; copyright 1920 by Edwin Arlington Robinson, renewed 1948 by Ruth Nivison. Reprinted by permission of Macmillan Publishing Co. Contrast Conrad Aiken's "Night falls with a shrill of horns; or is it daybreak" from "The Jig of Forslin."

[28] From "The Jig of Forslin" by Conrad Aiken. In *Collected poems*; copyright © 1953, 1970 by Conrad Aiken. Reprinted by permission of Oxford University Press.

from the system of delitescent meanings and connotations that the reader brings along.

This distinction between what might be called intrinsic and extrinsic synesthetic meaning is fundamental. *Intrinsic* synesthesia expresses what is already known, even if much of the time only implicitly known. The cross-modal associations are always present, ready to be tapped. *Extrinsic* synesthesia expresses correspondences that may not be already known, that certainly are not salient. When extrinsic synesthetic imagery makes the reader or listener aware of new relations between modalities, relations that can be accepted and appreciated, the poet is successful.

Any individual poet may, of course, either stick to a single type or indulge in both extrinsic and intrinsic cross-modal metaphors. Poe, I would contend, leaned toward using the defined, but intrinsic. In "the murmur of the gray twilight," the analogy between soft sound and slight darkness appears immediately to be appropriate. What about the darkness as "palpable and loud?" One might argue this also is intrinsic, that when darkness is greater, so is loudness. Very nearly the same analogies appear in W. S. Merwin's "The Annunciation." At the start

> *the darkness began: it brushed*
> *Just lightly first, like it might be the wing*
> *Of a bird.*[29]

But soon the darkness wells, as the soft touch of twilight yields to oncoming power

> *and the blackness*
> *Of their shadow growing as they came down*
> *Whirring and beating, cold and like thunder, until*
> *All the light was gone.*[30]

As I said, I interpret Poe's and Merwin's metaphors as intrinsic. This interpretation hinges on Poe's contrast between gray and darkness, on Merwin's contrast between darkness and blackness. Grayness, darkness, and blackness express different degrees of visual intensity, and because they do they have natural analogues in soft and loud sounds. That light colors as well as dark colors correspond to loud sounds means that the relation between brightness and loudness is not always monotonic. Intermediate grays are soft, but blackness as well as brightness or whiteness can be loud. Merwin's black shadow and Kipling's dawn both well up like thunder.

---

[29]From "The Annunciation" by W. S. Merwin. In *The first four books of poems*. Copyright © 1955, 1956, 1975 by W. S. Merwin. Reprinted by permission of Atheneum Publishers.
[30]*Ibid.*

This account should not be taken to imply that Poe's synesthetic metaphors are restricted completely to intrinsic connections, or even to analogous qualities of sound and light. One metaphor, at least, also found in "Al Aaraaf," lies so far to the other extreme as to be distinctly nondescriptive:

> Fair flowers, and fairy! to whose care is given
> To bear the Goddess' song, in odors, up to Heaven.

Little in the way of intrinsic synesthesia in this couplet! Indeed, the cross-modal similarity is so amorphous, its basis so obscure, the lines much resemble some of Shelley's—for instance, his

> old wild songs which in the air
> Like homeless odours floated.[31]

Yet despite occasional forays outside the realm of light and sound, the most significant of Poe's synesthetic metaphors explore the connections between the seen and the heard. Whether these connections were so prominent in Edgar Allen Poe's perceptual experience as to permit calling him synesthetic is really not so important. What is important is the fact that Poe's synesthetic metaphors, by and large, rely on fundamental intersensory relations that readily communicate to the reader.

After Baudelaire: Rimbaud, Huysmans, de Maupassant

It is appropriate here to point out again Arthur Rimbaud's (1854–1891) explicit statement about the colors of vowels. In his "Sonnet des Voyelles," Rimbaud charged each primary vowel with a different color: "A noir, E blanc, I rouge, U vert, O bleu." Now, it is true that people with sensory synesthesia often perceive vowel sounds as colored; but, as I have already noted, the particular associations that Rimbaud asserted do not match up very well with typical correspondences between vowels and colors encountered in synesthesia (compare Table 3.2, p. 88). It is somewhat difficult to know just how to interpret Rimbaud. Was he synesthetic? Where did he get vowel colors from? The associations he gives surely do not qualify as intrinsic or appropriate, because they are not generally acknowledged, not even by those synesthetic

---

[31]"The Revolt of Islam."

individuals who claim to perceive colors in vowels. Yet to call them extrinsic or defined seems to pervert the sense in which I have employed those terms, because even as defined the associations seem not to carry any special meaning. Perhaps the best guess is that Rimbaud was mostly playing a little game, exercising his imagination. In "Une Saison en Enfer," published in 1873, 2 years after "Sonnet des Voyelles," he not only restated the intersensory associations, but went on to say that the colors of the vowels were his *invention*

> I was inventing the colors of the vowels!—A black, E white, I red, O blue, U green—I controlled the form and movement of every consonant, and, with instinctive rhythms, it pleased me to invent a poetic language accessible, one day or other, for all the senses. I reserved translation [Rimbaud, 1937, p. 285].

Rimbaud's "invention" brings to mind a similar exercise—the nonsense verse of Antonin Artaud (1896–1948), which contains lines like "par ertin / tara / tara bulla / rara bulla / ra para hutin."[32] Artaud said that he wrote "in a language which is not French, but which everyone could read, whatever his nationality" (cited by Shattuck, 1976). Sounds, it seems, held within themselves secret meanings for Artaud, maybe as they did for Rimbaud.

At least small mention should be made of two *fin de siècle* French writers: Joris-Karl Huysmans (1848–1907) and Guy de Maupassant (1850–1893). Works of both display important synesthetic passages: Huysmans's fiction is replete with sensory imagery. Although one can find what may be called traditional, or at least Baudelairian, synesthetic language in some of his writing—for instance, his phrase about "the green sounds of harmonicas [Huysmans, 1895, p. 2]"—nevertheless the most famous of Huysmans's synesthetic passages is quite untraditional. This is his outrageous description of the musical synesthesia that tastes aroused in Jean des Esseintes, the "hero" of *A rebours* (1884):

> Each liquor corresponded, individually, by its taste, to an instrument's sound. Dry curaçao, for example, to a clarinet whose song was bitter and mellow; kummel to an oboe with sonorous and nasal tones; mint and anisette to a flute, at once sugary and peppery, piquant and sweet; and to complete the orchestra, kirsch rang furiously on the trumpet [p. 62].

The presumed analogies continue in subsequent paragraphs, as Huysmans explores the possible taste–music of quartets and quintets, of major and minor keys.

So striking a passage screams out for elucidation. Unfortunately,

---

[32] "Emission."

there is little to be said. It is bizarre, almost surely intentionally so. Auditory taste is far from being a common form of synesthesia, and the unusual associations perceived by des Esseintes strike no particularly responsive chord in the reader. The tone is mock-serious, which thwarts any willing suspension of disbelief, and whimsical, which makes the passage border on burlesque.

In marked contrast stands a synesthetic passage from Maupassant's *La vie errante* (1890), where, under intoxication, lights, sounds, odors all intermingle, but in a distinctly Baudelairian manner, with none of Huysmans's brashness:

> It was the land's wind that rose, laden with breaths from the coast, and that also carried out toward the open sea that vagabond harmony, mingling there with the odor of alpine plants.
>
> I remained gasping, so drunk of sensation, that the turmoil of that intoxication made my senses delirious. I truly no longer knew if I breathed music, or if I heard perfumes, or if I slept among the stars [p. 18].

The passage in itself shows Maupassant's debt to Baudelaire and Rimbaud; but if this is not enough, the indebtedness is demonstrated beyond any doubt in subsequent pages, where Maupassant quotes directly both "Correspondances" and "Sonnet des Voyelles." Here, in Maupassant's writing, however, the interrelations of color, sound, odor are not doctrinal, certainly not the way they are for Baudelaire. Synesthesia is an appendage instead of a vital organ, *logos* instead of philosophy, mere metaphor instead of metaphor.

Synesthetic Metaphors of Odor and Music—Percy Bysshe Shelley

Among the most extensive portrayals of the scents of music are those disclosed in the poems of Percy Shelley (1792–1822). For this reason, it is to Shelley that I shall now turn.

The poetry of nineteenth century England—especially the poetry of the so-called Romantics—reveals some of the finest examples of synesthetic metaphor in literature. And the poetry of Shelley reveals some of the finest examples of literary synesthesia in the English Romantic period. With Shelley, as with Baudelaire, odors play a signal role. Olfactory images abound in Shelley's verse and, not surprisingly, also in his synesthetic metaphor. The imagery is often vague, emotional in tone, and even then often emotional in only a general way. Where Shakespeare was specific, Shelley was diffuse. How does a strain of music appear? Like "the sweet south [wind] that breathes upon a bank of violets"? Not to Shelley. Instead, he writes

> *Such sounds as breathed around like odourous winds*
> *Of awakening spring arose,*
> *Filling the chamber and the moonlight sky.*[33]

The quintessential synesthetic image in Shelley's poetry plunges the reader into a mélange of sensations, where ingredients from several senses blend into an affective batter

> *And every motion, odour, beam, and tone*
> *With that deep music is in unison.*

This last couplet comes in the midst of a section in "Epipsychidion" that basks in perceptual imagery, including other synesthetic imagery, a section where Shelley lyrically recounts an imaginary island paradise, captivating in its beauty and unspoiled purity. In the couplet just quoted, a quadruplet of senses link together—kinesthesia (movement sense), smell, sight, hearing—but with no specific analogies. Everything corresponds.

The problem is, when everything corresponds, nothing corresponds. To say that anything corresponds is to acknowledge that something else does not.

To be sure, Shelley was able to be more specific, detailing at times what it is that corresponds

> *And the hyacinth purple, and white, and blue,*
> *Which flung from its bells a sweet peal anew*
> *Of music so delicate, soft, and intense,*
> *It was felt like an odour within the sense.*[34]

Here, the poet names colors, and the sounds of music are readily imaginable. Through defined synesthetic metaphor, some characteristics of the odor come through—fragrant, light rather than musky, yet compact. Even more specific, perhaps, are these musical scents that Shelley brews out of the nightingale's song

> *and soon her strain*
> *The nightingale began; now loud,*
> *Climbing in circles the windless sky,*
> *Now dying music; suddenly*

[33] "The Daemon of the World."
[34] "The Sensitive Plant."

'Tis scattered in a thousand notes,
And now to the hushed ear it floats
Like field smells known in infancy.[35]

The flight of sound first rises in a crescendo, then falls in a decrescendo that musters faint and familiar smells buried deep in memory.

I have already suggested that there is a relation between how specific or vague is a synesthetic metaphor, on the one hand, and how extrinsic or intrinsic it is, on the other. At one end stand wholly diffuse and unspecified intersensory associations, as when "every motion, odour, beam, and tone / With that deep music is in unison." Here, the rule goes: The more vague the metaphor, the more its effectiveness must rely on intrinsic correspondences. To communicate metaphorical meaning, reader and poet must share common ground, must agree— even if only implicitly—on the rules governing analogy across the senses. Otherwise, the intended meaning will not be communicated. (Of course, a poet is never guaranteed that the meaning will be communicated, just as a reader is never guaranteed that any meaning exists to be communicated.)

At the other extreme stand precisely specified intersensory associations. Given that the poet spells out the analogy, two possibilities emerge. For one, the analogy may conform to an intrinsic connection, as when Joseph Auslander's allusion to "the silver needle-note of a fife" taps a brightness common to sight, touch, and sound. Alternatively, the analogy may create an extrinsic association, as when Conrad Aiken's allusion to "flute notes seen / Now are red and now are green"[36] forges a relation between sound and color.

Whether synesthetic metaphor, like Gaul, is properly divided into three parts can only be conjecture at present. I do not submit the tripartite division as a complete account. One might argue, for instance, that synesthetic metaphors that are not specific can nonetheless be extrinsic. Without clear exposition of precisely what corresponds in different modalities, it may be difficult to be sure if intrinsic associations are intended, or even if they exist.

Back now to Shelley: Allusions to smells—to odor sensations and perceptions, to their qualities and the emotions they evoke—play a prominent role in his poetry in general and in his literary synesthesia in particular. His contemporary John Keats's (1795–1821) poetry, by way of contrast, displays a greater emphasis on taste, including taste synesthesia—as evidenced by phrases like "the same bright face I tasted

---

[35] "Rosalind and Helen."

[36] From "Music" by Conrad Aiken. In *Collected poems*; copyright © 1953, 1970 by Conrad Aiken. Reprinted by permission of Oxford University Press.

in my sleep,"[37] "to taste the gentle moon,"[38] and "taste the music of that vision pale,"[39] among others. The poetry of Shelley and of Keats, it might be argued, discloses an important development, namely increasing freedom from an informational poetry of two sense modalities and movement toward an affective poetry of many modalities. To the extent that perceptual images were important to the English poetry of the eighteenth century, the prime media were sight and hearing. These two modalities are, of course, the senses typically considered most important to daily commerce. There is no comparison between the trauma and terror that accompany blindness or deafness and the more benign reactions that accompany loss of smell or taste. Eyes and ears guide us through the world to such a degree that, it seems fair to say, for most of us the universe is formed largely of visual brick and auditory mortar. Other senses, especially active touch, can be important, but often in different ways and not really to the same extent.

What are the functions of smell, taste, temperature, pain? In large measure, we use these senses to help regulate important biological functions and maintain the body's health and integrity. Taste and smell channel eating and drinking, sensations of warmth and cold modulate the behavioral regulation of body temperature, pain mediates the avoidance of injury. Although the informational components of these senses are important to the way they function, it is not primarily the abstract information that is of overriding value, but instead the motivation induced by affect.

The poetry of Shelley and Keats serves generous helpings of imagery from the affective senses. The expanded use of gustatory and olfactory imagery was an important step historically, but that is not the concern here. What is, is the interrelation of sensory imagery, affect, and synesthesia. The affective component of synesthesia, both in its perceptual and in its literary forms, has already been noted. Analogies between senses can be imparted by innuendoes of pleasantness or unpleasantness. At the conclusion to Shelley's "To Jane: 'The Keen Stars Were Twinkling'," a common, unifying emotion bridges the gulf between sound and light

> *A tone*
> *Of some world far from ours,*
> *Where music and moonlight and feeling*
> *Are one.*

[37] "Endymion."
[38] *Ibid.*
[39] "Isabella."

There are several ways in which affect creeps into literary synesthesia. In one, the emotional mood or tone comes first, expressing itself
simultaneously in several sense modalities and by doing so providing
the source for the intersensory link. In another, the emotion comes
second, like an epiphenomenon to some other mode of correspondence.
Affect engenders synesthesia in a number of Shelley's metaphors. Consider

Sweet streams of sunny thought and flowers fresh-blowing
Are there, and weave their sounds and odours into one.[40]

It is the "sunny thought" that delineates the character of the sounds and
odors. Later in the same poem Shelley continues with a synesthesia
born in emotion, to which the poet then welds an added component of
almost playful delicateness

slowly there is heard
The music of a breath-suspending song,
Which, like the kiss of love when life is young,
Steeps the faint eyes in darkness sweet and deep;
With ever-changing notes it floats along,
Till on my passive soul there seemed to creep
A melody, like waves on wrinkled sands that leap.

To give one final example of this sort, consider the more vibrant and
potent emotions underlying

In thy dark eyes a power like light doth lie,
Even though the sounds which were thy voice, which burn
Between thy lips, are laid to sleep;
Within thy breath, and on thy hair, like odour, it is yet,
And from thy touch like fire doth leap.[41]

But as I said, even when common affective feelings permeate the
sensory correspondences, these feelings need not be the cause of the
link; instead, something else may be the primary cause, the feelings
only a by-product. To be sure, when sensory images that share intensity or brightness happen also to evoke similar pleasurable or un-
pleasurable responses, the link between the images will be that much
stronger. This is exemplified in the couplet

---

[40] "The Revolt of Islam."
[41] "To Constantia, Singing."

> *And odours warm and fresh fell from her hair*
> *Dissolving the dull cold in the frore air* [42]

and perhaps also in the lines

> *this is the mystic shell;*
> *See the pale azure fading into silver*
> *Lining it with a soft yet glowing light;*
> *Looks it not like lulled music sleeping there?* [43]

Actually, good examples of this second sort are harder to come by—in Shelley's poetry—than are examples of the first sort, where affect itself forms the link. For the sensory images are rarely specific in Shelley (as they almost always are specific in Keats). Moods frequently dominate Shelley's imagery, specific sensory attributes themselves hinted at, when hinted at at all, by those moods.

Let me return to the observation that odors turn up often in Shelley's synesthetic metaphors. Some idea of this may be gleaned from Table 8.1, which compiles the cross-modal associations found in 87 striking examples of synesthetic metaphor in his poetic language. Eighty-seven may seem a rather small number of excursions into cross-modal analogy, especially given the size of Shelley's output (in the Oxford edition of his poetry, a total of more than 20,000 lines—this in a life that spanned only three decades). These 87 do not necessarily constitute all of Shelley's synesthetic metaphors. The relatively small number may be attributed in part to my use of a stringent criterion for accepting a poetic image as synesthetic; had I used a looser criterion, the number would be much greater. For one thing, I specifically omitted all examples of synesthetically dead sensory adjectives like "sharp" and "sweet," though one might argue that these examples should be included. In addition, I rejected those verses that contain nothing more than conjunctions of several senses. An example of the latter is

> *The quivering vapours of the dim noontide,*
> *Which like a sea o'er the warm earth glide,*
> *In which every sound, and colour, and beam,*
> *Move, as reeds in a single stream.* [44]

This and others like it were omitted because in them the various senses coexist, but in no way interact, or even interrelate.

[42] "Epipsychidion."
[43] "Prometheus Unbound."
[44] "The Sensitive Plant."

Table 8.1

Cross-modality associations in the poetic metaphors of Percy Bysshe Shelley

Two-modality metaphors

	Vision	Hearing	Smell	Taste	Touch	Tempera-ture	Pain
Vision		38	3	0	1	12	0
Hearing			7	0	2	6	0
Smell				0	0	3	0
Taste					0	1	1

Three-modality metaphors
Vision–Hearing–Smell	4
Vision–Hearing–Touch	1
Vision–Hearing–Temperature	3
Vision–Hearing–Pain	1
Smell–Touch–Pain	1

Four-modality metaphors
Vision–Hearing–Smell–Temperature	1
Vision–Hearing–Touch–Temperature	1

Five-modality metaphor
Vision–Hearing–Smell–Touch–Temperature	1

As Table 8.1 shows, 20 of the 87 metaphors involve olfaction—whereas, by contrast, 7 involve touch and only 2 involve taste. What makes this most striking is the fact that, according to Ellis's (1892) concordance, variants of the word "odour" appear a total of only 67 times in all of Shelley's poetry. Of the 20 synesthetic metaphors involving smell, 15 actually mention the scents through variants of the word "odour." Hence a goodly portion of Shelley's images of odor are synesthetic.

Having said this, I feel obliged to point out that, in terms of absolute numbers, most of Shelley's synesthetic metaphors do not involve odors. It is their relative, not their absolute, frequency that attracts attention: One olfactory image adds texture, but two or three capture the reader's notice. In fact, most of Shelley's synesthetic images involve sight and sound, sans smell. To Shelley's ear, music and song seem to have conjured up vibrant visual cousins—in "Music" one hears the command to

> *Pour forth the sound like enchanted wine,*
> *Loosen the notes in a silver shower.*

The "silver shower" is a river through air, a rapid flow of brilliant, sharp notes.

Shelley's synesthetic imagery of sound and light attains perhaps its fullest expression in the ode "To a Skylark." That "blithe Spirit" the skylark soars up through the sky, free, like the poetic imagination itself, singing as it soars. Though the skylark flies so high it cannot even be seen, its voice reaches the earth with a rich intensity:

> *All the earth and air*
> > *With thy voice is loud,*
> *As, when night is bare,*
> > *From one lonely cloud*
> *The moon rains out her beams, and Heaven is overflowed.*

So loud and clear is the skylark's melody, it resembles the bright moon set out against the bare, black night. The same analogy is reinforced in the next stanza, where the poet convinces us that

> *From rainbow clouds there flow not*
> > *Drops so bright to see*
> *As from thy presence showers a rain of melody.*[45]

The analogy between song and light is no mere addition to the poem, but neither is the analogy itself the theme. Instead, the synesthesia of sound and light integrally relates to the theme—of freedom, of "illumination"; Fogle (1949) argued that the synesthetic imagery of Shelley, and that of Baudelaire, is a means to an end. The correspondence between sound and light in the "Skylark" ode appears to be totally natural, hardly forced or unusual, the epitome of expression of an intrinsic relationship between two modalities.

Light in Music, Music in Light—Algernon Charles Swinburne

When Shelley and Keats work synesthetic metaphors into their poetry, they use the metaphors judiciously and with control. In the poetry of Swinburne (1837–1909), control is all but lost as the imagery effervesces and bubbles over. The poetic language bespeaks intent:

---

[45] Compare George Meredith's "The Lark Ascending," where the skylark's song is a "silver chain of sound, . . . / As up he wings the spiral stair, / A song of light."

Both a seemingly self-conscious construction of individual images and a
pulling together of disparate ones pervade Swinburne's verse. There are
places, in "Thalassius," for instance, where the poet states directly the
cross-modal equivalence of sensory experiences, usually experiences of
sight and sound:

> And heard from above afar
> A noise of songs and wind enamoured wings
> And lutes and lyres of milder and mightier strings,
> And round the resonant radiance of his car
> Where depth is one with height,
> Light heard as music, music seen as light.

Swinburne's poetry is sometimes accused of being diffuse and
imprecise. Indeed, to T. S. Eliot's (1920/1950) thinking, this diffuseness
is one of Swinburne's glories. If this is so, then it would seem that
Swinburne reaches his pinnacle of glory when he waxes synesthetic. To
hear the light as music, to see the music as light, in and by itself
conveys virtually nothing additional in the way of meaning. Yet
analogies and, beyond analogies, syntheses of light and sound turn up
time and again, exhaling undefined, amorphous clouds—in "Dirae,"
the phrase "visible music," and in "Epilogue," its cousin "visible
sound, light audible." Sometimes, the vagueness suggests a unity of
the senses, where "light, sound and life are one,"[46] and where sense
modalities interconnect through a philosophic core, in a monism reminiscent of Shelley

> Summer, and noon, and a splendour of silence, felt,
> Seen, and heard of the spirit within the sense.[47]

It would be a serious error, though, to conclude too hastily that all
of Swinburne's synesthetic images are loosely put together, vague, and
poorly defined as to what sensory qualities correspond. On the contrary, many passages exemplify principles of the sort that have already
been considered. Swinburne was able to pinpoint, at least sometimes,
analogous qualities of light and sound, qualities that express intrinsic
perceptual correspondences. Brightness, an attribute common to both
sight and hearing, provides one transition from sense modality to sense
modality:

> And now the heaven is dark and bright and loud.[48]

[46] "On the Cliffs."
[47] "A Nympholept."
[48] "In the Bay."

The intersensory equivalences develop further: Music virtually dances as it takes on visual characteristics to marry the auditory

> *Music bright as the soul of light, for wings an eagle,*
> *for notes a dove,*
> *Leaps and shines from lustrous lines where through thy*
> *soul from afar above*
> *Shone and sang till darkness rang with light whose fire*
> *is the fount of love.*[49]

The common intersensory dimension that mediates the correspondence is, again, brightness.

Brightness was not Swinburne's only specific vehicle for synesthetic metaphor. In vision, brightness also equals intensity, and the mutual intensity of light and sound forms a basis for synesthetic analogy. In a passage reminiscent of Kipling's "dawn comes up like thunder," Swinburne wrote of daybreak:

> *Beneath a heavier light*
> *Of stormier day or night*
> *Began the music of the heaven of dawn;*
> *Bright sound of battle along the Grecian waves,*
> *Loud light of thunder above the Median graves.*[50]

Here sound and light are hopelessly intertwined, as the dawn sweeps up into the sky with a roar.

Swinburne's verse shows examples of other principles enunciated in the present work. One is the binding of different senses through a common affective quality or response. Light and scent combine with sound, and all join to sing in a multisensory harmony

> *Where the sound and light of sweetest songs still*
> *float and shine.*
> *Here the music seems to illume the shade, the light*
> *to whisper*
> *Song, the flower to put not odours only forth, but*
> *words*
> *Sweeter far than fragrance.*[51]

A significant feature of the poetic effect is the musical beauty of the verse itself, reinforcing the analogy among three senses.

Often, it is simply the two modes of sound and light whose similar-

---

[49] "Astrophel."
[50] "Birthday Ode."
[51] "Athens."

ity is expressed in terms of common affective or esthetic components. The auditory, Swinburne reminds us, like the visual can be lovely. In his "Birthday Ode," it is the "sounds of love-songs lovelier than the light"; earlier in the same poem he wrote of

> Sounds lovelier than the light
> And light more sweet than song from night's own bird.[52]

Let me point out an interesting fact. In these examples taken from Swinburne, and in previous examples taken from other poets, where senses are linked by means of an equivalent or common expression of affect, the affect or emotion has almost always been positive. Nearly always, it seems to be a feeling of pleasure that ties senses together. This need not be so; it is perfectly possible for negative emotions to bind together different senses. If "sweet streams of sunny thought and flowers fresh-blowing" can "weave their sounds and odours into one," if light can be "more sweet than song," then so can discords stink, and odors clash like sour notes. Negative tones can, and sometimes do, capture sensory qualities, as in the opening lines of Swinburne's "A Match," which contrast negative and positive:

> If love were what a rose is,
> And I were like the leaf,
> Our lives would grow together
> In sad or singing weather,
> Blown fields or flowerful closes
> Green pleasure or grey grief.

Because we are talking about the use of metaphor in poetry, the question is not whether or how often negative affect actually does serve as a basis for synesthesia in its perceptual form; instead, the question is why poets—or at least, those poets considered here—choose to use a preponderance of positive moods as links in their synesthetic images. Part of the answer doubtless lies in the subject matter. Poets write, much of the time, of pleasantries: It is not that they choose positive moods to enact synesthetic metaphors, but that they choose synesthetic metaphors to dramatize positive moods. But I suspect a full answer goes deeper than this. Frequently, there is a suggestion that the positive affect or pleasure underlying different sensory experiences is not just a subjective response or phenomenal appearance, but moreover that it manifests an intrinsic characteristic of the objects or events themselves, embodying an esthetic that transcends mere perception. As I have indicated, one way to interpret Baudelaire's poem "Correspondances"

---

[52] This harks back to Shelley's "Adonais," where "there is heard / His voice in all her music, from the moan / Of thunder, to the song of night's sweet bird."

is as a philosophical statement—that perfumes, sounds, and colors speak to one another at two levels: The synesthetic metaphor expresses not only unity of sensory experience, but unity at the level of some underlying reality. If Baudelaire's poem is a good model, then it suggests that a few instances, at least, where synesthetic metaphors come by way of positive affect can also be read as philosophical statements. Swinburne's "Hawthorne Dyke" gives an example, as the psychological merges into the philosophical; the poet, in his experience,

> Finds the radiant utterance perfect, sees the word
> Spoken, hears the light that speaks it. Far and near
> All the world is heaven; and man and flower and bird
> Here are one at heart with all things seen and heard.

The unity of nature through the unity of the senses is distinctly Baudelairian. According to McGann (1972), Swinburne's poetry tries to reveal the organization of nature through relationships. Given this view, we might say that synesthesia provides one means whereby interrelations reveal reality.

Before leaving Swinburne, I would like to mention his use of music in synesthetic metaphor. Often, when sounds serve as one component of synesthetic metaphor in poetry, the sounds are musical or described as if they are musical (just as music serves as one of the most potent stimuli for arousing synesthesia in perception). I have already cited, to give but two examples, Lanier's description of the "fluted note [that] / Somewhat, half song, half odor, forth did float" and Shelley's "pale azure fading into silver / Lining it with a soft yet glowing light / . . . like lulled music." In the former, music takes on qualities of odor; in the latter, a visual image takes on qualities of music.

As I just said, in people predisposed to experience synesthetic perception, music is an especially effective stimulus for stirring visual and other imagery. Karwoski, Odbert, and Osgood (1942) asked nonsynesthetic individuals to evaluate pieces of music, and found that the evaluations strongly resembled the relations underlying musical synesthesia. Nonsynesthetic people characterize music with "synesthetic" qualities. Music, then, appears to touch a highly responsive intersensory nerve.

The purpose of this brief review was to lead up to the following point—that poems about music can provide a rich vein of synesthetic ore. Consider Swinburne's brief ode on "Music." All three of its five-line stanzas begin with synesthetic metaphors. Two themes dominate them. The first is an analogy between music bursting forth out of silence and dawn bursting forth out of the night. Indeed, this is how the ode begins, with the rhetorical query

> Was it light that spake from the darkness, or music that shone
>   from the word,
> When the night was enkindled with sound of the sun or the
>   first-born bird?

Prominent here is the characteristic of intensity or perhaps brightness, not stated directly, but nevertheless clearly implied. The music "shone from the word," just as the night was "enkindled with sound." Music, the light of the sun, shoots forth its rays, showing itself to be closely related to Poe's light rays that fall like sound on the retina.

The metaphor repeats in the second stanza's opening lines

> Music, sister of sunrise, and herald of life to be,
> Smiled as dawn on the spirit of man

and again, in the third stanza's first phrase "Morning spake." But immediately the image changes, from day to night, from sun to moon

> and soft from the mounting moon
> Fell the sound of her splendour, heard as dawn's in the breath-
>   less night.

From here the poem moves to its second synesthetic theme, an analogy between visual and musical harmonies, suggesting another unity of sight and sound. As the ode concludes, harmony melts into the spirit of day and night

> And the song of it spake, and the light and the darkness
>   of earth were as chords in tune.

To summarize, light comes forth like a song, defining a spatial pattern of light and dark that mimics the harmony of a musical chord. Patterns of light flow one to another like a melody of chords. What is left unclear, however, is precisely what this pattern of light and dark is like. Does the poet mean a blending of one into the other, with soft, muted edges; or is it a crispness of outline, the flickering of shadowed forms that often pass their brief life in the morning air?

The Music of the Spheres

If a momentary pattern of light and shade, a static array that a snapshot can capture in full, suggests the harmony of music, what effect is produced by a dynamic pattern, a changing array that requires a motion picture? Spatial patterns moving through time, some say, re-semble melody as well as harmony. Indeed, this very analogy seems to possess the fancy of poets in virtually every generation, especially when they inspect a clear sky at night, a sky that looks almost alive with speckles of light. Pythagoras is usually credited with coining the phrase *the music of the spheres* to indicate the celestial pattern of planets, stars, and moons tumbling against the matte black night. The relative posi-tions of one orb to another—and the ways they change in location over time—are akin to the harmonies and melodies of music.

References to the music of the spheres—and embellishments on it—appear throughout world literature, from Chaucer and Dante through Shakespeare and Milton on down to Byron and Poe. Both melody and harmony of light were noted by Geoffrey Chaucer in *Parle-ment of foules*

> *And after shewede he hym the nyne speres;*
> *And after that the melodye herde he,*
> *That comyth of thilkè speres thryes thre,*
> *That welle is of musik and melodye*
> *In this world here and cause of armonye.*

The stars and planets course through the sky in a regular and systematic fashion, with the mathematical constraints of motion that also charac-terize the structure of music. To say this is to confess that the "music of the spheres" is not nearly so much a sensory similarity as it is a cognitive abstraction, that it is not so much a quality common to immediate experience of lights and tones as it is an appreciation of equivalent patterns and orderings. The abstract character of this simi-larity asserts itself in Sir Thomas Browne's (*Religio Medici,* 1642) elegant statement

> For there is musick wherever there is a harmony, order, or proportion; and thus far we may maintain the musick of the sphears; for those well-ordered motions and regular paces, though they give no sound unto the ear, yet to the understanding they strike a note most full of harmony.

The Music of Conrad Aiken

I want to return now to the more immediate, sensory qualities of music, so as to consider the synesthetic imagery of a contemporary poet—Conrad Aiken (1889–1973). Music pervades Aiken's verse on several levels, from the repeated allusions to music and its properties in the poetic texts to the very structural organization of some of the poems themselves. Themes weave musical patterns through the verse, one challenging and displacing another as in counterpoint. At the level of synesthetic metaphor, the reader discovers, amidst the images of music, a variety of analogies to other sense modalities. These run a wide gamut, ranging from relatively concrete associations between musical qualities and colors to more abstract relationships like some of those found in elaborations on the music of the spheres.

Aiken's "Music" exemplifies the concrete, with its opening lines describing the colors of musical notes

> The calyx of the oboe breaks,
> Silver and soft the flower it makes.
> And next, beyond, the flute-notes seen
> Now are white and now are green.[53]

Specific though they are, these images contrasting the silvery and soft notes of the oboe with the white and green notes of the flute, they are not characteristic of the way Aiken handles music in synesthetic metaphor. Only the last line intimates their quintessential property in his poetry, which is metamorphosis. By and large, the music of Conrad Aiken flows, the melodies rise and ebb in "intricate patterns." Music clearly plays a central role in the poetry, for music not only saturates the air, it actually saturates the poetic universe. If this musical current is epitomized anywhere, it is in the series of long poems called *The divine pilgrim*. "The Jig of Forslin" finds the poet ruminating how

> Things mused upon are, in the mind, like music,
> They flow, they have a rhythm, they close and open,
> And sweetly return upon themselves in rhyme.
> Against the darkness they are woven,
> They are lost for a little, and laugh again,
> They fall or climb.[54]

Music characterizes the process and content of thinking, especially of dreaming. "Mused" and "music" are close in sound, and brought close in meaning, despite their different roots. "We bear our dreams," wrote Aiken, "among us, bear them all, / Like hurdy-gurdy music they

---

[53]From "Music" by Conrad Aiken. In *Collected poems*; copyright © 1953, 1970 by Conrad Aiken. Reprinted by permission of Oxford University Press.
[54]From "The Jig of Forslin" by Conrad Aiken. In *Collected poems*; copyright © 1953, 1970 by Conrad Aiken. Reprinted by permission of Oxford University Press.

rise and fall." [55] The tapestry of mental life is like a complex music, a music of themes and variations that rise and fall in slow, rhythmic repetition and counterpoint, a music whose notes weave fine threads of multifarious color. Movements through time, rhythms and repetitions of music, parallel both the flow of the stream of consciousness and a braid of color laid out in space:

> *The violins were weaving a weft of silver,*
> *The horns were weaving a lustrous brede of gold.*[56]

Contrariety begets assimilation. The bright silver melody of the violins contrasts with the mellow golden song of the horns, yet both are woven music, woof and braid. Things thought of, like music, are woven against the blackness: Rain falling through night air can be heard "weaving in silver an intricate pattern of pain." When, near the end of "The Jig of Forslin" Forslin sits alone, meditating as

> *The music weaves about him, gold and silver;*
> *The music chatters, the music sings,*
> *The music sinks and dies*[57]

it is, again, time and change that predominate. The world is born in music and dies in music, the golden song of day is transformed, transmuted into the silver melody of night, in what the poem described previously as an "alchemy of sound."

Aiken's music is dynamic, never static. Even a stationary visual scene emerges in musical motion; when

> *The world lay luminous;*
> *Every petal and cobweb trembled music,*[58]

the visible glow is heard as tremolo. This is symptomatic. Earlier in the

---

[56] *Ibid*. How much more precise than Shelley's homologous lines in "Alastor": "Her voice was like the voice of his own soul / Heard in the calm of thought, its music long, / Like woven sounds of streams and breezes, held / His inmost sense suspended in its web / Of many-coloured woof and shifting hues."

[58] *Ibid*.

poem, a voice is described as "a breaking of golden ripples." Not any motion, not just change for its own sake, but regular motions, the rhythms of the mental universe, speak in music, these rhythms "that take the blood with magic, / Smoothing it out in silver," rhythms that "die in the brain's dark chambers / Like a blowing fragrance."

Correspondences between sound and light, between patterns in music and patterns in color, play a thematic role. Yet neither sound nor light alone truly dominates the poetry, for neither vision nor hearing emerges as the major modality. If there is a primary modality it is not a sensory one at all, but instead imagination or consciousness. Sound—especially music—generates sight by way of the sine qua non, creative imagination; but it is the imagination itself that gives the impetus, shaping sound into form:

> The music, as you lie sleeping,
> Builds a world of hills and stars about you,
> Cities of silver in forests of blue![59]

Perhaps there is some parallel here to Baudelaire, to the notion of an underlying reality—in Aiken, the creative springs of the mind—that symbolically expresses itself through a synesthetic unity of the senses.

The Metaphorical Imperative

One thing is clear: Synesthetic metaphor in poetry far transcends the relative simplicity of perceptual synesthesia. Another thing is equally clear: Metaphor in poetry far transcends the relative simplicity of everyday synesthetic language. Yet these connect one to another, synesthesia to synesthetic language to metaphor. Fundamental to cognitive activity, to the process of thinking, is that we extend the limits of our comprehension. Metaphor is a main means to this end, if it is not an end in itself. Metaphor is a means to disclose new analogies and equivalences. As Wallace Stevens wrote, "The proliferation of resemblances extends an object [1951, p. 78]." Metaphor snares independent threads and weaves them into a coherent fabric. Mind follows a metaphorical imperative, seeking out relationships that entwine disparate phenomena and events.

Metaphor's secret lies in the fact that once an analogy is made between A and B, a whole gamut of associated meanings also become

---

[59]From "The Pilgrimage of Festus" by Conrad Aiken. In *Collected poems*; copyright © 1953, 1970 by Conrad Aiken. Reprinted by permission of Oxford University Press.

available. Not only is B like A in a certain way, but any and all of A's properties now become fair game to be absorbed into B. And so the process of metaphorization may proceed, through C, D, E, and so on, linking together formal and abstract as well as concrete aspects of phenomena that formerly were disparate.

It is tempting to try to account for the process of metaphorization by means of a well-established psychological principle, namely, stimulus generalization. Such an account, however, merely restates the facts without explicating them. To be sure, metaphor implies equivalence, and the process of stimulus generalization implies that a common response is made to external events that are, by definition, partially equivalent; but the crux of the matter is how to derive the equivalence itself. Stimulus generalization provides not an explanation but a name. Two essential questions remain: Why metaphor? Why particular metaphors?

I shall not presume to try to explain metaphor. What I shall try, though, is to indicate briefly some significant psychological features of metaphor. How do meanings transfer synesthetically from one sensory modality to another?

Undaunted by the matter-of-fact way that the world is laid out, the creative understanding—the imagination, if you will—asserts its cognitive control by participating actively in the process of comprehending. It measures reality by testing resemblances. Much as scientists seek to examine nature by confronting it empirically and constructing models (metaphors) of the outcome of these confrontations, so children seek to comprehend their world through whatever cognitive skills they have available. It is convenient to utilize here Bruner's (1964) characterization of mental growth. An infant tests the simple properties of the physical world, such as the permanence of objects, by reaching, grasping, pushing, and by doing so measures how self-generated motor acts influence the environment; a young child tests by perceiving, by transforming perceptions into images, and by operating on these iconic representations; an older child tests by listening and speaking, and by manipulating the symbolic representations that words provide.

Because more children than adults exhibit sensory synesthesia, it is likely that many synesthetic children lose their synesthesia when they grow up. This makes me suspect that synesthesia is a characteristic of the processes that dominate cognitive growth's perceptual or iconic stage. Like perception in general, synesthesia is a direct and economical means of cognitive organization. But it is limited by being inflexible, as well as poorly discriminating and imprecise. Though the meanings borne by synesthesia are salient, they are at the same time restrictive and intractable. Flexibility requires symbolization, that is, language; so, as mental structures develop—and symbolic, linguistic abilities increase—the connections between senses transfer from synesthetic perception to synesthetic language.

A price is paid for this: As language becomes more and more significant, and cognition comes to rely more and more on verbal signs, perceptual relations decrease in salience. Lost is much of the richness of synesthetic perception, gained is an increased capacity for manipulating symbols and making metaphors. The natural correspondences governed by the unity of the senses provide one basis for discovering potential interrelations, for "extending objects." No longer must analogies be limited to fixed, synesthetic relationships.

The verve with which children use language to explore the latent structure of reality strikingly reveals itself in Kenneth Koch's *Wishes, lies, and dreams* (1970). Koch recounts his endeavor to engage elementary-school children in writing poetry. Comparisons and metaphors play a prominent role in children's verbal explorations, these no doubt galvanized by the poet Koch's impetus. It is particularly notable how readily children grasp the possibilities made available through synesthetic transfer of meaning:

> In giving the Color Poem, for instance, I asked them to close their eyes; then clapped my hands and asked them what color that was. Almost everyone raised his hand: "Red!" "Green!" "White!" [p. 30].

The children often put synesthesia into their poems, using images such as "red as a beating of drums" and "white as screaming out." Also clearly demonstrated was a sensitivity to nuances of sound—sound symbolism—as evidenced by Koch's remark that "I asked them to close their eyes and listen while I said 'night' and then '*la noche.*' I asked them what color each word was, and which was darker (*La noche* turned out to be darker, and more purple) [p. 45]."

The synesthetic, like the metaphoric in general, expands the horizon of knowledge by making actual what were before only potential meanings. What makes both synesthesia and metaphor potent and cogent is their succinctness, the fact that they provide a dense cognitive code, a shorthand that captures some kernel of resemblance and at the same time opens gates to a host of additional relationships. The economy of synesthesia, to which I referred in an earlier study (Marks, 1975), is reminiscent of Freud's (1905) homologous analysis of wit, which, he concluded, always consists of saying something in too few words, with an "economy of expenditure." Meanings, whether synesthetic or otherwise, are dynamic, in flux, metamorphosizing—

"desiring the exhilarations of changes," to use Wallace Stevens's phrase—for the end point of the search for signification usually, maybe necessarily, is unknown. From this derives the impulse to seek

> the hammer
> Of red and blue, the hard sound—
> Steel against intimation—the sharp flash,
> The vital, arrogant, fatal, dominant X.[60]

To discover synesthesia among the roots of metaphor is not surprising. Sensory qualities are concrete, and thus specific, yet they contain a nugget of the general—or at least what can be generalized. The unity of the senses creates a network of suprasensory attributes, of dimensions common to all senses, that enter first in the act of perception, then in the act of linguistic representation.

The story is almost ended. I have tried to uncover the path, sometimes hidden, that traces the course of the unity of the senses from sensation and perception to verbal expressions of synesthetic metaphor, and I have tried to show how synesthetic metaphor might serve more generally as a model for metaphor. The steps are exposed and bared, revealing the fabric of the mental tapestry richly woven in form and color, sound, taste, touch, and scent.

[60]From "The Motive for Metaphor" by Wallace Stevens. Copyright 1948 by Wallace Stevens. Reprinted from *The collected poems of Wallace Stevens*, by permission of Alfred A. Knopf, Inc.

References

Abbott, T. K. *Sight and touch: An attempt to disprove the received (or Berkelian) theory of vision.* London: Longman, Green, Longman, Roberts & Green, 1864.

Abravanel, E. The development of intersensory patterning with regard to selected spatial dimensions. *Monographs of the Society for Research in Child Development,* 1968, *33,* Whole No. 18.

Abravanel, E. Active detection of solid-shape information by touch and vision. *Perception and Psychophysics,* 1971, *10,* 358–360. (a)

Abravanel, E. The synthesis of length within and between perceptual systems. *Perception and Psychophysics,* 1971, *9,* 327–328. (b)

Abravanel, E. How children combine vision and touch when perceiving the shape of objects. *Perception and Psychophysics,* 1972, *12,* 171–175.

Adrian, E. D. The all-or-none principle in nerve. *Journal of Physiology,* 1914, *47,* 460–474.

Adrian, E. D. The impulses produced by sensory nerve endings. Part I. *Journal of Physiology,* 1926, *61,* 49–72.

Adrian, E. D., & Matthews, R. The action of light on the eye. Part 1:The discharge of impulses in the optic nerve and its relation to the electric changes in the retina. *Journal of Physiology,* 1927, *63,* 378–414.

Aiken, C. *Collected poems.* New York: Oxford University Press, 1953.

Aitkin, L. M. Medial geniculate body of the cat: Responses to tonal stimuli of neurons in the medial division. *Journal of Neurophysiology,* 1973, *36,* 275–283.

Albe-Fessard, D., & Besson, J. M. Convergent thalamic and cortical projections—The non-specific system. In A. Iggo (Ed.), *Handbook of sensory physiology,* Vol. II. *Somatosensory systems.* Berlin: Springer-Verlag, 1973. Pp. 489–560.

257

Alexander, K. R., & Shansky, M. S. Influence of hue, value, and chroma on the perceived heaviness of colors. *Perception and Psychophysics*, 1976, *19*, 70–74.

Allen, W. F. Formatio reticularis and reticulo-spinal tracts, their visceral functions and possible relationships to tonicity and clonic contractions. *Journal of the Washington Academy of Sciences*, 1932, *22*, 490–495.

Amoore, J. E. Evidence for the chemical olfactory code in man. In W. S. Cain (Ed.), *Odors: Evaluation, Utilization, and Control. Annals of the New York Academy of Sciences*, 1974, *237*, 137–143.

Anschütz, G. Untersuchungen zur Analyse musikalischer Photismen. *Archiv für die Gesamte Psychologie*, 1925, *51*, 155–218.

Anschütz, G. Untersuchungen über komplexe musikalische Synopsie. *Archiv für die Gesamte Psychologie*, 1926, *54*, 129–273.

Anstis, S. M., & Loizos, C. M. Cross-modal judgments of small holes. *American Journal of Psychology*, 1967, *80*, 51–58.

Argelander, A. *Das Farbenhören und der synästhetische Faktor der Wahrnehmung*. Jena: Fischer, 1927.

Aristotle. *The works of Aristotle*, edited by W. D. Ross. Oxford: Clarendon Press, 1931.

Arnheim, R. *Visual thinking*. Berkeley: University of California Press, 1969.

Aronson, E., & Rosenbloom, S. Space perception in early infancy: Perception within a common auditory-visual space. *Science*, 1971, *172*, 1161–1163.

Asch, S. E. On the use of metaphor in the description of persons. In H. Werner (Ed.), *On expressive language*. Worcester, Massachusetts: Clark University Press, 1955. Pp. 29–38.

Attneave, F., & Benson, B. Spatial coding of tactual stimulation. *Journal of Experimental Psychology*, 1969, *81*, 216–222.

Atweh, S. F., Banna, N. R., Jabbur, S. J., & To'mey, G. F. Polysensory interactions in the cuneate nucleus. *Journal of Physiology*, 1974, *238*, 343–355.

Auerbach, C., & Sperling, P. A common auditory–visual space: Evidence for its reality. *Perception and Psychophysics*, 1974, *16*, 129–135.

Austin, J. L. *Sense and sensibilia*. Oxford: Clarendon Press, 1962.

Balzac, H. de. *Séraphita*, 1835. In *Oeuvres complètes*, Tome 21. Paris: Le Prat, 1961. Pp. 41–164.

Baratoux, J. De l'audition colorée. *Le Progrès Médical*, 1887, *6*, 495–496, 515–517, 538–539.

Barber, C. L. An essay on the sonnets. In *The sonnets of William Shakespeare*. New York: Dell, 1960.

Barlow, H. B. Retinal noise and absolute threshold. *Journal of the Optical Society of America*, 1956, *46*, 634–639.

Barlow, H. B. Single units and sensation: A neuron doctrine for perceptual psychology? *Perception*, 1972, *1*, 371–394.

Baudelaire, C. *L'art romantique*, 1846. In *Oeuvres complètes de Charles Baudelaire*, Tome 4. Paris: Gallimard, 1923.

Baudelaire, C. *Les fleurs du mal*. Paris: Calmann-Lévy, 1857.

Baudelaire, C. *Les paradis artificiels*, 1860. In *Oeuvres complètes de Charles Baudelaire*, Tome 3. Paris: Gallimard, 1923.

Baudelaire, C. *Salon de 1846*. In *Curiosités esthétiques*. Paris: Calmann-Lévy, 1889.

Baudelaire, C. *Correspondance général*, 1833–1856. In J. Crépet (Ed.), *Oeuvres complètes de Charles Baudelaire*, Tome 1. Paris: Conard, 1947.

Beaunis, H., & Binet, A. Sur deux cas d'audition colorée. *Revue Philosophique*, 1892, *33*, 448–460.

Behar, I., & Bevan, W. The perceived duration of auditory and visual intervals: Cross-modal comparison and interaction. *American Journal of Psychology,* 1961, 74, 17–26.

Békésy, G. von. Human skin perception of traveling waves similar to those on the cochlea. *Journal of the Acoustical Society of America,* 1955, 27, 830–841.

Békésy, G. von. Neural volleys and the similarity between some sensations produced by tones and by skin vibrations. *Journal of the Acoustical Society of America,* 1957, 29, 1059–1069. (a)

Békésy, G. von. Sensations on the skin similar to directional hearing, beats and harmonics of the ear. *Journal of the Acoustical Society of America,* 1957, 29, 489–501. (b)

Békésy, G. von. Funneling in the nervous system and its role in loudness and sensory intensity on the skin. *Journal of the Acoustical Society of America,* 1958, 30, 399–412.

Békésy, G. von. Similarities between hearing and skin senses. *Psychological Review,* 1959, 66, 1–22. (a)

Békésy, G. von. Synchronism of neural discharges and their demultiplication in pitch perception on the skin and in hearing. *Journal of the Acoustical Society of America,* 1959, 31, 338–349. (b)

Békésy, G. von. *Experiments in hearing.* New York: McGraw-Hill, 1960.

Békésy, G. von. Pitch sensation and its relation to the periodicity of the stimulus. Hearing and skin vibrations. *Journal of the Acoustical Society of America,* 1961, 33, 341–348.

Békésy, G. von. Lateral inhibition of heat sensations on the skin. *Journal of Applied Physiology,* 1962, 17, 1003–1008.

Békésy, G. von. Interaction of paired sensory stimuli and conduction in peripheral nerves. *Journal of Applied Physiology,* 1963, 18, 1276–1284.

Békésy, G. von. Olfactory analogue to directional hearing. *Journal of Applied Physiology,* 1964, 19, 369–373. (a)

Békésy, G. von. Rhythmical variations accompanying gustatory stimulation observed by means of localization phenomena. *Journal of General Physiology,* 1964, 47, 809–825. (b)

Békésy, G. von. Mach band type lateral inhibition in different sense organs. *Journal of General Physiology,* 1967, 50, 519–532. (a)

Békésy, G. von. *Sensory inhibition.* Princeton: Princeton University Press, 1967. (b)

Békésy, G. von. Similarities of inhibition in the different sense organs. *American Psychologist,* 1969, 24, 707–719.

Békésy, G. von. Auditory backward inhibition in concert halls. *Science,* 1971, 171, 529–536.

Bentley, M., & Varon, E. J. An accessory study of "phonetic symbolism." *American Journal of Psychology,* 1933, 45, 76–86.

Berkeley, G. *An essay toward a new theory of vision.* Dublin: Pepyat, 1709.

Berkeley, G. *A treatise concerning the principles of human knowledge.* Dublin: Pepyat, 1710.

Bignall, K. E., & Imbert, M. Polysensory and cortico-cortical projections to frontal lobe of squirrel and rhesus monkeys. *Electroencephalography and Clinical Neurophysiology,* 1969, 26, 206–215.

Binet, A., & Philippe, J. Étude sur un nouveau cas d'audition colorée. *Revue Philosophique,* 1892, 33, 461–464.

Birch, H. G., & Lefford, A. Intersensory development in children. *Monographs of the Society for Research in Child Development,* 1963, 128, Whole No. 89.

Björkman, M. Relations between intra-modal and cross-modal matching. *Scandinavian Journal of Psychology,* 1967, 8, 65–80.

Black, M. *Models and metaphors: Studies in language and philosophy.* Ithaca, New York: Cornell University Press, 1962.

Blakeslee, P., & Gunter, R. Cross-modal transfer of discrimination learning in cebus monkeys. *Behaviour,* 1966, 26, 76–90.

Blank, M., & Bridger, W. H. Cross-modal transfer in nursery-school children. *Journal of Comparative and Physiological Psychology,* 1964, *58,* 277–282.

Blank, M., & Klig, S. Dimensional learning across sensory modalities in nursery school children. *Journal of Experimental Child Psychology,* 1970, *9,* 166–173.

Bleuler, E., & Lehmann, K. *Zwangsmässige Lichtempfindungen durch Schall und verwandte Erscheinungen.* Leipzig: Fues' Verlag, 1881.

Börnstein, W. On the functional relations of the sense organs to one another and to the organism as a whole. *Journal of General Psychology,* 1936, *15,* 117–131.

Börnstein, W. S. Perceiving and thinking: Their interrelationship and organismic organization. *Annals of the New York Academy of Sciences,* 1970, *169,* 673–682.

Borg, G., Diamant, H., Ström, L., & Zotterman, Y. The relation between neural and perceptual intensity. A comparative study on the neural and psychophysical response to taste stimuli. *Journal of Physiology,* 1967, *192,* 13–20.

Boring, E. G. An operational restatement of G. E. Müller's psychophysical axioms. *Psychological Review,* 1941, *48,* 457–464.

Boring, E. G., & Stevens, S. S. The nature of tonal brightness. *Proceedings of the National Academy of Sciences,* 1936, *22,* 514–521.

Bornstein, M. H. Qualities of color vision in infancy. *Journal of Experimental Child Psychology,* 1975, *19,* 401–419.

Bouman, M. A. Peripheral contrast thresholds of the human eye. *Journal of the Optical Society of America,* 1950, *40,* 824–832.

Bouman, M. A., & van der Velden, H. A. The two-quanta explanation of the dependence of the threshold values and visual acuity on the visual angle and the time of observation. *Journal of the Optical Society of America,* 1947, *37,* 908–919.

Bower, T. G. R., Broughton, J. M., & Moore, M. K. The coordination of visual and tactual input in infants. *Perception and Psychophysics,* 1970, *8,* 51–53.

Boynton, R. B., & Onley, J. W. A critique of the special status assigned by Brindley to "psychophysical linking hypotheses" of "Class A." *Vision Research,* 1962, *2,* 383–390.

Brindley, G. S. *Physiology of the retina and visual pathway.* London: Arnold, 1960.

Brown, R. W., Black, A. H., & Horowitz, A. E. Phonetic symbolism in natural languages. *Journal of Abnormal and Social Psychology,* 1955, *50,* 388–393.

Brown, R., & McNeill, D. The "tip of the tongue" phenomenon. *Journal of Verbal Learning and Verbal Behavior,* 1966, *5,* 325–337.

Brown, R., & Nuttall, R. Method in phonetic symbolism experiments. *Journal of Abnormal and Social Psychology,* 1959, *59,* 441–445.

Browne, T. *Religio Medici.* London: Crooke, 1642.

Brugge, J. F., & Merzenich, M. M. Patterns of activity of single neurons of the auditory cortex in monkey. In A. R. Moller (Ed.), *Basic mechanisms in hearing.* New York: Academic Press, 1973. Pp. 745–766.

Bruner, J. S. The course of cognitive growth. *American Psychologist,* 1964, *195,* 1–15.

Bruner, J. S., & Koslowski, B. Visually preadapted constituents of manipulatory action. *Perception,* 1972, *1,* 3–14.

Bryant, P. E., Jones, P., Claxton, V., & Perkins, G. M. Recognition of shapes across modalities by infants. *Nature,* 1972, *240,* 303–304.

Buffardi, L. Factors affecting the filled-duration illusion in the auditory, tactual, and visual modalities. *Perception and Psychophysics,* 1971, *10,* 292–294.

Bujas, Z. La mesure de la sensibilité différentielle dans le domaine gustatif. *Acta Instituti Psychologica, Universitatis Zagrebensis,* 1937, *11,* 3–18.

Bullough, E. On the apparent heaviness of colours. *British Journal of Psychology,* 1907, *2,* 111–152.

Buranelli, V. *Edgar Allan Poe*. New York: Twayne, 1961.

Burton, D., & Ettlinger, G. Cross-modal transfer of training in monkeys. *Nature*, 1960, *186*, 1071–1072.

Buser, P., & Imbert, M. Sensory projections to the motor cortex in cats: A microelectrode study. In W. A. Rosenblith (Ed.), *Sensory communication*. New York: Wiley, 1961. Pp. 607–626.

Butters, N., & Brody, B. A. The role of the left parietal lobe in the mediation of intra- and cross-modal associations. *Cortex*, 1968, *4*, 328–343.

Cain, W. S. Differential sensitivity for smell: "Noise" at the nose. *Science*, 1977, *195*, 796–798.

Carlson, K. R., & Eibergen, R. Factors influencing the acquisition of tactual random figure discriminations by rhesus monkeys. *Animal Learning and Behavior*, 1974, *2*, 133–137.

Carreras, M., & Andersson, S. A. Functional properties of neurons of the anterior ectosylvian gyrus of the cat. *Journal of Neurophysiology*, 1963, *26*, 100–126.

Cashdan, S. Visual and haptic form discrimination under conditions of successive stimulation. *Journal of Experimental Psychology*, 1968, *76*, 215–218.

Cassirer, E. *The philosophy of symbolic forms*, Vol. 1. *Language*. New Haven, Connecticut: Yale University Press, 1953.

Castel, L.-B. Clavecin par les yeux, avec l'art de Peindre les sons, & toutes sortes de Pieces de Musique. *Mercure de France*, 1725, n.v., 2552–2577.

Castel, L.-B. Nouvelles experiences d'Optique & d'Acoustique. *Mémoires pour l'Histoire des Sciences et des Beaux Arts*, 1735, n.v., 1444–1482; 1619–1666; 1807–1839; 2018–2053; 2335–2372; 2642–2768.

Cattell, J. M. On errors of observations. *American Journal of Psychology*, 1893, *5*, 285–293.

Chaix, M.-A. *La correspondance des arts dans la poésie contemporaire*. Paris: Alcan, 1919.

Chandler, K. A. The effect of monaural and binaural tones of different intensities on the visual perception of verticality. *American Journal of Psychology*, 1961, *74*, 260–265.

Claparède, E. Persistance de l'audition colorée. *Comptes Rendus de la Société de Biologie*, 1903, *55*, 1257–1259.

Clavière, J. L'audition colorée. *L'Année Psychologique*, 1898, *5*, 161–178.

Clynes, M. Sentography: Dynamic forms of communication of emotion and qualities. *Computers in Biology and Medicine*, 1973, *3*, 119–130.

Cohen, N. E. Equivalence of brightnesses across modalities. *American Journal of Psychology*, 1934, *46*, 117–119.

Coleridge, S. T. *Biographia literaria*, Vol. II. London: Pickering, 1847.

Collins, M. A case of synaesthesia. *Journal of General Psychology*, 1929, *2*, 12–27.

Connolly, K., & Jones, B. A developmental study of afferent-reafferent integration. *British Journal of Psychology*, 1970, *61*, 259–266.

Coriat, I. H. A case of synesthesia. *Journal of Abnormal Psychology*, 1913, *8*, 38–43. (a).

Coriat, I. H. An unusual case of synesthesia. *Journal of Abnormal Psychology*, 1913, *8*, 109–112. (b)

Craig, J. C. Vibrotactile loudness addition. *Perception and Psychophysics*, 1966, *1*, 185–190.

Craig, J. C. Difference threshold for intensity of tactile stimuli. *Perception and Psychophysics*, 1972, *11*, 150–152.

Craig, J. C. Vibrotactile difference thresholds for intensity and the effect of a masking stimulus. *Perception and Psychophysics*, 1974, *15*, 123–127.

Crocker, E. C., & Henderson, L. F. Analysis and classification of odors. *American Pefumery*, 1927, *22*, 325–327, 356.

Crozier, W. J., & Holway, A. H. On the law for minimal discrimination of intensities. I. *Proceedings of the National Academy of Sciences*, 1937, *23*, 23–28.

Czurda, M. Beziehungen zwischen Lautcharakter und Sinneseindrücken. *Wiener Archiv für Psychologie, Psychiatrie, und Neurologie,* 1953, *3,* 73–84.

Davenport, R. K., & Rogers, C. M. Intermodal equivalence of stimuli in apes. *Science,* 1970, *168,* 279–280.

Davenport, R. K., & Rogers, C. M. Perception of photographs by apes. *Behaviour,* 1971, *39,* 318–320.

Davis, H. Peripheral coding of auditory information. In W. A. Rosenblith (Ed.), *Sensory communication.* New York: Wiley, 1961. Pp. 119–141.

Davis, H. Relations of peripheral action potentials and cortical evoked potentials to the magnitude of sensation. In H. R. Moskowitz, B. Scharf, & J. C. Stevens (Eds.), *Sensation and measurement: Papers in honor of S. S. Stevens.* Dordrecht, Netherlands: Reidel, 1974. Pp. 37–47.

Davis, H., Bowers, C., & Hirsh, S. K. Relations of the human vertex potential to acoustic input: Loudness and masking. *Journal of the Acoustical Society of America,* 1967, *43,* 431–438.

Davis, H., & Kranz, F. W. International audiometric zero. *Journal of the Acoustical Society of America,* 1964, *36,* 1450–1454.

Davis, H., Osterhammel, P. A., Wier, C. C., & Gjerdingen, D. B. Slow vertex potentials: Interactions among auditory, tactile, electric and visual stimuli. *Electroencephalography and Clinical Neurophysiology,* 1972, *32,* 537–545.

Davis, R. The fitness of names to drawings. *British Journal of Psychology,* 1961, *26,* 259–268.

Delattre, P., Liberman, A. M., Cooper, F. S., & Gerstman, L. J. An experimental study of the acoustic determinants of vowel color; Observations on one- and two-formant vowels synthesized from spectrographic patterns. *Word,* 1952, *8,* 195–210.

Delay, J., Gérard, H.-P., & Racamier, P.-C. Les synesthésies dans l'intoxication mescalinique. *L'Encéphale,* 1951, *40,* 1–10.

De Rochas, A. L'audition colorée. *La Nature,* 1885, Pt. 1, 306–307, 406–408; Pt. 2, 274–275.

Deutsch, B. *This modern poetry.* New York: Norton, 1935.

De Vries, H., & Stuiver, M. The absolute sensitivity of the sense of smell. In W. A. Rosenblith (Ed.), *Sensory communication.* New York: Wiley, 1961. Pp. 159–167.

Dowling, J. E. The site of visual adaptation. *Science,* 1967, *155,* 273–279.

Downey, J. E. A case of colored gustation. *American Journal of Psychology,* 1911, *22,* 528–539.

Downey, J. E. Literary synesthesia. *Journal of Philosophy, Psychology, and Scientific Methods,* 1912, *9,* 490–498.

Dubner, R. Interaction of peripheral and central input in the main sensory trigeminal nucleus in the cat. *Experimental Neurology,* 1967, *17,* 186–202.

Dubner, R. T., & Rutledge, L. T. Recording and analysis of converging input upon neurons in cat association cortex. *Journal of Neurophysiology,* 1964, *27,* 620–634.

Dudycha, G. J., & Dudycha, M. M. A case of synesthesia: Visual-pain and visual-audition. *Journal of Abnormal and Social Psychology,* 1935, *30,* 57–69.

Efron, R. Conservation of temporal information by perceptual systems. *Perception and Psychophysics,* 1973, *14,* 518–530.

Eijkman, E., & Vendrik, A. J. H. Can a sensory system be specified by its internal noise? *Journal of the Acoustical Society of America,* 1965, *37,* 1102–1109.

Eliot, T. S. Swinburne as poet, 1920. In *Selected essays.* New York: Harcourt, Brace and World, 1950.

Ellis, F. S. *A lexical concordance to the poetical works of Percy Bysshe Shelley.* London: Quaritch, 1892.

Empson, W. *Seven types of ambiguity* (Revised Ed.). New York: New Directions, 1947.

Erhardt-Siebold, E. von. Harmony of the senses in English, German, and French Romanticism. *Publications of the Modern Language Association,* 1932, *47,* 577–592.

Ettlinger, G. Cross-modal transfer of training in monkeys. *Behaviour,* 1960, *16,* 56–65.

Ettlinger, G. Learning in two sense-modalities. *Nature,* 1961, *191,* 398.

Ettlinger, G., & Blakemore, C. B. Cross-modal matching in the monkey. *Neuropsychologia,* 1967, *5,* 147–154.

Exner, S. Experimentelle Untersuchung der einfachsten psychischen Processe. *Pflügers Archiv für die Gesammte Physiologie,* 1875, *11,* 403–432.

Fechner, G. T. *Elemente der Psychophysik.* Leipzig: Breitkopf und Härtel, 1860.

Fechner, G. T. *Vorschule der Aesthetik.* Leipzig: Breitkopf und Härtel, 1876.

Féré, C. *La pathologie des emotions.* Paris: Alcan, 1892.

Fessard, A. The role of neuronal networks in sensory communications within the brain. In W. A. Rosenblith (Ed.), *Sensory communication.* New York: Wiley, 1961. Pp. 585–606.

Field, G. *Aesthetics, or the analogy of the sensible sciences indicated; with an appendix on light and colors.* London: 1820.

Fischer, O. Über Verbindung von Farbe und Klang. Eine literar-psychologische Untersuchung. *Zeitschrift für Ästhetik,* 1907, *2,* 501–534.

Fishman, M. C., & Michael, C. R. Integration of auditory information in the cat's visual cortex. *Vision Research,* 1973, *13,* 1415–1419.

Flournoy, T. L'audition colorée. *Archives des Sciences Physiques et Naturelles,* 1892, *28,* 505–508.

Flournoy, T. *Des phénomènes de synopsie.* Paris: Alcan, 1893.

Fogle, R. H. *The imagery of Keats and Shelley.* Chapel Hill: University of North Carolina Press, 1949.

Folkins, C., & Lenrow, P. An investigation of the expressive values of graphemes. *Psychological Record,* 1966, *16,* 193–200.

Forbes, A., & Gregg, A. Electrical studies in mammalian reflexes: II. The correlation between strength of stimulation and the direct and reflex nerve response. *American Journal of Physiology,* 1915, *39,* 172–235.

Ford, J. M., Roth, W. T., Dirks, S. J., & Kopell, B. S. Evoked potential correlates of signal recognition between and within modalities. *Science,* 1973, *181,* 465–466.

Foster, J. L. On translating Hieroglyphic love songs—I. *Chicago Review,* 1971, *23*(2), 70–94; *23*(3), 95–112.

Freeman, K. *Ancilla to the pre-Socratic philosophers.* Oxford: Blackwell, 1948.

Freud, S. *Der Witz und seine Beziehung zum Unbewussten.* Leipzig und Wien: Deuticke, 1905.

Frye, N. *Anatomy of criticism.* Princeton: Princeton University Press, 1957.

Fuortes, M. G. F. Generation of responses in receptor. In W. R. Lowenstein (Ed.), *Handbook of sensory physiology,* Vol. I. *Principles of receptor physiology.* Berlin: Springer-Verlag, 1971, Pp. 243–268.

Galambos, R. The human auditory evoked response. In H. R. Moskowitz, B. Scharf, & J. C. Stevens (Eds.), *Sensation and measurement: Papers in honor of S. S. Stevens.* Dordrecht, Netherlands: Reidel, 1974. Pp. 215–221.

Galambos, R., & Davis, H. The response of single auditory-nerve fibers to acoustic stimulation. *Journal of Neurophysiology,* 1943, *6,* 39–57.

Galileo Galilei. *Il Saggiatore nel quale con bilancia esquisita e qiusta si ponderano le cose contenute uella Libra astronomica. . . .* Roma: Giacomo Mascardi, 1623.

Galton, F. *Inquiries into human faculty and its development.* London: Macmillan, 1883.

Garner, W. R. Effect of frequency spectrum on temporal integration in the ear. *Journal of the Acoustical Society of America*, 1947, *19*, 808–815.

Garver, L. N., Gleason, J. M., & Washburn, M. F. The source of affective reactions to articulate sounds. *American Journal of Psychology*, 1915, *26*, 292–295.

Gautier, T. Le Club des Hachichins. *Revue des Deux Mondes*, 1846, *13*, 520–535.

Gaydos, H. F. Intersensory transfer in the discrimination of form. *American Journal of Psychology*, 1956, *69*, 107–110.

Geldard, F. A. The saltatory effect in vision. *Sensory Processes*, 1976, *1*, 77–86.

Geldard, F. A., & Sherrick, C. E. The cutaneous "rabbit": A perceptual illusion. *Science*, 1972, *178*, 178–179.

Gescheider, G. Auditory and cutaneous temporal resolution of successive brief stimuli. *Journal of Experimental Psychology*, 1967, *75*, 570–572.

Gescheider, G. A., & Niblette, R. K. Cross-modality masking for touch and hearing. *Journal of Experimental Psychology*, 1967, *74*, 313–320.

Geschwind, N. Disconnexion syndromes in animals and man. *Brain*, 1965, *88*, 237–294.

Gibson, E. J. *Principles of perceptual learning and development.* New York: Appleton-Century-Crofts, 1969.

Gibson, J. J. Adaptation, after-effect, and contrast in the perception of curved lines. *Journal of Experimental Psychology*, 1933, *16*, 1–31.

Gibson, J. J. Observations on active touch. *Psychological Review*, 1962, *69*, 477–491.

Gibson, J. J. *The senses considered as perceptual systems.* Boston: Houghton Mifflin, 1966.

Ginsberg, L. A case of synaesthesia. *American Journal of Psychology*, 1923, *34*, 582–589.

Goethe, J. W. von. *Zur Farbenlehre.* Tübingen: J. G. Cotta, 1810.

Goldstein, J. L. Is the power law simply related to the driven spike response rate from the whole auditory nerve? In H. R. Moskowitz, B. Scharf, & J. C. Stevens (Eds.), *Sensation and measurement: Papers in honor of S. S. Stevens.* Dordrecht, Netherlands: Reidel, 1974. Pp. 223–229.

Goldstone, S., & Goldfarb, J. Judgment of filled and unfilled durations: Intersensory effects. *Perceptual and Motor Skills*, 1963, *17*, 763–774.

Gordon, B. Receptive fields in deep layers of cat superior colliculus. *Journal of Neurophysiology*, 1972, *1*, 157–178.

Gordon, G., & Manson, J. R. Cutaneous receptive fields of single nerve cells in the thalamus of the cat. *Nature*, 1967, *215*, 597–599.

Grafé, A. Sur un cas à rattacher à ceux d'audition colorée. *Revue de Médecine*, 1898, *18*, 225–228.

Graham, C. H., & Kemp, E. H. Brightness discrimination as a function of the duration of the increment in intensity. *Journal of General Physiology*, 1938, *21*, 635–650.

Grammont, M. La psychologie et la phonétique. *Journal de Psychologie Normale et Pathologique*, 1930, *27*, 544–613.

Gregory, R. L. Origin of eyes and brains. *Nature*, 1967, *213*, 369–372.

Gregory, R. L., & Wallace, J. G. Recovery from early blindness: A case study. *Experimental Psychology Society Monograph*, 1963, No. 2.

Gregson, R. A. M. Representation of taste mixture cross-modal matching on a Minkowski R-metric. *Australian Journal of Psychology*, 1965, *17*, 195–204.

Grinspoon, L. *Marihuana reconsidered.* Cambridge, Massachusetts: Harvard University Press, 1971.

Gross, C. G., Bender, D. B., & Rocha-Miranda, C. E. Visual receptive fields of neurons in inferotemporal cortex of the monkey. *Science*, 1969, *166*, 1303–1306.

Hall, G. S. The contents of children's minds. *Princeton Review*, 1883, n.v., 249–272.

Harrington, T., & Merzenich, M. M. Neural coding in the sense of touch: Human sensations of skin indentation compared with the responses of slowly adapting mechanoreceptive afferents innervating the hairy skin of monkeys. *Experimental Brain Research*, 1970, *10*, 251–264.

Harris, C. S. Perceptual adaptation to inverted, reversed, and displaced vision. *Psychological Review*, 1965, *72*, 419–444.

Harris, J. D. *Some relations between vision and audition*. Springfield, Illinois: Thomas, 1950.

Hartley, D. *Observations on man, his frame, his duty, and his expectations*. London and Bath: Hitch and Austen, and Leake and Frederick, 1749.

Hartline, H. K. Inhibition of activity of visual receptors by illuminating nearby retinal areas in the Limulus eye. *Federation Proceedings*, 1949, *8*, 69.

Hartmann, G. W. *Gestalt psychology*. New York: Ronald Press, 1935.

Hartshorne, C. *The philosophy and psychology of sensation*. Chicago: University of Chicago Press, 1934.

Hayek, F. A. *The sensory order*, London: Routledge & Kegan Paul, 1952.

Hecht, S., Schlaer, S., & Pirenne, M. H. Energy, quanta, and vision. *Journal of General Physiology*, 1942, *25*, 819–840.

Helmholtz, H. L. F. von. *Die Thatsachen in der Wahrnehmung*. Berlin: Hirschwald, 1879.

Henning, H. *Der Geruch*. Leipzig: Barth, 1916. (a)

Henning, H. Die Qualitätenreihe des Geschmacks. *Zeitschrift für Psychologie*, 1916, *74*, 203–219. (b)

Henning, H. Eine neuartige Komplexsynästhesie und Komplexzuordnung. *Zeitschrift für Psychologie*, 1923, *92*, 149–160.

Hevner, K. An experimental study of the affective value of sounds in poetry. *American Journal of Psychology*, 1937, *49*, 419–434.

Hirsh, I. J., & Sherrick, C. E., Jr. Perceived order in different sense modalities. *Journal of Experimental Psychology*, 1961, *62*, 423–432.

Hobbes, T. *Leviathan; or the matter, forme, and power of a commonwealth, ecclesiasticall and civill*. London: Ckooke [sic], 1651.

Hobbes, T. *Elements of philosophy*. London: Crooke, 1656.

Holland, M. K., and Wertheimer, M. Some physiognomic aspects of naming, or, maluma and takete revisited. *Perceptual and Motor Skills*, 1964, *119*, 111–117.

Holmgren, G. L., Arnoult, M. D., & Manning, W. H. Intermodal transfer in a paired-associates learning task. *Journal of Experimental Psychology*, 1966, *71*, 254–259.

Holton, G. On the role of themata in scientific thought. *Science*, 1975, *188*, 328–334.

Horn, G. The effect of somaesthetic and photic stimuli on the activity of units in the striate cortex of unanaesthetized, unrestrained cats. *Journal of Physiology*, 1965, *179*, 263–277.

Horn, G., Stechler, G., & Hill, R. M. Receptive fields in the visual cortex of the cat in the presence and absence of bodily tilt. *Experimental Brain Research*, 1972, *15*, 113–132.

Hornbostel, E. M. von. Die Einheit der Sinne. *Melos, Zeitschrift für Musik*, 1925, *4*, 290–297. Translated as: The unity of the senses. *Psyche*, 1927, *7*, 83–89.

Hornbostel, E. M. von. Über Geruchshelligkeit. *Pflügers Archiv für die Gesamte Physiologie*, 1931, *227*, 517–538.

Hornbostel, E. M. von, & Wertheimer, M. Über die Wahrnehmung der Schallrichtung. *Sitzungsberichte der Preusslichen Akademie der Wissenschaften*, Berlin, 1920, *20*, 388–396.

Hubel, D. H., & Wiesel, T. N. Receptive fields, binocular interaction and functional architecture in the cat's visual cortex. *Journal of Physiology*, 1962, *160*, 106–154.

Hubel, D. H., & Wiesel, T. N. Receptive fields and functional architecture of monkey striate cortex. *Journal of Physiology*, 1968, *195*, 215–243.

Hug-Hellmuth, H. von. Über Farbenhören. *Imago*, 1912, *1*, 228–264.

Hume, D. *A treatise of human nature: Being an attempt to introduce the experimental method of reasoning into moral subjects*. London: 1739.

Huxley, A. *Point counter point*. London: Chatto and Windus, 1928.

Huysmans, J.-K. *À rebours*. Paris: Charpentier, 1884.

Huysmans, J.-K. *En route*. Paris: Tresse et Stock, 1895.

Irwin, E. *Colour terms in Greek poetry*. Toronto: Hakkert, 1974.

Jassik-Gerschenfeld, D. Activity of somatic origin evoked in the superior colliculus of the cat. *Experimental Neurology*, 1966, *16*, 104–118.

Jastrow, J. The perception of space by disparate senses. *Mind*, 1886, *11*, 539–554.

Jeddi, E. Confort du contact et thermoregulation comportementale. *Physiology and Behavior*, 1970, *5*, 1487–1493.

Jeffress, L. A. A place theory of sound localization. *Journal of Comparative and Physiological Psychology*, 1948, *41*, 35–39.

Johnson, R. C., Suzuki, N. S., & Olds, W. K. Phonetic symbolism in an artificial language. *Journal of Abnormal and Social Psychology*, 1964, *69*, 233–236.

Johnson, S. *The lives of the most eminent English poets with critical observations on their works*, Vol. 4. London: Bathurst *et alia*, 1778.

Jones, B., & Connolly, K. Memory effects in cross-modal matching. *British Journal of Psychology*, 1970, *61*, 267–270.

Joyce, J. *Ulysses*. New York: Random House, 1934.

Juhász, A. Über eine neue Eigenschaft der Geruchsempfindungen. *Bericht über den IX. Kongress für experimentelle Psychologie in München*, 1926, *9*, 178–179.

Kandinsky, W. *Über das Geistige in der Kunst, inbesondere in der Malerei*. München: Piper, 1912.

Kant, I. *Kritik der reinen Vernunft*. Riga: Hartknoch, 1781.

Karwoski, T. F., & Odbert, H. S. Color-music. *Psychological Monographs*, 1938, *50*, Whole No. 222.

Karwoski, T. F., Odbert, H. S., & Osgood, C. E. Studies in synesthetic thinking. II. The role of form in visual responses to music. *Journal of General Psychology*, 1942, *26*, 199–222.

Kearney, G. F. Hue preferences as a function of ambient temperatures. *Australian Journal of Psychology*, 1966, *18*, 271–275.

Kelvin, R. P. Discrimination of size by sight and touch. *Quarterly Journal of Experimental Psychology*, 1954, *6*, 25–34.

Kinney, J. A. S., & Luria, S. M. Conflicting visual and tactual-kinesthetic stimulation. *Perception and Psychophysics*, 1970, *8*, 189–192.

Kirman, J. H. Tactile apparent movement: The effects of interstimulus onset interval and stimulus duration. *Perception and Psychophysics*, 1974, *15*, 1–6.

Klinckowström, A. Trois cas d'audition colorée dans la même famille. *Biologiska Föreningens i Stockholm Förhandlingar*, 1890, *3*, 117–118.

Koch, K. *Wishes, lies, and dreams: Teaching children to write poetry*. New York: Random House, 1970.

Köhler, W. *Gestalt psychology*. New York: Liveright, 1947.

Kolers, P. A. *Aspects of motion perception*. Oxford: Pergamon Press, 1972.

Krantz, D. H. A theory of magnitude estimation and cross-modality matching. *Journal of Mathematical Psychology*, 1972, *9*, 168–199.

Krauthamer, G. Form perception across sensory modalities. *Neuropsychologia*, 1968, *6*, 105–113.

Krohn, W. D. Pseudo-chromesthesia, or the association of colors with words, letters, and sounds. *American Journal of Psychology*, 1892, *5*, 20–41.

Külpe, O. *Grundriss der Psychologie.* Leipzig: Engelmann, 1893.

Laignel-Lavastine (sic). Audition colorée familiale. *Revue Neurologique,* 1901, *9,* 1152–1162.

Langenbeck, K. Die akustisch-chromatischen Synopsien. *Zeitschrift für Sinnesphysiologie,* 1913, *47,* 159–181.

Langer, S. *Mind: An essay on human feeling,* Vol. I. Baltimore: Johns Hopkins Press, 1967.

Lauret and Duchaussoy (sic). Un cas héréditaire d'audition colorée. *Revue Philosophique,* 1887, *23,* 222–224.

Leakey, F. W. *Baudelaire and nature.* Manchester, England: The University Press, 1969.

Lechelt, E. C. Some stimulus parameters of tactile numerousness perception. In F. A. Geldard (Ed.), *Conference on cutaneous communications systems and devices.* Austin, Texas: Psychonomic Society, 1974. Pp. 1–5.

Lehman, R. S. A multivariate model of synesthesia. *Multivariate Behavioral Research,* 1972, *7,* 403–439.

Leibniz, G. W. von. *New essays concerning human understanding,* 1704. New York: Macmillan, 1896.

Leibniz, G. W. von. Considérations sur le principe de vie, et sur les natures plastiques, par l'auteur de l'Harmonie Préétablie. *Histoire des Ouvrages des Savans,* 1705. Translated in P. P. Wiener (Ed.), *Leibniz selections.* New York: Scribner's, 1951. Pp. 190–199.

Lemaitre, A. Un cas d'audition colorée hallucinatoire. *Archives de Psychologie,* 1904, *3,* 164–177.

Levine, M. V. Geometric interpretations of some psychophysical results. In D. H. Krantz, R. C. Atkinson, R. D. Luce, & P. Suppes (Eds.), *Contemporary developments in mathematical psychology,* Vol. 2. San Francisco: Freeman, 1974. Pp. 200–235.

Linker, E., Moore, M. E., & Galanter, E. Taste thresholds, detection models, and disparate results. *Journal of Experimental Psychology,* 1964, *67,* 59–66.

Lipetz, L. E. The relation of physiological and psychological aspects of sensory intensity. In W. R. Loewenstein (Ed.), *Handbook of sensory physiology,* Vol. I. *Principles of receptor physiology.* Berlin: Springer-Verlag, 1971. Pp. 191–225.

Lobb, H. Vision *versus* touch in form discrimination. *Canadian Journal of Psychology,* 1965, *19,* 175–187.

Lobb, H. Asymmetrical transfer of form discrimination across sensory modalities in human adults. *Journal of Experimental Psychology,* 1970, *86,* 350–354.

Locke, J. *An essay concerning humane understanding.* London: Basset, 1690. Oxford: Clarendon Press, 1894.

Lomer, G. Beobachtungen über farbiges Hören (auditio colorata). *Archiv für Psychiatrie und Nervenkrankheiten,* 1905, *40,* 593–601.

Love, J. A., & Scott, J. W. Some response characteristics of cells of the magnocellular division of the medial geniculate body of the cat. *Canadian Journal of Physiology and Pharmacology,* 1969, *47,* 881–888.

Luria, A. R. *The mind of a mnemonist.* New York: Basic Books, 1968.

Macdermott, M. M. *Vowel sounds in poetry: Their music and tone-colour.* London: Kegan Paul, 1940.

Mach, E. Über die physiologische Wirkung räumliche verheilter Lichtreise. *Sitzungsberichte der Mathematisch-naturwissenschaftlichen Classe der Kaiserlichen Akadamie der Wissenschaften,* Wien, 1868, *57,* 11–19.

MacIntyre, C. F. (Trans.). *French symbolist poetry.* Berkeley and Los Angeles: University of California Press, 1958.

MacKay, D. M. Psychophysics of perceived intensity: A theoretical basis for Fechner's and Stevens' laws. *Science,* 1963, *139,* 1213–1216.

Magoun, H. W. *The waking brain* (2nd ed.). Springfield, Illinois: Thomas, 1963.

Mahling, F. Das Problem der "Audition colorée." *Archiv für die Gesamte Psychologie*, 1926, *57*, 165–302.

Mallarmé, S. Crise de vers. *Divagations*. Paris: Charpentier, 1935.

Mansfield, R. J. W. Measurement, invariance, and psychophysics. In H. R. Moskowitz, B. Scharf, & J. C. Stevens (Eds.), *Sensation and measurement: Papers in honor of S. S. Stevens*. Dordrecht, Netherlands: Reidel, 1974. Pp. 113–128.

Marchland, H. Phonetic symbolism in English word-formation. *Indogermanische Forschungen*, 1958, *64*, 146–168, 256–277.

Margis, P. Die Synästhesien bei E. T. A. Hoffmann. *Zeitschrift für Ästhetik*, 1910, *5*, 91–99.

Marinesco, G. Contribution à l'étude des synesthésies particulièrement de l'audition colorée. *Journal de Psychologie Normale et Pathologique*, 1912, *9*, 385–422.

Marks, L. E. Visual brightness: Some applications of a model. *Vision Research*, 1972, *12*, 1409–1421.

Marks, L. E. On associations of light and sound: The mediation of brightness, pitch, and loudness. *American Journal of Psychology*, 1974, *87*, 173–188. (a)

Marks, L. E. *Sensory processes: The new psychophysics*. New York: Academic Press, 1974. (b)

Marks, L. E. On colored-hearing synesthesia: Cross-modal translations of sensory dimensions. *Psychological Bulletin*, 1975, *82*, 303–331.

Marks, L. E. Phonion: Translation and annotations concerning loudness scales and the processing of auditory intensity. In N. J. Castellan & F. Restle (Eds.), *Cognitive theory*, Vol. 3. Hillsdale, New Jersey: Erlbaum, 1978. Pp. 7–31.

Marks, L. E., & Stevens, J. C. Individual brightness functions. *Perception and Psychophysics*, 1966, *1*, 17–24.

Marks, L. E., & Stevens, J. C. Spatial summation of warmth: Influence of duration and configuration of the stimulus. *American Journal of Psychology*, 1973, *86*, 251–267.

Martin, L. J. Über ästhetische Synästhesie. *Zeitschrift für Psychologie*, 1909, *53*, 1–60.

Mashhour, M., & Hosman, J. On the new "psychophysical law": A validation study. *Perception and Psychophysics*, 1968, *3*, 367–375.

Masson, D. I. Synesthesia and sound spectra. *Word*, 1952, *8*, 39–41.

Masson, D. I. Vowel and consonant patterns in poetry. *Journal of Aesthetics and Art Criticism*, 1953, *12*, 213–227.

Matin, L. Critical duration, the differential luminance threshold, critical flicker frequency and visual adaptation: A theoretical treatment. *Journal of the Optical Society of America*, 1968, *58*, 404–415.

Maupassant, G. de. *La vie errante*. Paris: Ollendorff, 1890.

McGann, J. J. *Swinburne: An experiment in criticism*. Chicago: University of Chicago Press, 1972.

McGill, W. J., & Goldberg, J. P. A study of the near-miss involving Weber's law and pure-tone intensity discrimination. *Perception and Psychophysics*, 1968, *4*, 105–109.

McGurk, H., & Lewis, M. Space perception in early infancy: Perception within a common auditory-visual space? *Science*, 1974, *186*, 649–650.

McMurray, G. Meaning associated with the phonetic structure of unfamiliar foreign words. *Canadian Journal of Psychology*, 1960, *14*, 166–174.

Melamed, L. E. The role of response processes in the formation of cross-modality assimilation effects. *Perception and Psychophysics*, 1970, *8*, 185–188.

Mill, J. S. *An examination of Sir William Hamilton's philosophy*. London: Longman, Green, Longman, Roberts & Green, 1865.

Miller, G. A. Sensitivity to changes in the intensity of white noise and its relation to loudness and masking. *Journal of the Acoustical Society of America*, 1947, *19*, 609–619.

Mills, A. W. On the minimum audible angle. *Journal of the Acoustical Society of America*, 1958, *30*, 237–246.

Milner, A. D., & Bryant, P. E. Cross-modal matching by young children. *Journal of Comparative and Physiological Psychology*, 1970, *71*, 453–458.

Moffett, A., & Ettlinger, G. Opposite responding in two sense modalities. *Science*, 1966, *153*, 205–206.

Mogensen, M. F., & English, H. B. The apparent warmth of colors. *American Journal of Psychology*, 1926, *37*, 427–428.

Morgan, G. A., Goodson, F. E., & Jones, T. Age differences in the associations between felt temperatures and color choices. *American Journal of Psychology*, 1975, *88*, 125–130.

Morrell, F. Visual system's view of acoustic space. *Nature*, 1972, *238*, 44–46.

Moul, E. R. An experimental study of visual and auditory thickness. *American Journal of Psychology*, 1930, *42*, 544–560.

Moynihan, W. T. The auditory correlative. *Journal of Aesthetics and Art Criticism*, 1958, *17*, 93–102.

Mudge, E. L. The common synaesthesia of music. *Journal of Applied Psychology*, 1920, *4*, 342–345.

Mueller, C. G. Frequency of seeing functions for intensity discrimination at various levels of adapting intensity. *Journal of General Physiology*, 1951, *34*, 463–474.

Müller, G. E. Zur Psychophysik der Gesichtsempfindungen. *Zeitschrift für Psychologie*, 1896, *10*, 1–82.

Müller, J. *Handbuch der Physiologie des Menschen*, Band V. Coblenz: Hölscher, 1838.

Murata, K., Cramer, H., & Bach-y-Rita, P. Neuronal convergence of noxious, acoustic, and visual stimuli in the visual cortex of the cat. *Journal of Neurophysiology*, 1965, *28*, 1223–1239.

Nabokov, V. Portrait of my mother. *New Yorker*, 1949, *25*(7), 33–37.

Nabokov, V. *King, queen, knave*. New York: McGraw-Hill, 1968.

Nachmias, J., & Steinman, R. M. Study of absolute visual detection by the rating-scale method. *Journal of the Optical Society of America*, 1963, *53*, 1206–1212.

Nafe, J. P. The psychology of felt experience. *American Journal of Psychology*, 1927, *39*, 367–389.

Nafe, J. P. A quantitative theory of feeling. *Journal of General Psychology*, 1929, *2*, 199–210.

Nerval, G. de. *Aurélia*, 1855. Paris: Flammarion, 1897.

Newman, S. S. Further experiments in phonetic symbolism. *American Journal of Psychology*, 1933, *45*, 53–75.

Newton, I. *Opticks: or, A treatise of the reflexions, refraxions, inflexions and colours of light.* London: Smith and Walford, 1704.

O'Connor, N., & Hermelin, B. Seeing and hearing in space and time. *Perception and Psychophysics*, 1972, *11*, 46–48.

O'Malley, G. Literary synesthesia. *Journal of Aesthetics and Art Criticism*, 1957, *15*, 391–411.

Ortmann, O. Theories of synesthesia in the light of a case of color-hearing. *Human Biology*, 1933, *5*, 155–211.

Osgood, C. E. The cross-cultural generality of visual-verbal synesthetic tendencies. *Behavioral Science*, 1960, *5*, 146–169.

Osgood, C. E. Semantic differential technique in the comparative study of cultures. *American Anthropologist*, 1964, *66*, 171–200.

Osgood, C. E., May, W. H., & Miron, M. S. *Cross-cultural universals of affective meaning.* Urbana, Illinois: University of Illinois Press, 1974.

Osgood, C. E., Suci, G. J., & Tannenbaum, P. H. *The measurement of meaning*. Urbana, Illinois: University of Illinois Press, 1957.

Owen, D. H., & Brown, D. R. Visual and tactual form complexity: A psychophysical approach to perceptual equivalence. *Perception and Psychophysics*, 1970, *7*, 225–228. (a)

Owen, D. H., & Brown, D. R. Visual and tactual form discrimination: Psychophysical comparison within and between modalities. *Perception and Psychophysics*, 1970, *7*, 302–306. (b)

Oxford English dictionary. Oxford: Oxford University Press, 1971.

Pedrono (sic). De l'audition colorée. *Annales d'Oculistique*, 1882, *88*, 224–237.

Petrides, M., & Iversen, S. D. Cross-modal matching and the primate frontal cortex. *Science*, 1976, *192*, 1023–1024.

Philippe, J. Résumé d'une observation d'audition colorée. *Revue Philosophique*, 1893, *36*, 330–334.

Pick, A. D., Pick, H. L., Jr., & Thomas, M. L. Cross-modal transfer and improvement of form discrimination. *Journal of Experimental Child Psychology*, 1966, *3*, 279–288.

Pick, H. L., Jr., Warren, D. H., & Hay, J. C. Sensory conflict in judgments of spatial direction. *Perception and Psychophysics*, 1969, *6*, 203–205.

Pierce, A. H. Gustatory audition; a hitherto undescribed variety of synaesthesia. *American Journal of Psychology*, 1907, *18*, 341–352.

Piéron, Mme. H. Contribution expérimentale à l'étude des phénomènes de transfert sensoriel: La vision et la kinésthesie dans la perception des longueurs. *L'Année Psychologique*, 1922, *23*, 76–124.

Pikler, J. *Schriften zur Anpassungstheorie des Empfindungsvorganges*, Band IV. *Theorie der Empfindungsqualität als Abbild des Reizes*. Leipzig: Barth, 1922.

Plato. *The collected dialogues*, edited by E. Hamilton & H. Cairns. New York: Pantheon, 1961.

Poe, E. A. *The complete tales and poems of Edgar Allan Poe*. New York: Random House, 1938.

Poncelet, P. *Chimie du guot et de l'odorat, ou principes pour composer facilement, & à peu de frais, les liqueurs à boire, & les eaux de senteurs*. Paris: Le Mercier, 1755.

Quincke, H. Ueber Mitempfindungen und verwandte Vorgänge. *Zeitschrift für Klinische Medizin*, 1890, *17*, 429–451.

Raab, D. H. Backward masking. *Psychological Bulletin*, 1963, *60*, 118–129.

Ratliff, F., & Hartline, H. K. The response of limulus optic nerve fibers to patterns of illumination on the receptor mosaic. *Journal of General Physiology*, 1959, *42*, 1241–1255.

Reese, T. S., & Brightman, M. W. Olfactory surface and central olfactory connexions in some vertebrates. In G. E. W. Wolstenholme & J. Knight (Eds.), *Taste and smell in vertebrates*. London: Churchill, 1970. Pp. 115–149.

Reichard, G., Jakobson, R., & Werth, E. Language and synesthesia. *Word*, 1949, *5*, 224–233.

Reid, T. *An inquiry into the human mind, on the principles of common sense*. Edinburgh: Millar, 1764.

Révész, G. Über audition colorée. *Zeitschrift für Angewandte Psychologie*, 1923, *21*, 308–332.

Rich, G. J. A study of tonal attributes. *American Journal of Psychology*, 1919, *30*, 121–164.

Riggs, L. A., & Karwoski, T. Synaesthesia. *British Journal of Psychology*, 1934, *25*, 29–41.

Rimbaud, A. Une saison en enfer, 1873. In *Oeuvres de Arthur Rimbaud*. Paris: Mercure de France, 1937.

Roblee, L., & Washburn, M. F. The affective values of articulate sounds. *American Journal of Psychology*, 1912, *23*, 579–583.

Rock, I. *An introduction to perception*. New York: Macmillan, 1975.

Rock, I., & Victor, J. Vision and touch: An experimentally created conflict between the two senses. *Science*, 1964, *143*, 594–596.

Roffler, S. K., & Butler, R. A. Localization of tonal stimuli in the vertical plane. *Journal of the Acoustical Society of America*, 1968, *43*, 1260–1266.

Rogers, G. A. J. The veil of perception. *Mind*, 1975, *84*, 210–224.

Ronco, P. G. An experimental quantification of kinesthetic sensation: Extent of arm movement. *Journal of Psychology*, 1963, *55*, 227–238.

Rose, S. A., Blank, M. S., & Bridger, W. H. Intermodal and intramodal retention of visual and tactual information in young children. *Developmental Psychology*, 1972, *6*, 482–486.

Rosner, B. S., & Goff, W. R. Electrical responses of the nervous system and subjective scales of intensity. In W. D. Neff (Ed.), *Contributions to sensory physiology*, Vol. 2. New York: Academic Press, 1967. Pp. 169–221.

Rudel, R. G., & Teuber, H.-L. Decrement of visual and haptic Müller-Lyer illusion on repeated trials: A study of crossmodal transfer. *Quarterly Journal of Experimental Psychology*, 1963, *15*, 125–131.

Rudel, R. G., & Teuber, H.-L. Crossmodal transfer of shape discrimination by children. *Neuropsychologia*, 1964, *2*, 1–8.

Rushton, W. A. H. Visual adaptation. *Proceedings of the Royal Society*, London, 1965, *162B*, 20–46.

Sapir, E. A study of phonetic symbolism. *Journal of Experimental Psychology*, 1929, *12*, 225–239.

Schacknow, P. N., & Raab, D. H. Intensity discrimination of tone bursts and the form of the Weber function. *Perception and Psychophysics*, 1973, *14*, 449–450.

Schiffman, S. S. Physicochemical correlates of olfactory quality. *Science*, 1974, *185*, 112–117.

Schiffman, S. S., & Erickson, R. P. A psychophysical model for gustatory quality. *Physiology and Behavior*, 1971, *7*, 617–633.

Schiller, P. von. Intersensorielle Transposition bei Fischen. *Zeitschrift für Vergleichende Physiologie*, 1933, *19*, 304–309.

Schiller, P. von. Interrelation of different senses in perception. *British Journal of Psychology*, 1935, *25*, 465–469.

Schmitt, F. O., Dev, P., & Smith, B. H. Electrotonic processing of information by brain cells. *Science*, 1976, *193*, 114–120.

Schneider, D. The sex-attractant receptor of moths. *Scientific American*, 1974, *231(1)*, 28–35.

Scholtz, D. A. Die Grundsätze der Gestaltwahrnehmung in der Haptik. *Acta Psychologica*, 1958, *13*, 299–333.

Schultze, E. Krankafter Wandertrieb räumlich beschränkte Taubheit für bestimmte Töne und "tertiäre" Empfindungen bei einem Psychopathen. *Zeitschrift für die Gesamte Neurologie und Psychiatrie*, 1912, *10*, 399–419.

Semb, G. The detectability of the odor of butanol. *Perception and Psychophysics*, 1968, *4*, 335–340.

Senden, M. von. *Raum- und Gestaltauffassung bei operierten Blindgebornen von und nach der Operation*. Leipzig: Barth, 1932.

Shaffer, R. W., & Ellis, H. C. An analysis of intersensory transfer of form. *Journal of Experimental Psychology*, 1974, *102*, 948–953.

Shaffer, R. W., & Howard, J. The transfer of information across sensory modalities. *Perception and Psychophysics*, 1974, *15*, 344–348.

Shattuck, R. Review of *Antonin Artaud: Selected writings* by S. Sontag. *New York Review of Books*, 1976, 23(18), 17–23.

Shelley, P. B. *The complete poetical works of Percy Bysshe Shelley*, edited by T. Hutchinson. London: Oxford University Press, 1905.

Sherrick, C. E., Jr. Effects of background noise on the auditory intensive difference limen. *Journal of the Acoustical Society of America*, 1959, 31, 239–242.

Sherrick, C. E., & Rogers, R. Apparent haptic movement. *Perception and Psychophysics*, 1966, 1, 175–180.

Siebold, E. von. Synästhesien in der englischen Dichtung des 19. Jahrhunderts. *Englische Studien*, 1919, 53, 196–334.

Silz, W. Heine's synesthesia. *Publications of the Modern Language Association*, 1942, 57, 469–488.

Simpson, L., & McKellar, P. Types of synesthesia. *Journal of Mental Science*, 1955, 101, 141–147.

Simpson, R. H., Quinn, M., & Ausubel, D. P. Synesthesia in children: Association of colors with pure tone frequencies. *Journal of Genetic Psychology*, 1956, 89, 95–103.

Sitwell, E. *The collected poems of Edith Sitwell.* New York: Vanguard Press, 1954.

Sivian, L. J., & White, S. D. On minimum audible sound fields. *Journal of the Acoustical Society of America*, 1933, 4, 288–321.

Skinner, B. F. A quantitative estimate of certain types of sound-patterning in poetry. *American Journal of Psychology*, 1942, 30, 64–79.

Skramlik, E. von. *Handbuch der Physiologie der niederen Sinne*, Band I. *Die Physiologie des Geruchs- und Geschmackssinnes.* Leipzig: Thienne, 1926.

Slawson, A. W. Vowel quality and musical timbre as functions of spectrum envelope and fundamental frequency. *Journal of the Acoustical Society of America*, 1968, 43, 87–101.

Sperling, G., & Sondhi, M. M. Model for visual luminance discrimination and flicker detection. *Journal of the Optical Society of America*, 1968, 58, 1133–1145.

Stein, B. E., Magalhães-Castro, B., & Kruger, L. Superior colliculus: Visuotopic-somatotopic overlap. *Science*, 1975, 189, 224–226.

Steinhardt, J. Intensity discrimination in the human eye. I. The relation of $\Delta I/I$ to intensity. *Journal of General Physiology*, 1936, 20, 185–209.

Stelzner, H.-F. Ein Fall von akustisch-optischer Synästhesie. *Albrecht von Graefes Archiv für Ophthalmologie*, 1903, 55, 549–563.

Stern, W. *General psychology from the personalistic standpoint.* New York: Macmillan, 1938.

Stevens, J. C. *A comparison of ratio scales for the loudness of white noise and the brightness of white light.* Unpublished doctoral dissertation, Harvard University, 1957.

Stevens, J. C., & Hall, J. W. Brightness and loudness as functions of stimulus duration. *Perception and Psychophysics*, 1966, 1, 319–327.

Stevens, J. C., Mack, J. D., & Stevens, S. S. Growth of sensation on seven continua as measured by force of handgrip. *Journal of Experimental Psychology*, 1960, 59, 60–67.

Stevens, J. C., & Marks, L. E. Cross-modality matching of brightness and loudness. *Proceedings of the National Academy of Sciences*, 1965, 54, 407–411.

Stevens, S. S. On the psychophysical law. *Psychological Review*, 1957, 64, 153–181.

Stevens, S. S. Some similarities between hearing and seeing. *The Laryngoscope*, 1958, 68, 508–527.

Stevens, S. S. Cross-modality validation of subjective scales for loudness, vibration, and electric shock. *Journal of Experimental Psychology*, 1959, 57, 201–209.

Stevens, S. S. The psychophysics of sensory function. In W. A. Rosenblith (Ed.), *Sensory communication.* New York: Wiley, 1961. Pp. 1–33.

Stevens, S. S. Power-group transformations under glare, masking, and recruitment. *Journal of the Acoustical Society of America*, 1966, 39, 725–735.

Stevens, S. S. Neural events and the psychophysical law. *Science,* 1970, *170,* 1043–1050.

Stevens, S. S. A neural quantum in sensory discrimination. *Science,* 1972, *177,* 749–762.

Stevens, S. S., & Davis, H. Psychophysiological acoustics: Pitch and loudness. *Journal of the Acoustical Society of America,* 1936, *8,* 1–13.

Stevens, S. S., & Greenbaum, H. B. Regression effect in psychophysical judgment. *Perception and Psychophysics,* 1966, *1,* 439–446.

Stevens, S. S., & Guirao, M. Subjective scaling of length and area and the matching of length to loudness and brightness. *Journal of Experimental Psychology,* 1963, *66,* 177–186.

Stevens, S. S., & Newman, E. B. The localization of actual sources of sound. *American Journal of Psychology,* 1936, *48,* 297–306.

Stevens, S. S., & Stone, G. Finger span: Ratio scale, category scale, and jnd scale. *Journal of Experimental Psychology,* 1959, *57,* 91–95.

Stevens, W. *The necessary angel.* New York: Knopf, 1951.

Stevens, W. *Opus posthumus.* New York: Knopf, 1957.

Stone, H., & Bosley, J. J. Olfactory discrimination and Weber's law. *Perceptual and Motor Skills,* 1965, *20,* 657–665.

Stout, G. F. *A manual of psychology,* New York: Hinds, Noble, and Eldredge, 1915.

Suarez de Mendoza, F. *L'audition colorée.* Paris: Octave Doin, 1890.

Sully, J. Harmony of colours. *Mind,* 1879, *4,* 172–191.

Swedenborg, E. *Heavenly arcana,* 1751. Boston: New Church Printing Society, 1840.

Swets, J. A., Tanner, W. P., & Birdsall, T. G. Decision processes in perception. *Psychological Review,* 1961, *68,* 301–340.

Swinburne, A. C. *Poems.* Philadelphia: McKay, undated.

Syka, J., & Straschill, M. Activation of superior colliculus neurons and motor responses after electrical stimulation of the inferior colliculus. *Experimental Neurology,* 1970, *28,* 384–392.

Tart, C. T. *On being stoned: A psychological study of marijuana intoxication.* Palo Alto: Science and Behavior Books, 1971.

Teghtsoonian, M., & Teghtsoonian, R. Seen and felt length. *Psychonomic Science,* 1965, *3,* 465–466.

Teghtsoonian, R. On the exponents in Stevens' law and the constant in Ekman's law. *Psychological Review,* 1971, *78,* 71–80.

Teghtsoonian, R., & Teghtsoonian, M. Two varieties of perceived length. *Perception and Psychophysics,* 1970, *8,* 389–392.

Theophrastus. *De sensibus.* In G. M. Stratton, *Theophrastus and the Greek physiological psychology before Aristotle.* London: Allen and Unwin, 1917.

Thompson, R. F., Johnson, R. H., & Hoopes, J. J. Organization of auditory, somatic sensory, and visual projection to association fields of cerebral cortex in the cat. *Journal of Neurophysiology,* 1963, *26,* 343–364.

Thompson, R. F., Mayers, K. S., Robertson, R. T., & Patterson, C. J. Number coding in association cortex of the cat. *Science,* 1970, *168,* 271–273.

Tieck, J. L. *Schriften,* Band 10. Berlin: Reimer, 1828.

Titchener, E. B. *Experimental psychology of the thought-processes.* New York: Macmillan, 1909.

Treisman, M. Noise and Weber's law: The discrimination of brightness and other dimensions. *Psychological Review,* 1964, *71,* 314–330.

Troland, L. T. *Principles of psychophysiology,* Vol. 2. *Sensation.* New York: Van Nostrand, 1930.

Tsuru, S., & Fries, H. S. A problem in meaning. *Journal of General Psychology,* 1933, *8,* 281–284.

Ulich, E. Synästhesie und Geschlecht. *Zeitschrift für Experimentelle und Angewandte Psychologie*, 1957, *4*, 31–57.

Ullmann, S. L'art de la transposition dans la poésie de Théophile Gautier. *Le Français Moderne*, 1947, *15*, 265–286.

Ullmann, S. *The principles of semantics*. Glasgow: Jackson, 1951.

Ulrich, A. Phénomènes de synesthésies chez un épileptique. *Revue Philosophique*, 1903, *56*, 181–187.

Urbantschitsch, V. Ueber den Einfluss einer Sinneserregung auf die übrigen Sinnesempfindungen. *Pflügers Archiv für die Gesamte Physiologie*, 1888, *42*, 154–182.

van Bergeijk, W. A. The evolution of vertebrate hearing. In W. D. Neff (Ed.), *Contributions to sensory physiology*, Vol. 2. New York: Academic Press, 1967. Pp. 1–49.

Vendrik, A. J. H. Psychophysics of the thermal sensory system and statistical detection theory. In J. D. Hardy, A. P. Gagge, & J. A. J. Stolwijk (Eds.), *Physiological and behavioral temperature regulation*. Springfield, Illinois: Thomas, 1970. Pp. 819–830.

Vernon, P. E. Synaesthesia in music. *Psyche*, 1930, *10*, 22–40.

Verrillo, R. T. Effect of spatial parameters on the vibrotactile threshold. *Journal of Experimental Psychology*, 1966, *71*, 570–575.

Voss, W. Das Farbenhören bei Erblindeten. *Archiv für die Gesamte Psychologie*, 1929, *73*, 407–524.

Waller, A. D. Points relating to the Weber-Fechner law. Retina; muscle; nerve. *Brain*, 1895, *18*, 200–216.

Walter, W. G. The convergence and interaction of visual, auditory, and tactile responses in human nonspecific cortex. *Annals of the New York Academy of Sciences*, 1964, *112*, 320–361.

Wapner, S., Werner, H., & Chandler, K. A. Experiments on sensori-tonic field theory of perception. I. Effect of extraneous stimulation on the visual perception of verticality. *Journal of Experimental Psychology*, 1951, *42*, 341–345.

Waterman, C. N., Jr. Hand-tongue space perception. *Journal of Experimental Psychology*, 1917, *2*, 289–294.

Watson, C. S., & Gengel, R. W. Signal duration and signal frequency in relation to auditory sensitivity. *Journal of the Acoustical Society of America*, 1969, *46*, 989–997.

Weber, E. H. *De pulsu, resorptione, auditu et tactu: Annotationes anatomicae et physiologicae.* Leipzig: Koehler, 1834.

Weimer, W. B., & Palermo, D. S. (Eds.) *Cognition and the symbolic process*. Hillsdale, New Jersey: Erlbaum, 1974.

Wepsic, J. F. Multimodal sensory activation of cells in the magnocellular medial geniculate nucleus. *Experimental Neurology*, 1966, *15*, 299–318.

Werner, G., & Mountcastle, V. B. Neural activity in mechanoreceptive cutaneous afferents: Stimulus-response relations, Weber functions, and information transmission. *Journal of Neurophysiology*, 1965, *28*, 359–397.

Werner, H. L'unité des sens. *Journal de Psychologie Normale et Pathologique*, 1934, *31*, 190–205.

Werner, H. *Comparative psychology of mental development*. New York: Harper, 1940.

Werner, H., & Kaplan, B. *Symbol formation: An organismic-developmental approach to language and the expression of thought*. New York: Wiley, 1963.

Werner, H., & Wapner, S. Sensory-tonic field theory of perception. *Journal of Personality*, 1949, *18*, 88–107.

Wheeler, R. H. The synaesthesia of a blind subject. *University of Oregon Publications*, 1920, No. 5.

White, C. T., & Cheatham, P. G. Temporal numerosity: IV. A comparison of the major senses. *Journal of Experimental Psychology*, 1959, *58*, 441–444.

Whitfield, I. C. Coding in the auditory nervous system. *Nature,* 1967, *213,* 756–760.

Whorf, B. L. *Language, thought, and reality.* Cambridge, Massachusetts: Technology Press, 1956.

Wickelgren, B. G. Superior colliculus: Some receptive field properties of bimodally responsive cells. *Science,* 1971, *173,* 69–72.

Wicker, F. W. Mapping the intersensory regions of perceptual space. *American Journal of Psychology,* 1968, *81,* 178–188.

Williams, J. M. Synaesthetic adjectives: A possible law of semantic change. *Language,* 1976, *52,* 461–478.

Willmann, R. R. An experimental investigation of the creative process in music. *Psychological Monographs,* 1944, *57,* Whole No. 261.

Wilska, A. Eine Methode zur Bestimmung der Hörschwellenamplituden des Trommelfells bei verschiedenen Frequenzen. *Skandinavisches Archiv für Physiologie,* 1935, *72,* 161–165.

Wilska, A. On the vibrational sensitivity in different regions of the body surface. *Acta Physiologica Scandinavica,* 1954, *31,* 285–289.

Wilson, G. D. Arousal properties of red versus green. *Perceptual and Motor Skills,* 1966, *23,* 947–949.

Wilson, W. A., Jr. Intersensory transfer in normal and brain-operated monkeys. *Neuropsychologia,* 1965, *3,* 363–370.

Wilson, W. A., Jr., & Shaffer, O. C. Intermodality transfer of specific discriminations in the monkey. *Nature,* 1963, *197,* 107.

Witkin, H. A., Wapner, S., & Leventhal, T. Sound localization with conflicting visual and auditory cues. *Journal of Experimental Psychology,* 1952, *43,* 58–67.

Wittgenstein, L. *Philosophical investigations,* translated by G. E. M. Anscombe. Oxford: Blackwell, 1953.

Wittgenstein, L. *Zettel,* edited by G. E. M. Anscombe & G. H. von Wright. Oxford: Blackwell, 1967.

Woods, P. J., & Campbell, B. A. Relative aversiveness of white noise and cold water. *Journal of Comparative and Physiological Psychology,* 1967, *64,* 493–495.

Woodward, W. R. Fechner's panpsychism: A scientific solution to the mind-body problem. *Journal of the History of the Behavioral Sciences,* 1972, *8,* 367–385.

Wright, B., & Rainwater, L. The meanings of color. *Journal of General Psychology,* 1962, *67,* 89–99.

Wundt, W. *Beiträge zur Theorie der Sinneswahrnehmung.* Leipzig und Heidelberg: Winter, 1862.

Wundt, W. *Grundzüge der physiologischen Psychologie.* Leipzig: Engelmann, 1874.

Yeats, W. B. The symbolism of poetry. *Essays.* London: Macmillan, 1924.

Yilmaz, H. Perceptual invariance and the psychophysical law. *Perception and Psychophysics,* 1967, *2,* 533–538.

Yoshida, M. Dimensions of tactual impressions (1), (2). *Japanese Psychological Research,* 1968, *10,* 123–137, 153–173.

Zigler, M. J. Tone shapes: A novel type of synaesthesia. *Journal of General Psychology,* 1930, *3,* 277–287.

Zigler, M. J., & Northrup, K. M. The tactual perception of form. *American Journal of Psychology,* 1926, *37,* 391–397.

Zwicker, E., Flottorp, G., & Stevens, S. S. Critical band width in loudness summation. *Journal of the Acoustical Society of America,* 1957, *29,* 548–557.

Name Index

277

Subject Index

A

Adaptation, 138–139
  physiological basis, 172–173
Affect, 74–75
  in sound symbolism, 200–201, 208–209
  in synesthetic metaphor, 75, 181, 216–
    218, 221–222, 231, 236–237, 239–241,
    245–246
All-or-none law, 167
Analogy, 189–190, 252–253, *see also*
    Metaphor; Resemblance; Similarity;
    Synesthetic metaphor
Apparent movement, 126–127, 149
Associationism, 166–167, 186

B

Bloch's law, 136–137
Brightness, perception of, 56–61, 63, 146
  cross-modality matching, 56–57, 61,
    68–69
  versus intensity, 58

physiological basis, 58, 146, 152–153
in sound symbolism, 78–80, 202–208
in synesthesia, 58, 89–92, 99–100, 103
in synesthetic metaphor, 212–214, 218,
    232, 238, 240, 242–245, 248, 251
Brightness contrast, 69

C

Cattell's law, 121
Causal theory of perception, 41, *see also*
    Secondary quality
Common sense, *see Sensus communis*
Common sensible attribute, 4, 11–14, 26,
    40, 50, 228, *see also* specific attribute
  physiological basis, 146, 160, 164
  and primary quality, 13, 21, 34–35, 37–38
Constructionist theory of perception,
    39–40, 41–42
Correspondence
  between perception and reality, 47–48,
    50–51, 71, 86, 224–229, 246–247, 252,
    see also Resemblance